DISEASES OF POULTRY

Diseases of Poultry

Editor:

Sarika Garg

Delve Publishing

www.delvepublishing.com

Diseases of Poultry

Editor: **Sarika Garg**

708 3rd Avenue, 6th Floor
New York, NY 10017
United States of America
www.delvepublishing.com

ISBN: 978-1-68095-862-1

Library of Congress Control Number: 2016951615

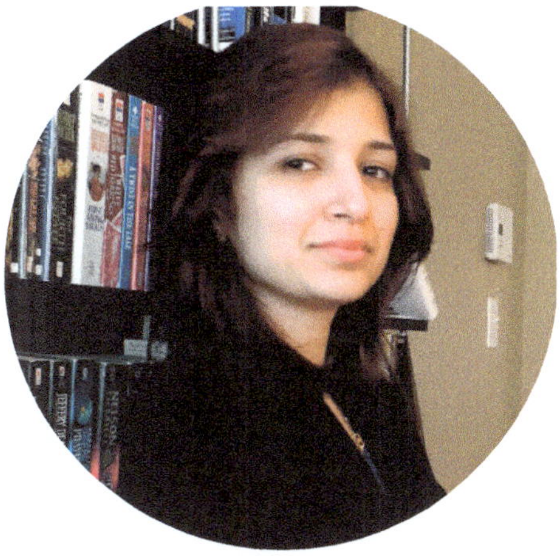

About the Editor

Sarika Garg

Ph.D. Montreal, Canada

Sarika Garg procured her doctoral degree at the Max Planck Unit For Structural Molecular Biology, University of Hamburg, Germany in 2011. This was followed by Postdoctoral Scientist position at University of Saskatchewan, Canada. Later, she moved to CRCHUM, University of Montreal for her second Postdoc. She has diverse research interests and has contributed immensely in many research fields viz. Enzyme Technology, Environmental Science, and Neuroscience. She has numerous research papers and review articles to her credit. She has coauthored two books 'Enzymes & Enzyme Technology'; and 'Biochemical Tests: Principles and Protocols'. She has also contributed several chapters in various books including a chapter on Regulation of Gene Expression in Encyclopedia of Molecular Cell Biology and Molecular Medicine. She is a recipient of 2012 SHRF Postdoctoral Fellowship Award and 2012 Laura E. Chapman Research Award. She is currently working as a Career Counselor in her very own venture 'higherstudiescounseling.com', Montreal, Canada and as a freelancer science writer.

Contents

List of Contributors

Freitas ES de
MercoLab Laboratórios Ltda Brazil

A Back
MercoLab Laboratórios Ltda Brazil

Ibrahim Thabet Hagag[1,2]
[1] Department of Virology, Faculty of Veterinary Medicine, Zagazig University, Zagazig, Egypt
[2] Department of Veterinary and Biomedical Sciences, College of Veterinary Medicine, University of Minnesota, Twin Cities, Saint Paul, Minnesota, United States of America

Shimaa M. G. Mansour
Department of Virology, Faculty of Veterinary Medicine, Zagazig University, Zagazig, Egypt

Zerui Zhang
The State Key Laboratory of Pharmaceutical Biotechnology and Medical School, Nanjing University, Nanjing, China

Ahmed A. H. Ali
Department of Virology, Faculty of Veterinary Medicine, Zagazig University, Zagazig, Egypt

El-Bakry M. Ismaiel
Department of Virology, Faculty of Veterinary Medicine, Zagazig University, Zagazig, Egypt

Ali A. Salama
Department of Virology, Faculty of Veterinary Medicine, Zagazig University, Zagazig, Egypt

Carol J. Cardona
Department of Veterinary and Biomedical Sciences, College of Veterinary Medicine, University of Minnesota, Twin Cities, Saint Paul, Minnesota, United States of America

James Collins
Veterinary Diagnostic Laboratory, College of Veterinary Medicine, University of Minnesota, Twin Cities, Saint Paul, Minnesota, United States of America

Zheng Xing
Department of Veterinary and Biomedical Sciences, College of Veterinary Medicine, University of Minnesota, Twin Cities, Saint Paul, Minnesota, United States of America
The State Key Laboratory of Pharmaceutical Biotechnology and Medical School, Nanjing University, Nanjing, China

Ilse D. Jacobsen
Department for Microbial Pathogenicity Mechanisms, Leibniz Institute for Natural Product Research and Infection Biology, Jena, Germany

Katharina Große
Department for Microbial Pathogenicity Mechanisms, Leibniz Institute for Natural Product Research and Infection Biology, Jena, Germany

Angela Berndt
Institute of Molecular Pathogenesis, Friedrich-Loeffler-Institut (Federal Research Institute for Animal Health), Jena, Germany

Bernhard Hube
Department for Microbial Pathogenicity Mechanisms, Leibniz Institute for Natural Product Research and Infection Biology, Jena, Germany
Friedrich Schiller University, Jena, Germany

S. M. Lutful Kabir
Graduate School of Life and Environmental Sciences, Osaka Prefecture University, Osaka, Japan
Department of Microbiology and Hygiene, Faculty of Veterinary Science, Bangladesh Agricultural University, Mymensingh-2202, Bangladesh

Silva PS da
DVM, Poultry Health Laboratory of Bahia (LASAB)/UFBA

Batinga T de B
DVM, Poultry Health Laboratory of Bahia (LASAB)/UFBA

Sales TS
DVM, graduate student in Tropical Animal Science, School of Veterinary Medicine / UFBA

Herval EFG
DVM, graduate student in Tropical Animal Science, School of Veterinary Medicine / UFBA

Ramos I
DVM, Poultry Health Laboratory of Bahia (LASAB)/UFBA

Maia PCC
DVM, M. Sc. in Animal Pathology, Professor of the Departament of Preventive Veterinary Medicine, School of Veterinary Medicine /UFBA

Fernandes LMB
DVM, Ph.D. in Immunology, Professor of the Departament of Preventive Veterinary Medicine, School of Veterinary Medicine/ UFBA, coordinator of the Poultry Health Laboratory of Bahia (LASAB)/UFBA

Faruku Bande
Department of Veterinary Pathology and Microbiology, Faculty of Veterinary Medicine, Universiti Putra Malaysia (UPM), 43400 Serdang, Selangor, Malaysia
Department of Veterinary Services, Ministry of Animal Health and Fisheries Development, PMB 2109, Usman Faruk Secretariat, Sokoto 840221, Sokoto State, Nigeria

Siti Suri Arshad
Department of Veterinary Pathology and Microbiology, Faculty of Veterinary Medicine, Universiti Putra Malaysia (UPM), 43400 Serdang, Selangor, Malaysia

Abdul Rahman Omar
Department of Veterinary Pathology and Microbiology, Faculty of Veterinary Medicine, Universiti Putra Malaysia (UPM), 43400 Serdang, Selangor, Malaysia
Laboratory of Vaccine and Immunotherapeutics, Institute of Bioscience, Universiti Putra Malaysia (UPM), 43400 Serdang, Selangor, Malaysia

Mohd Hair Bejo
Department of Veterinary Pathology and Microbiology, Faculty of Veterinary Medicine, Universiti Putra Malaysia (UPM), 43400 Serdang, Selangor, Malaysia
Laboratory of Vaccine and Immunotherapeutics, Institute of Bioscience, Universiti Putra Malaysia (UPM), 43400 Serdang, Selangor, Malaysia

Muhammad Salisu Abubakar
Department of Veterinary Pathology and Microbiology, Faculty of Veterinary Medicine, Universiti Putra Malaysia (UPM), 43400 Serdang, Selangor, Malaysia

Yusuf Abba
Department of Veterinary Pathology and Microbiology, Faculty of Veterinary Medicine, Universiti Putra Malaysia (UPM), 43400 Serdang, Selangor, Malaysia

Katherine E Atkins
Centre for Infectious Diseases, University Of Edinburgh, West Mains Road, EH9 3JT, UK
Department of Epidemiology and Public Health, Yale School of Medicine, New Haven

Andrew F Read
Center for Infectious Disease Dynamics, Departments of Biology and Entomology, 208 Mueller Laboratory, The Pennsylvania State University, University Park, PA 16802, USA

Nicholas J Savill
Centre for Infectious Diseases, University Of Edinburgh, West Mains Road, EH9 3JT, UK

Katrin G Renz
Centre for Animal Health and Welfare, School of Environmental and Rural Science, The University of New England, Armidale NSW 2351, Australia

Stephen W Walkden-Brown
Centre for Animal Health and Welfare, School of Environmental and Rural Science, The University of New England, Armidale NSW 2351, Australia

Mark EJ Woolhouse
Centre for Infectious Diseases, University Of Edinburgh, West Mains Road, EH9 3JT, UK

Xinyu Zhuang[1]
[1] Ministry of Education Key Laboratory for Avian Preventive Medicine, Yangzhou University, No. 12 East Wenhui Road, Yangzhou, Jiangsu 225009, P.R. China

Haitao Zou
Ministry of Education Key Laboratory for Avian Preventive Medicine, Yangzhou University, No. 12 East Wenhui Road, Yangzhou, Jiangsu 225009, P.R. China

Huoying Shi
Ministry of Education Key Laboratory for Avian Preventive Medicine, Yangzhou University, No. 12 East Wenhui Road, Yangzhou, Jiangsu 225009, P.R. China
Key Laboratory of Jiangsu Preventive Veterinary Medicine, Yangzhou University, Yangzhou 225009, P.R. China
Jiangsu Co-innovation Center for the Prevention and Control of Important Animal Infectious Diseases and Zoonoses, Yangzhou 225009, P.R. China.

Hongxia Shao
Ministry of Education Key Laboratory for Avian Preventive Medicine, Yangzhou University, No. 12 East Wenhui Road, Yangzhou, Jiangsu 225009, P.R. China
Key Laboratory of Jiangsu Preventive Veterinary Medicine, Yangzhou University, Yangzhou 225009, P.R. China
Jiangsu Co-innovation Center for the Prevention and Control of Important Animal Infectious Diseases and Zoonoses, Yangzhou 225009, P.R. China.

Jianqiang Ye
Ministry of Education Key Laboratory for Avian Preventive Medicine, Yangzhou University, No. 12 East Wenhui Road, Yangzhou, Jiangsu 225009, P.R. China
Key Laboratory of Jiangsu Preventive Veterinary Medicine, Yangzhou University, Yangzhou 225009, P.R. China
Jiangsu Co-innovation Center for the Prevention and Control of Important Animal Infectious Diseases and Zoonoses, Yangzhou 225009, P.R. China

Ji Miao
Key Laboratory of Jiangsu Preventive Veterinary Medicine, Yangzhou University, Yangzhou 225009, P.R. China

Genghua Wu
Key Laboratory of Jiangsu Preventive Veterinary Medicine, Yangzhou University, Yangzhou 225009, P.R. China

Aijian Qin
Ministry of Education Key Laboratory for Avian Preventive Medicine, Yangzhou University, No. 12 East Wenhui Road, Yangzhou, Jiangsu 225009, P.R. China
Key Laboratory of Jiangsu Preventive Veterinary Medicine, Yangzhou University, Yangzhou 225009, P.R. China
Jiangsu Co-innovation Center for the Prevention and Control of Important Animal Infectious Diseases and Zoonoses, Yangzhou 225009, P.R. China

Haque E
Faculty of Animal Science and Veterinary Medicine, Patuakhali Science and Technology University, Dumki, Patuakhali, Bangladesh

Uddin G
Department of Microbiology, University of Chittagong, Bangladesh

Akter S
Faculty of Animal Science and Veterinary Medicine, Patuakhali Science and Technology University, Dumki, Patuakhali, Bangladesh

Bahram Shojadoost
Department of Clinical Sciences, Faculty of Veterinary Medicine, University of Tehran, Tehran, Iran

Andrew R Vince
Department of Pathobiology, University of Guelph, Guelph, Ontario N1G 2W1, Canada

John F Prescott
Department of Pathobiology, University of Guelph, Guelph, Ontario N1G 2W1, Canada

Delesa Damena Mulisa
National Animal Health Diagnostic and Investigation Center, Sebeta, Ethiopia

Menbere Kidane W/Kiros
National Animal Health Diagnostic and Investigation Center, Sebeta, Ethiopia

Redeat Belaineh Alemu
National Animal Health Diagnostic and Investigation Center, Sebeta, Ethiopia

Melaku Sombo Keno
National Animal Health Diagnostic and Investigation Center, Sebeta, Ethiopia

Alice Furaso
Research and Innovation Department, Istituto Zooprofilattico Sperimentale delle Venezie, OIE/FAO and National Reference Laboratory for Newcastle Disease and Avian Influenza,OIE collaborating Center for Diseases at the Human-Animal Interface, Legnaro, Padova, Italy

Alireza Heidari
Research and Innovation Department, Istituto Zooprofilattico Sperimentale delle Venezie, OIE/FAO and National Reference Laboratory for Newcastle Disease and Avian Influenza,OIE collaborating Center for Diseases at the Human-Animal Interface, Legnaro, Padova, Italy

Tesfaye Rufael Chibsa
National Animal Health Diagnostic and Investigation Center, Sebeta, Ethiopia

Hassen Chaka Chunde
National Animal Health Diagnostic and Investigation Center, Sebeta, Ethiopia

A. H. Jibril
Department of Veterinary Physiology, Faculty of Veterinary Medicine, Usmanu Danfodiyo University, Sokoto P.M. B 2346, Nigeria

J. U. Umoh
Department of Veterinary Public Health and Preventive Medicine, Ahmadu Bello University, Zaria, Nigeria

J. Kabir[2]
[2]Department of Veterinary Public Health and Preventive Medicine, Ahmadu Bello University, Zaria, Nigeria

L. Saidu
Ahmadu Bello University Veterinary Teaching Hospital, Zaria, Nigeria

A. A. Magaji
Department of Veterinary Physiology, Faculty of Veterinary Medicine, Usmanu Danfodiyo University, Sokoto P.M. B 2346, Nigeria

M. B. Bello
Department of Veterinary Physiology, Faculty of Veterinary Medicine, Usmanu Danfodiyo University, Sokoto P.M. B 2346, Nigeria

A. A. Raji
Department of Veterinary Physiology, Faculty of Veterinary Medicine, Usmanu Danfodiyo University, Sokoto P.M. B 2346, Nigeria

Marie F Mutryn
Department of Animal and Food Sciences, University of Delaware, 531 South College Ave, Newark, DE 19716, USA

Erin M Brannick
Department of Animal and Food Sciences, University of Delaware, 531 South College Ave, Newark, DE 19716, USA

Weixuan Fu
Department of Animal and Food Sciences, University of Delaware, 531 South College Ave, Newark, DE 19716, USA

William R Lee
Maple Leaf Farms, Leesburg, IN, USA

Behnam Abasht
Department of Animal and Food Sciences, University of Delaware, 531 South College Ave, Newark, DE 19716, USA

Toby G. Knowles
School of Veterinary Science, University of Bristol, Langford, Bristol, United Kingdom

Steve C. Kestin
School of Veterinary Science, University of Bristol, Langford, Bristol, United Kingdom

Susan M. Haslam
School of Veterinary Science, University of Bristol, Langford, Bristol, United Kingdom

Steven N. Brown
School of Veterinary Science, University of Bristol, Langford, Bristol, United Kingdom

Laura E. Green
Ecology and Epidemiology Group, Biological Sciences, University of Warwick, Coventry, United Kingdom

Andrew Butterworth
School of Veterinary Science, University of Bristol, Langford, Bristol, United Kingdom

Stuart J. Pope
School of Veterinary Science, University of Bristol, Langford, Bristol, United Kingdom

Dirk Pfeiffer
The Royal Veterinary College, Royal College Street, London, United Kingdom

Christine J. Nicol
School of Veterinary Science, University of Bristol, Langford, Bristol, United Kingdom

Khaled Kaboudi
Department of Poultry Farming and Pathology, National School of Veterinary Medicine, Tunisia

Sajid Umar
National Veterinary School of Toulouse, 31300 Toulouse, France
Department of Pathobiology, PMAS, Arid Agriculture University, Rawalpindi, Pakistan

Muhammad Tanveer Munir
Nantes Atlantic National College of Veterinary Medicine, Food Science and Engineering (ONIRIS), Nantes, France

Lengmei Wang
Institute of Preventive Veterinary Medicine, College of Animal Sciences, Zhejiang University, Hangzhou, Zhejiang 310058, PR China

Xue Xue
Institute of Preventive Veterinary Medicine, College of Animal Sciences, Zhejiang University, Hangzhou, Zhejiang 310058, PR China

Jianqiu Li
Hangzhou College of Commerce, Zhejiang Gongshang University, Hangzhou, Zhejiang 310012, PR China

Qianjin Zhou
Faculty of Life Science and Technology, Ningbo University, Ningbo, Zhejiang 315211, PR China

Yingchao Yu
Institute of Preventive Veterinary Medicine, College of Animal Sciences, Zhejiang University, Hangzhou, Zhejiang 310058, PR China

Aifang Du
Institute of Preventive Veterinary Medicine, College of Animal Sciences, Zhejiang University, Hangzhou, Zhejiang 310058, PR China

Beata Dolka
Department of Pathology and Veterinary Diagnostics, Faculty of Veterinary Medicine, Warsaw University of Life Sciences-SGGW, Nowoursynowska 159c St., 02-776 Warsaw, Poland

Artur Żbikowski
Department of Pathology and Veterinary Diagnostics, Faculty of Veterinary Medicine, Warsaw University of Life Sciences-SGGW, Nowoursynowska 159c St., 02-776 Warsaw, Poland

Izabella Dolka
Department of Pathology and Veterinary Diagnostics, Faculty of Veterinary Medicine, Warsaw University of Life Sciences-SGGW, Nowoursynowska 159c St., 02-776 Warsaw, Poland

Piotr Szeleszczuk
Department of Pathology and Veterinary Diagnostics, Faculty of Veterinary Medicine, Warsaw University of Life Sciences-SGGW, Nowoursynowska 159c St., 02-776 Warsaw, Poland

Na Yang
College of Animal Science and Veterinary Medicine, Shenyang Agricultural University, Shenyang, Liaoning Province 110866, China

Ming-Yang Mu
College of Animal Science and Veterinary Medicine, Shenyang Agricultural University, Shenyang, Liaoning Province 110866, China

Hong-Kui Li
Liaoning Center for Animal Disease Control and Prevention, Shenyang, Liaoning Province 110164, China

Miao Long
College of Animal Science and Veterinary Medicine, Shenyang Agricultural University, Shenyang, Liaoning Province 110866, China

Jian-Bin He
College of Animal Science and Veterinary Medicine, Shenyang Agricultural University, Shenyang, Liaoning Province 110866, China

Oddvar Fossum
Department of Animal Health and Antimicrobial Strategies, National Veterinary Institute (SVA), SE-751 89 Uppsala, Sweden

Désirée S Jansson
Department of Animal Health and Antimicrobial Strategies, National Veterinary Institute (SVA), SE-751 89 Uppsala, Sweden

Pernille Engelsen Etterlin
Department of Pathology and Wildlife Diseases, National Veterinary Institute (SVA), SE-751 89 Uppsala, Sweden

Ivar Vågsholm
Office of Science and Quality, National Veterinary Institute (SVA, SE-751 89 Uppsala, Sweden

Preface

Poultry is retained world-wide for various rationales. They can be maintained by masses including commercial farmers for meat and eggs, small farmers, and even by the families in the backyard. They are one of the economical sources of meat. Despite its role in elevating emoluments and trimming poverty in the developing countries, its production is curbed by vast range of constraints, including diseases. Poultry is affected by four main types of diseases: metabolic and nutritional diseases, infectious diseases, parasitic diseases, and behavioral diseases.

Poultry production can be made victorious by taking preventive measures to eradicate the diseases. Key step for the poultry men is to understand rigorously the basis of the disease(s) to which domestic birds are susceptible to. Many scientists are allocating their time to study the diseases among poultry and to understand the factors contributing to the disease. As an editor, my aim is to elaborate the scientific side of the subject. In this book, efforts have been done to combine a vast range of published research studies on diseases among poultry.

An infectious disease is a disease induced by seizure of a host by a pathogen which eventually multiplies in the body. Infectious diseases are often transmittable. These include Avian Encephalomyelitis, Avian Influenza, Candidiasis, Colibacillosis, Salmonellosis, Fowl Pox, Infectious Bronchitis, Marek's disease, Mycoplasmosis, Necrotic Enteritis, Newcastle disease, etc. These diseases are described in first 12 Chapters of this book. Metabolic and nutritional diseases are conditions caused by a deficiency or a disturbance of metabolic functions through insufficient nutrition. These include Wooden breast disorder, Leg disorders and so on. These diseases are discussed in the following two Chapters. A parasitic disease is caused by invasion of parasitic organisms. These include Coccidiosis, Cryptosporidiosis, Histomoniasis, Toxoplasmosis etc. These diseases are reported in Chapters 15-18. Abnormal behavioral patterns of the birds can lead to behavioral diseases. This is reported in the last Chapter of the book.

I hope that this book will be beneficial for students, researchers, teachers, and poultry men. It will help in recognising the fact that the disease cannot be controlled by mere disinfection and treatment of ill birds, but involves many important matters such as the selection of flock, smart feeding, proper housing and environment, and successful management.

Editor
Sarika Garg, Ph.D.
Montreal, Canada

CHAPTER 1

NEW OCCURANCE OF AVIAN ENCEPHALOMYELITIS IN BROILER - IS THIS AN EMERGING DISEASE?

Freitas ES de[1], A Back[1]

[1]MercoLab Laboratórios Ltda Brazil

ABSTRACT

Avian encephalomyelitis is caused by an Hepatovirus and primarily affects chickens. Chickens of all ages are susceptible to the virus, but the nervous symptoms are manifested only in young chicks, between one to five weeks of age. During the last thirty years, avian encephalomyelitis appeared to be well controlled by breeder vaccination. However, the increase of the number of cases is causing concern in the poultry industry. In the present study, we performed a retrospective analysis of the cases presenting histological lesions compatible with avian encephalomyelitis in broilers. The evaluated cases affected broilers from one to 35 days old from the southern region of Brazil. Only cases with compatible microscopic lesions and associated with clinical symptoms in the field were considered. In addition the histopathological diagnosis, sera were tested by ELISA (Enzyme-Linked Immunosorbent Assay). Considering the clinical, histopathological, and serological evidences, the disease was confirmed, showing an increase in outbreaks from the last quarter of 2012, extending through 2013. The cause of this increase is not clear, although we suspect vaccine or vaccination error. Enhancing vaccinated breeders flocks monitoring before the beginning of egg production and/or using a protocol with two vaccinations is recommended.

INTRODUCTION

Avian encephalomyelitis is an infectious disease of poultry caused by*Hepatovirus*, belonging to the genus*Enterovirus*. Chickens are primarily affected, but turkeys and other species of birds have also been reported as natural hosts (Calnek, 2008; Vilarreal, 2009). The transmission of the virus is both vertical and horizontal. Vertical transmission tends to cause higher losses because day-old chicks are affected. This happens when breeders with no immunity are infected during the egg production period and transmit the virus to progeny. The virus is horizontally transmitted by the ingestion of feed, litter, or contaminated water (Back, 2010;Calnek, 2008, Calnek, 1998). In this case, the disease is less severe and tends to affect older chickens.

Although poultry of all ages are susceptible, under natural conditions, symptoms are manifested only in chicks from one to three weeks of age. The clinical signs are predominantly neurological and are variable. Chicks show ataxia, incoordination, paralysis, and prostration (Back, 2010). Fast tremors, particularly in the head and neck, are the classic clinical sign of the disease (Martins & Silva, 2009). Surviving birds may become blind due to corneal opacity. According to Taylor *et al.* (1955), breeder hens may present egg production drop; however, they do not develop neurological clinical signs.

Citation: Freitas Es De, A Back, New Occurance of Avian Encephalomyelitis in Broiler - is this an Emerging Disease?, Http://Dx.Doi. Org/10.1590/1516-635X1703399-404.

According to [Calnek (2008)], the only gross lesions observed in outbreaks that affect young chickens are pale areas in the proventriculus and gizzard muscles, but no bigger than a pinhead. Presumptive diagnosis is based on clinical signs presented in chicks. However, the disease is only definitively confirmed by laboratory exams. Among the available techniques, histopathology is considered of essential, and provides the definitive diagnosis of the disease, as demonstrated by the pathognomonic lesions in various tissues, such as the central nervous system, pancreas, proventriculus, gizzard, and heart ([Swayne, 2008; Randall, 1991]). The microscopic lesions in the central nervous system are found in the brain (cerebral peduncle, cerebellum, brain stem) and in the spinal cord and consist of degeneration and necrosis of neurons, perivascular lymphocytic cuffing, and gliosis with formation of glial nodules. In the cerebellum, there are areas of necrosis or loss of Purkinje cells and replacement by glial nodules that extend into the molecular layer of the gray matter. Neuronal lesions of central chromatolysis, shrinkage and increased basophilia, satellitosis, and neuronophagia are typically found in neuron clusters (nuclei) in the brain stem, arbor vitae of the cerebellum, and lateral horn (gray matter) of the spinal cord. Central chromatolysis of neurons is characterized by rounding of the cell contour and displacement of the Nissl granules to the cell periphery. Dorsal root ganglia may present multifocal nodular collections of lymphocytes ([Martins & Silva, 2009; Roy et al, 2009; Villareal, 2009; Calnek, 2008; Swayne, 2008; Taylor et al, 1995; Randall, 1991]). Furthermore, serological tests may also contribute for the diagnosis of the disease, as well as virus isolation ([Calnek, 2008]).

The presence of neutralizing antibodies in the serum of chickens has long been recognized as a major determinant of resistance to infection by avian encephalomyelitis virus ([Tannock & Shafren, 1994]). It was demonstrated that maternal antibodies in the chick yolk sac are fully absorbed between the second and third week post-hatch ([Szabó, 2012]). Therefore, the detection of antibodies against AEV in a flock of chickens with 21 days of age or older indicates field infection.

The best way to prevent and to control the disease is vaccinating breeder flocks during their grow-out period, preventing the infection of breeders during the egg production period, and thereby, virus transmission to the progeny. Moreover, breeder vaccination provides good immunization of progeny, ensuring protection against virus infection during the first weeks of life, when they are most susceptible to the virus ([Back, 2010; Calnek, 2008; Martins & Silva, 2009; Roy *et al*, 2009]).

In Brazil, the avian encephalomyelitis virus appeared to be very well controlled by breeder vaccination for many years ([Back, 2010]). However, the recent increase in the number of cases of avian encephalomyelitis has been a cause of concern in the poultry industry. Therefore, the aim of this study was to evaluate the occurrence of that disease in southern Brazil in the last five years.

MATERIAL AND METHODS

This study evaluated the results of histopathological diagnosis and serology tests performed by MercoLab Laboratórios Ltda., Cascavel, state of Paraná, Brazil. Data from broilers with between one to 35 days of age were studied. Samples derived from poultry farms located in southern Brazil and with suspected evidence of avian encephalomyelitis. Typically, the clinical history reported neurological symptoms such as paralysis, incoordination, neck tremors, and mortality rates ranging from moderate to high (1 to 10%). Data for this study were obtained from January 2009 to December 2013. During that period, 103 broiler flocks suspected of having the disease were evaluated.

The received samples (organs fixed in 10% formalin and serum) were collected by the veterinarian on the farm and submitted to the laboratory. Live birds with clinically suspected signs of the disease were occasionally taken to the laboratory for sample collection. For histopathological analyses, tissue fragments were processed according to routine techniques, including paraffin embedding and staining with hematoxylin-eosin (HE). Briefly, tissues were dehydrated in graded alcohol series (70% alcohol to absolute alcohol), cleared in xylene, and embedded in paraffin. Subsequently, 2- to 4-µm thick sections of the pancreas, brain, gizzard, proventriculus, and heart were cut using an automatic microtome (Leica RM 2125 NT). After deparaffinization in an oven at 60 °C overnight, tissue samples were hydrated in decreasing alcohol series and stained with hematoxylin and eosin (HE).

Encephalon, pancreas, proventriculus, gizzard and heart samples were examined under light microscopy by a veterinary pathologist for the microscopic observation of pathognomonic histopathological lesions of AE. Histopathological analysis results were only included if the observed microscopic lesions were compatible with avian encephalomyelitis and associated with clinical symptoms in the field. The evolution of the group of cases was evaluated per month and per year. Data were analyzed with the aid of likesoftware programs (Excel, Microsoft) and graphs and charts were created to illustrate the results.

In addition to the histopathological evaluation, the sera of broilers older than 21 days were tested by ELISA (Enzyme Linked Immunosorbent Assay) to determine antibody titers against the avian encephalomyelitis virus. Flocks were considered negative when not presenting seroconversion for the pathogen and positive when seroconversion was detected after 21 days of life. All samples were analyzed under the same conditions using a commercial kit (IDEXX) and according to the manufacturer's recommendations. Only the sera of broilers older than 21 days were analyzed in order to prevent any possible interference of maternal antibodies.

RESULTS AND DISCUSSION

The results of this study are shown on the tables, figures and graphs below. Avian encephalomyelitis diagnosis was carried out based on the histopathological changes described by [Swayne (2008)] and on the symptoms observed in the field (Figure 1).

The histopathological sections of the central nervous system showed an accumulation of lymphocytic cells in the perivascular space (perivascular cuffing) in multifocal areas, as well as neuronal necrosis, central chromatolysis and severe gliosis (Figures 2A and B). The muscle layer of the proventriculus, gizzard, and myocardium and the pancreatic interstitium revealed a large number of clusters of lymphocytic inflammatory infiltrate (Figures 3 A, B, C and D). These microscopic findings are considered pathognomonic of avian encephalomyelitis and are consistent with the findings of [Martins & Silva (2009)], [Roy et al. (2009)], [Calnek (2008)], [Swayne (2008)], [Taylor et al. (1995)], [Randall (1991)], and [Butterfield et al. (1969)].

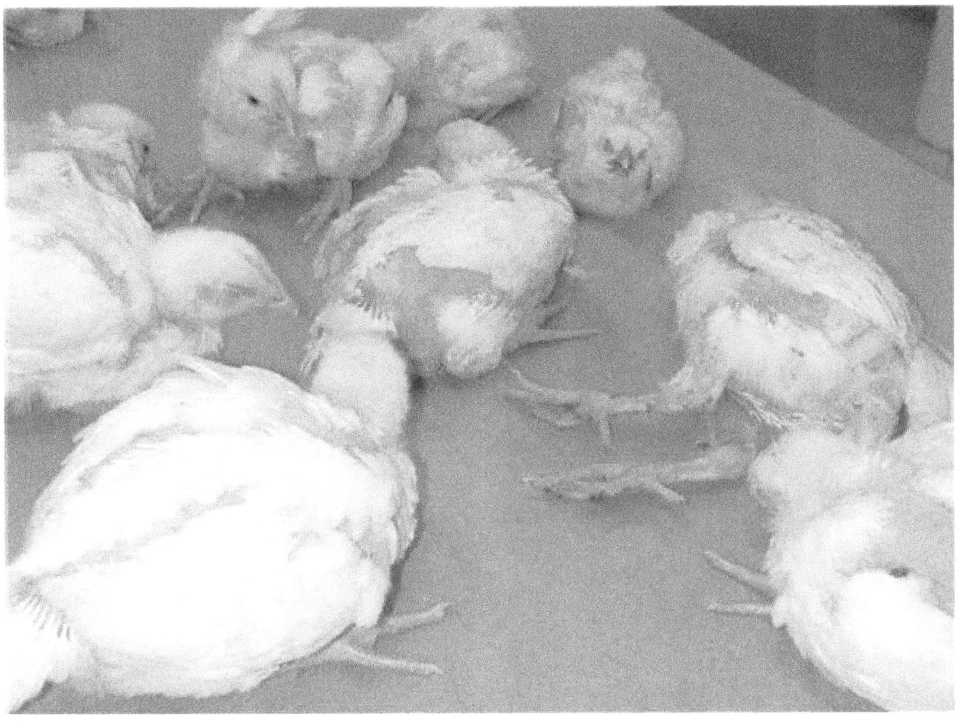

Figure 1: Two-week-old broiler presenting neurological signs of avian encephalomyelitis virus infection.

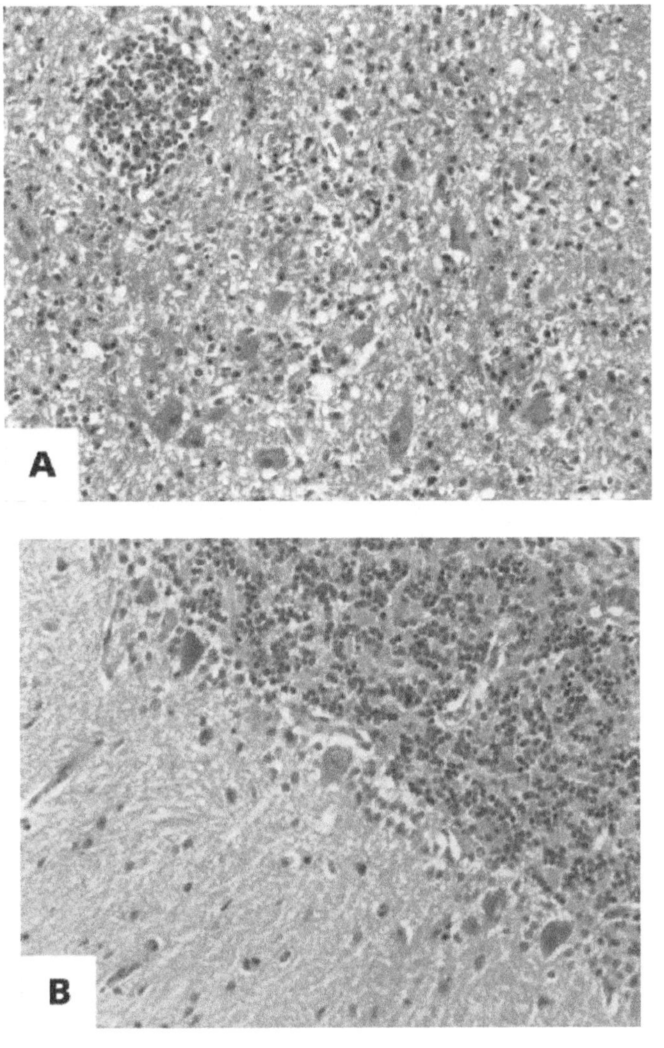

Figure 2: Central nervous system of a two-week-old broiler with avian encephalomyelitis. A) Perivascular cuffs showing marked multifocal gliosis. B) Degeneration and necrosis of neurons with central chromatolysis.

The histological changes presented in Figures 2and 3 are considered pathognomonic for the diagnosis of avian encephalomyelitis, according to Calnek (2008).

In addition to the histopathological findings, high levels of antibodies against the avian encephalomyelitis virus were detected in sera of broilers older than 21 days. Considering that the maternal antibodies transmitted to the progeny do not last longer than two to three weeks after hatching (Szabó, 2012; Kowalczyk et al, 1985; Gharaibehet al, 2008), it is concluded that the detection of antibodies confirms that the chickens had previous contact with the field virus (Graph 1).

The monitoring data of avian encephalomyelitis cases of 2012, and especially of 2013, caught our attention. As shown in Table 1 and Graph 2, the histopathological results reveal a significant increase in the frequency of the disease from the last quarter of 2012 and peaked in May and August of 2013. In 2009 and 2010, no cases of avian encephalomyelitis were detected. These findings support the results described in literature (Calnek, 2008), which demonstrate that, overall, vaccines work very well and prevent the infection, unless breeder immunization mistakes are made (related to the vaccine or vaccination). Immunization errors during the rearing period allow breeder infection during the egg production period, and consequently transmission of the virus to the progeny and manifestation of the disease during the first two weeks of life. Considering the current outbreaks detected in the present study, our hypothesis is that there was a vaccination failure as well as possible low capacity of the virus to induce full immunity.

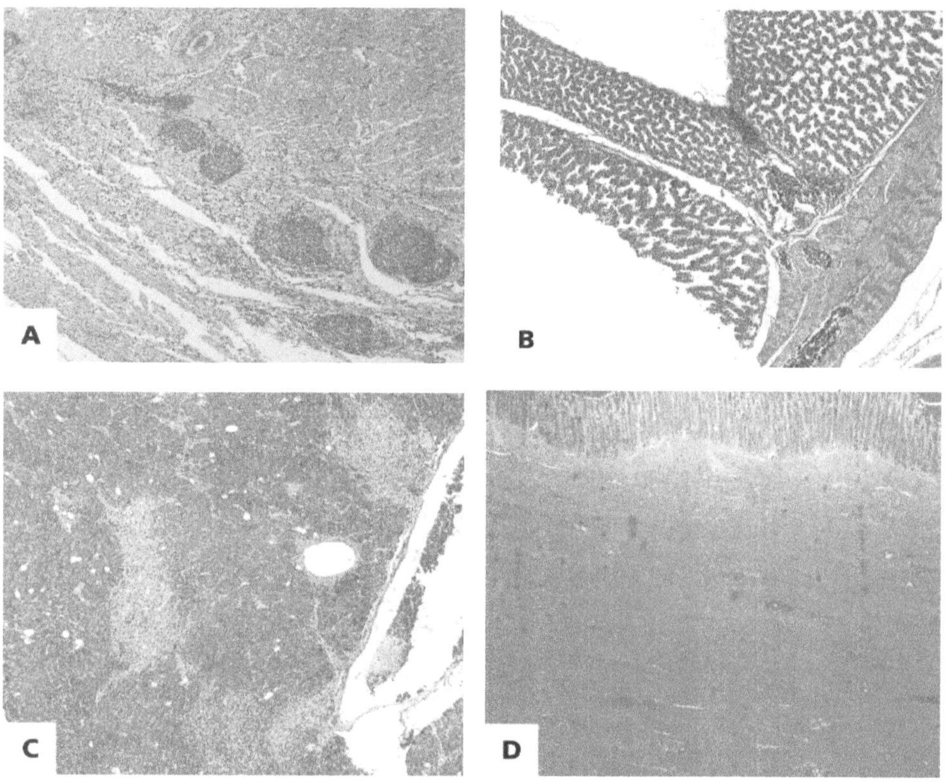

Figure 3: Two-week-old broiler showing lymphocytic inflammatory infiltrate in: A) Heart, B) Proventriculus, C) Pancreas, D) Gizzard.

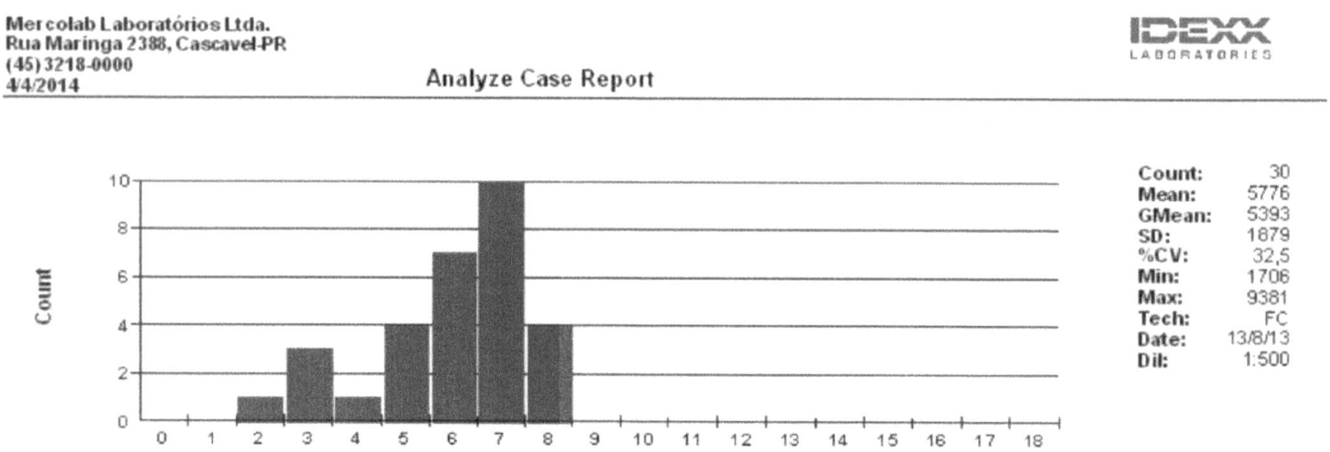

Graph 1: Serology results (ELISA) of 3-week-old broilers, showing seroconversion for the avian encephalomyelitis virus. The serum titers are shown in the x axis and the number of serum samples in the y axis.

Table 1: Number of cases of avian encephalomyelitis diagnosed by histopathology between January 2009 and December 2013 and the number of poultry companies involved

Year/Month	Cases diagnosed by histopathology	Companies involved
January to December/2009	0	0
January to December /2010	0	0
May/2011	4	4
October/2012	8	2
November/2012	6	3
December/2012	1	1
January/2013	5	3
February/2013	5	5
April/2013	9	5
May/2013	15	3
July/2013	6	3
August/2013	14	5
December/2013	4	1

Graph 2 shows that there were no cases of avian encephalomyelitis in 2009 and 2010, and that just a few cases were observed in 2011; however, these numbers started to increase in the last quarter of 2012, with 15 cases distributed in four companies. These numbers increased nearly four times in 2013, totaling 58 cases distributed among 25 poultry companies in southern Brazil. The peak occurred in May and August 2013, with 15 and 14 cases, respectively.

These results show that the problem has spread to several companies in a short time and in a large region. Considering the large number of cases, it appears that the cause was not a single mistake, but a wide range of factors, reaching several states and a large number of poultry companies, may contributed. The possibility of the emergence of new strain of *Enterovirus* and that the current vaccine strains are no longer protecting the flocks is speculated. However, literature and epidemiological data have not shown any evidences for that support such hypotheses. By monitoring the outbreak, it appears that these cases of avian encephalomyelitis are most likely due to vaccine or vaccination failures. These could be related to vaccine viral seed changes, virus attenuation, vaccine titer changes, vaccine conservation errors, errors in vaccination procedures, and vaccination program changes. It seems that breeders were not adequately immunized during the rearing period and became infected during the egg production period, thereby transmitting the virus to the progeny during a certain time, which resulted in disease in the field. Further studies are required to elucidate possible predisposing factors for these outbreaks. Meanwhile, we suggest the monitoring of breeders after vaccination to ensure their contact with the vaccine virus and that they produce antibodies before the egg production period. In case of weak response, revaccinate the breeders to guarantee good protection and transference of immunity to the progeny.

CONCLUSION

The clinical, histopathological, and serological evidences obtained in the present study showed a significant increase of cases of avian encephalomyelitis in broilers from the last quarter of 2012 until the end of 2013. The cause of this increase is not yet clear, but vaccine or vaccination failures are suspected. The monitoring of breeders before the beginning of egg production and the application of two vaccinations, if necessary, are suggested.

REFERENCES

1. Asasi K, Farzinpour A, Tafti AK. Clinico-Pathological Studies on Avian Encephalomyelitis in Shiraz, Iran. Turkish Journal of Veterinary and Animal Sciences 2008;3(3):229 - 231.
2. Back A. Encefalomielite aviária. In: Back A. Manual de doenças de aves. 2ª ed. Cafelândia : Editora Integração; 2010. p. 70-2.
3. Butterfield, W.K., Helmboldt, C.F., Luginbuhl, R.E. Studies on avian encephalomyelitis. IV. Early incidence and longevity of histopathological lesions in chickens. Avian Diseases 1969;13:53-57
4. Calnek BW. Avian encephalomyelitis. In: Saif YM. Diseases of poultry. 12th ed, Iowa: Blackwell; 2008. p. 430 - 41.
5. Calnek BW. Control of avian encephalomyelitis: a historical account. Avian Diseases1998;42:632 -647.
6. Gharaibeh S, Mahmoud K. Decay of maternal antibodies in broiler chickens. Poultry Science 2013; 92:2333 - 2336.
7. Gharaibeh S, Mahmoud K, Al-Natour M. Field evaluation of maternal antibody transfer to a group of pathogens in meat-type chickens. Poultry Science2008;87:1550 -55.
8. Kowalczyk K, Daiss J, Halpern J, Roth TF. Quantification of maternal-fetal IgG transport in the chicken. Immunology 1985;54:755- 62.
9. Martins PC, Silva PL. Encefalomielite aviária. In: Berchieri Jr A, Silva EN, Di Fábio J, Sesti L, Zuanase MAF. Doença das aves. 2th ed Campinas: Facta; 2009. p.763 - 74.
10. Randall CJ. Diseases and disorders of the domestic fowl and turkey. 2th ed. Barcelona: Mosby-Wolfe; 1991. p.66-68.

11. Roy P, Hemalatha S, Vairamuthu S, Purushothaman V, Chandramohan A, Karunamurthy G, Koteeswaran, A, Muralimanohar, B. An outbreak of avian encephalomyelitis in Tamil Nadu State of India. West Indian Veterinary Journal 2009;9 2):8 -10.

12. Swayne DE. Nervous system. In: Fletcher OJ. Avian histopathology. 3rd ed. Jacksonville: AAAP; 2008. p.58-79.

13. Szabó C. Transport of IGY from egg-yolk to the chicken embryo. Journal of Microbiology, Biotechnology and Food Sciences 2012;2(3):612 -20.

14. Tannock GA, Shafren DR. Avian encephalomyelitis: a review. Avian Pathology 1994;23:603 - 620.

15. Taylor LW, Lowry DC, Raggi LG. Effects of an outbreak of avian encephalomyelitis (epidemic tremor) in a breeding flock. Poultry Science1995;34:1036-45.

16. Villareal L. Encefalomielite aviária. In: Revolledo L, Ferreira AJP. Patologia aviária. Barueri: Manole; 2009. p. 234 - 39.

CHAPTER 2

PATHOGENICITY OF HIGHLY PATHOGENIC AVIAN INFLUENZA VIRUS H5N1 IN NATURALLY INFECTED POULTRY IN EGYPT

Ibrahim Thabet Hagag[1,2], Shimaa M. G. Mansour[1], Zerui Zhang[4], Ahmed A. H. Ali[1], El-Bakry M. Ismaiel[1], Ali A. Salama[1], Carol J. Cardona[2], James Collins[3], Zheng Xing[2,4]

[1] Department of Virology, Faculty of Veterinary Medicine, Zagazig University, Zagazig, Egypt

[2] Department of Veterinary and Biomedical Sciences, College of Veterinary Medicine, University of Minnesota, Twin Cities, Saint Paul, Minnesota, United States of America

[3] Veterinary Diagnostic Laboratory, College of Veterinary Medicine, University of Minnesota, Twin Cities, Saint Paul, Minnesota, United States of America

[4] The State Key Laboratory of Pharmaceutical Biotechnology and Medical School, Nanjing University, Nanjing, China

ABSTRACT

Highly pathogenic avian influenza virus (HPAIV) H5N1 has been endemic in Egypt since 2006, and there is increasing concern for its potential to become highly transmissible among humans. Infection by HPAIV H5N1 has been described in experimentally challenged birds. However, the pathogenicity of the H5N1 isolated in Egypt has never been reported in naturally infected chickens and ducks. Here we report a 2013 outbreak of HPAIV H5N1 in commercial poultry farms and backyards in Sharkia Province, Egypt. The main symptoms were ecchymosis on the shanks and feet, cyanosis of the comb and wattles, subcutaneous edema of the head and neck for chickens, and nervous signs (torticollis) for ducks. Within 48-72 hrs of the onset of illness, the average mortality rates were 22.8-30% and 28.5-40% in vaccinated chickens and non-vaccinated ducks, respectively. Tissue samples of chickens and ducks were collected for analyses with cross-section immunohistochemistry and real-time RT-PCR for specific viral RNA transcripts. While viral RNA was detected in nearly all tissues and sera collected, viral nucleoprotein was detected almost ubiquitously in all tissues, including testis. Interestingly, viral antigen was also observed in endothelial cells of most organs in chickens, and clearly detected in the trachea and brain in particular. Viral nucleoprotein was also detected in mononuclear cells of various organs, especially pulmonary tissue. We performed phylogenetic analyses and compared the genomic sequences of the hemagglutinin (HA) and nonstructural proteins (NS) among the isolated viruses, the HPAIV circulated in Egypt in the past and currently, and some available vaccine strains. Further analysis of deduced amino acids of both HA and NS1 revealed that our isolates carried molecular determinants of HPAIV, including the multibasic amino acids (PQGERRRK/KR*GLF) in the cleavage site in HA and glutamate at position 92 (D92E) in NS1. This is the first report of the pathogenicity of the HPAIVH5N1 strain currently circulating in naturally infected poultry in Egypt, which may provide unique insights into the viral pathogenesis in HPAIV-infected chickens and ducks.

INTRODUCTION

Highly pathogenic avian influenza virus (HPAIV) H5N1 persists in natural reservoirs of aquatic birds and waterfowl. In 1996 it was discovered that infected wild geese in Southern China were responsible for transmitting the virus to poultry [1]. In 2003, HPAIV H5N1 began to spread from Southeast Asia to other regions, and in the past decade it has caused numerous outbreaks on poultry farms in over 60 countries in Asia, Africa, and Europe. While the virus remains highly pathogenic to poultry and humans, it has also evolved to become pathogenic to domestic ducks beginning in 2002, and has killed wild

Citation: Hagag IT, Mansour SMG, Zhang Z, Ali AAH, Ismaiel E-BM, Salama AA, et al. (2015) Pathogenicity of Highly Pathogenic Avian Influenza Virus H5N1 in Naturally Infected Poultry in Egypt. PLoS ONE 10(5): e0120061. doi:10.1371/journal.pone.0120061.

waterfowl beginning with the outbreaks in Qinghai Lake in 2005 [2–5]. HPAIV H5N1 has caused severe agricultural and economic burdens with hundreds of millions of poultry culled, and poses a serious public health threat with over 370 human deaths reported since 2003 [6, 7].

HPAIV H5N1 was first transmitted to Africa in 2006 and spread quickly, with outbreaks reported in Nigeria, Egypt, Cameroon, and other African countries [8]. Notably, since then it has become endemic only in Egypt, which is the largest poultry producing country of the Arab nations [9], with regularly reported outbreaks, enormous economic losses in poultry industry, and confirmed human cases with high mortality [10]. While breeders' farms may have strict biosecurity, most commercial farms and household backyards, which comprise the majority of poultry producers in the country, practice poor biosecurity measures [11]. In addition, Egyptian customers rely heavily on live bird markets, where birds of different species and ages and from various locations are offered for trade and slaughter, providing numerous opportunities for viral transmission [12]. Since early control plans including culling infected birds, implementing quarantine measures, and movement restrictions have failed to contain the virus since its emergence in early 2006, control strategies have shifted to massive vaccination programs with inactivated H5N1 or H5N2 viruses, virus surveillance in poultry sectors, and preemptive culling of infected birds [11–13]. These new strategies have significantly reduced outbreaks in recent years. However, surveillance data reveal continuous and wide circulation of the virus in vaccinated and non-vaccinated commercial farms, household backyards, and live bird markets [14]. In addition, the virus may be undergoing genetic divergence, evolving into multiple genotypes. Remarkably, the H5N1 isolates circulating in Egypt that originated from the Qinghai Lake H5N1 viruses possess several critical genetic hallmarks, including the mutations in HA154-156, where a glycosylation site is missing, and PB2627K [15, 16]. The first renders the virus capable of transmission in mammals, and the second increases viral replication in humans, causing concern that HPAIV H5N1 variants may emerge in Egypt with increased potential for transmissibility in mammals [17].

The HPAIV H5N1 viruses circulating in Egypt since 2006 are highly pathogenic to chickens and can be lethal to ducks [12]. Since becoming endemic in Egypt, the virus has spread from farm to farm, even under immune pressure produced from vaccinated H5 viruses, which may lead to its evolution and mutation [14]. There is limited understanding of the viral pathogenicity and pathogenesis of the current Egyptian H5N1 viruses, the most common cause of outbreaks in poultry in the country.

In this study we report a recent outbreak of the HPAIV H5N1 in commercial poultry farms and backyards in Sharkia Province, Egypt. Our data indicate that the mortality rates were 22.8–30% in broilers and layers that were vaccinated once with inactivated H5 vaccines, in contrast to the mortality rate of 0.14% in layers which were vaccinated twice. The mortality rates for two backyard flocks of ducks were 28.5 and 40%, respectively, and none of the ducks were vaccinated. Using immunohistochemistry staining we detected viral nucleoprotein in multiple organs and tissues, including trachea, lung, brain, spleen, pancreas, liver, proventriculus, bursa of Fabricius, and testis. The resultant HPAI H5N1 viruses A/chicken/Egypt/IT-1/2013, A/chicken/Egypt/IT-2/2013, and A/duck/Egypt/IT-3/2013 were isolated, and their HA and NS genes analyzed by comparing with the H5N1 viruses previously isolated in Egypt, neighboring countries and worldwide.

MATERIALS AND METHODS

Viruses

HPAIV H5N1 strains were isolated from chicken and duck tissue samples in commercial poultry farms or backyards in Sharkia Province, Egypt, from February to May 2013. Tissue samples were collected and ground in DMEM cultural medium and centrifuged at 500xg for 10 min. The supernatants were collected and inoculated into 9- to 11-old embryonated chicken eggs, which were then incubated at 37°C. Allantoic fluids were collected and tested with a standard hemagglutination (HA) assay. For HA positive samples, viral RNA was extracted and viral subtypes were identified by reverse transcriptase-polymerase chain reaction (RT-PCR) using a set of subtype-specific primers for viral genes (Table 1), and then further confirmed using nucleotide sequencing. The viruses were aliquoted and stored at -80°C. All animal work was performed with accomplice to the rules and approved ahead by the ethics committee for animal studies at Zagazig University, Egypt.

Table 1: Sequences of the Oligonucleotide Primers Used in the Study

Target Gene	Primer Forward (5'→3')	Primer Reverse (5'→3')	Product Size (bp)	References
H5	H5-kha-1	H5-kha-3	~317	[18]
	CCTCCAGARTATGCMTAYAAAATTGTC	TACCAACCGTGTACCATKCCYTG		
N1	N1-84F	N1-288R	~245	[19]
	TCARTCTGYATGRTAAYTGG	[illegible]		
NS	Bm-NS-1	Bm-NS-890R	890+29	[20]
	TATTCGTCTCAGGGAGCAAAAGCAGGGTG	ATATCGTCTCGTATTAGTAGAAACAAGGGTGTTTT		
M	M+25F	M-124R	-	[22]
	AGATGAGTCTTCTAACCGAGGTCG	TGCAAAAACATCTTCAAGTCTCTG		
M Gene Probe	M+64probe FAM-TCAGGCCCCCTCAAAGCCGA-TAMRA		-	[22]

doi:10.1371/journal.pone.0[illegible].t001

RNA Extraction, RT-PCR, and Realtime RT-PCR

Viral RNA was extracted from allantoic fluids with Blood/ Liquid Sample Total RNA Rapid Extraction Kit (Bioteke Corporation, China) following manufacturer's instructions. Approximately 1 μg of RNA (5 μl) was reverse transcribed to cDNA using cDNA DiaStarRT Kit (Solgent Co., Korea) according to the manufacturer's protocol. The cDNA were used as templates for PCR with specific primers to H5 and N1 [18, 19], which was carried out for 35 cycles. PCR amplicons were subjected to electrophoresis in a 1.5% agarose gel, and fragments of H5 subtype HA and N1 subtype neuraminidase (NA) genes of expected sizes were detected (Fig 1F).

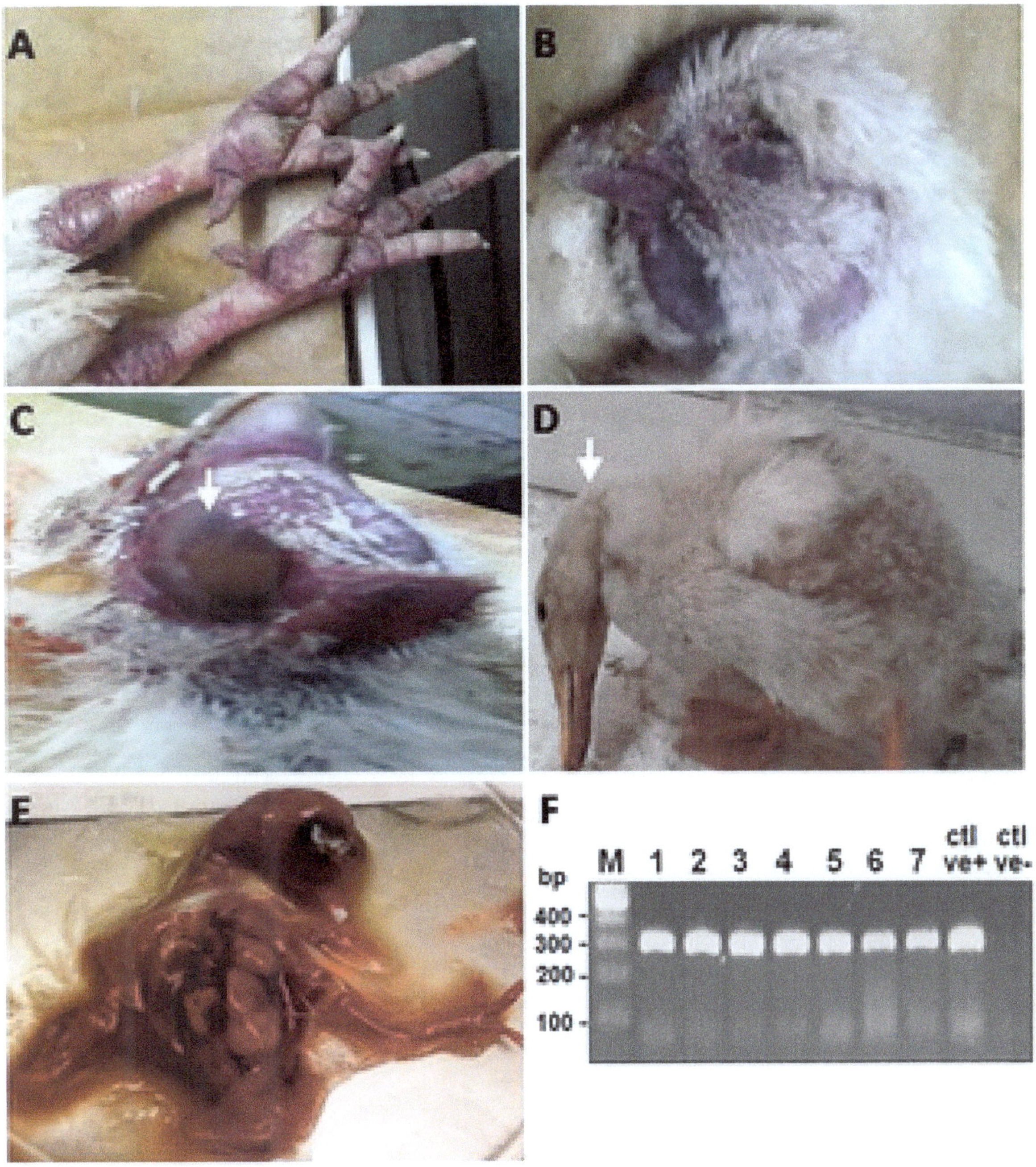

Figure 1: Naturally infected chickens and ducks by HPAIV H5N1.

(**A**) Chickens: subcutaneous hemorrhages in non-feathered skin. (**B**) Chickens: cyanosis of comb & wattles. (**C**) Chickens: facial edema. (**D**) Ducks: nervous signs, torticollis. (**E**) Infected chicken embryos: chicken embryos were inoculated with supernatants of homogenized testicular tissue of naturally infected layer chickens; the inoculated embryos died within 48hrs with severe congestion and hemorrhages after the first passage. (**F**) PCR amplification for HA gene showing bands of 317bp in size. First lane: Molecular marker of 100 bp, Lane 1–7: Positive samples, Ctrl +ve: Positive AIV subtype H5N1, Ctrl-ve: Negative control.

For realtime RT-PCR, total RNA were prepared from various tissue and serum samples and reverse transcribed to cDNA. TaqMan-based realtime RT-PCR (Applied Biosystems, USA) was performed with 1 μl of cDNA in a volume of 25 μl to measure viral M gene transcripts in the tissues using a set of M gene specific primers and probe (Table 1). The probe was labeled with 5'-FAM and 3'-TAMRA. The reaction was run with ABI 7500 and each assay was repeated three times with positive and negative controls included with the tested samples.

Viral Gene Cloning, Sequencing, and Phylogenetic Analysis

Viral RNA extracted from the allontoic fluids was reverse transcribed with Superscript III Reverse Transcriptase (Invitrogen, USA) and a Uni-12 primer [20]. The cDNA was amplified by PCR with Taq DNA polymerase (Takara, Japan) and primers specific for influenza virus gene segment [20]. PCR products were cloned into a TA cloning vector (Invitrogen, USA) and the nucleotide sequences determined by DNA sequencing.

Phylogenetic analyses of the HA and NS gene were based on nucleotides 791–1100 (309 bases) of HA and 39–704 (666 bases) of NS. All gene sequence data of known H5N1 strains were collected from the NCBI Influenza Database. Multiple alignments were constructed using ClustalW Multiple Alignment with the MegAlign module of DNAStar software (Lasergene version 7.2, DNASTAR, Madison, WI, USA). The neighbor-joining method with Kimura two-parameter distances was used for constructing the phylogenetic tree using the Mega 5.0, and the tree was rooted to the A/goose/ Guangdong/1/1996 virus sequence. The reliability of the internal branches was assessed by the p-distance substitution model and 1000 bootstrap replications. The HA and NS genotypes was determined using the Influenza A Virus FluGenome web server, (http://www.flugenome.org/) [21].

Immunohistochemistry

Freshly collected tissues were fixed by 10% formalin and embedded in paraffin. For histopathology, cross-sections were prepared at 5 µm and stained with hematoxylin and eosin (HE). For immunohistochemistry (IHC) staining, a duplicate 4-µm section was cut, mounted on positively charged SuperFrost Plus microscope slides, dewaxed, and rehydrated. Antigen retrieval was performed by pressure-cooking for 25 mins in pH 6 citrate buffer. Endogenous peroxidases were blocked using 3% H_2O_2 for 15 mins. Non-specific bindings were blocked using normal goat serum at 1:10 in TBS for 15 mins. Slides were incubated overnight at 4°C with primary rabbit anti-influenza A nucleoprotein (NP) polyclonal antibody (Catalog ID19382; LifeSpan Biosciences, WA) at 1:50 dilution. The EnVision AP (DAKO K1396, Carpinteria, CA) detection system and nuclear fast red (DAKO K1396) were used as chromogens. Sections were counterstained with Mayer's hematoxylin. Positive and negative control sections were included in each IHC run. All tissues were systematically screened for microscopic lesions. The intensity of viral antigen staining in each section was also scored as following: (-), no antigen staining; (+), infrequent; (++), common; and (+++), widespread staining.

Statistical Analysis

Data were collected and continuous variables were analyzed using one-way analysis of variance (*ANOVA*), then comparison of means was carried out with Duncan's multiple range tests (*DMRT*) and summarized as mean ± standard deviation.

RESULTS

Outbreaks of HPAIV H5N1 in commercial poultry farms and backyards

Beginning in February 2013, chickens and ducks in commercial poultry farms and backyards in Sharkia Province, Egypt, became sick with symptoms including ecchymosis on the shanks and feet, cyanosis of the comb and wattles, subcutaneous edema of head and neck in chickens, and nervous signs (torticollis) in ducks, characteristics of HPAIV infection, as shown in Fig 1A–1D. Birds began to die within 48–72 hrs of the onset of illness. The mortality rates for two unvaccinated backyard flocks of ducks consisting of 14 and 20 birds were 28.5 and 40%, respectively (Table 2). On the other hand, the mortality rates were 22.8 to 30% in broilers and layers that were vaccinated once with inactivated H5 vaccines, and 0.14% in layers that were vaccinated twice (Table 2). The flock sizes of the commercial chicken farms ranged from 3,900 to 5,000 for both broilers and layers.

Table 2: The Outbreaks of HPAIV H5N1 in the Egyptian Commercial Poultry Farms and the Virus Identification

Flock No.	Species	Rearing System/ Breed	Age/ Days	Clinical Characteristics	Average Mortality Rates	No. of Sampled Birds	No. of H5N1 +ve Birds	Results of HPAI H5N1 Infected Flocks			
								Viral isolation	Routine HA	RT-PCR	IHC
1	Ducks	Backyard/ Mallard	25	Greenish diarrhea and nervous signs	28.50%	1	1	+ve	+ve	+VE	+VE
2	Ducks	Backyard/ Muscovy	30	(Torticollis)	40.00%	3	3	+ve	+ve	+VE	N/A
3	Chicken broilers	Commercial/ Cobb 500*	32		22.85%	9	9	+ve	+ve	+VE	+ve
4	Chicken broilers	Commercial/ Cobb 500*	37	Respiratory signs	30.00%	6	6	+ve	+ve	+VE	+ve
5	Chicken broilers	Commercial/ Cobb 500*	35	Cyanosis of the head, comb and wattles Subcutaneous edema of head and neck with ecchymoses on the shanks and feet	24.10%	9	9	+ve	+ve	+VE	N/A
6	Chicken layers	Commercial/ Hyline*	105		24.60%	6	6	+ve	+ve	+VE	+ve
7	Chicken layers	Commercial/ Hyline**	108		0.14%	6	3	+ve	+ve	+VE	+ve
Total	Ducks	-	-	-	-	4	4	-	-	-	-
	Chickens	-	-	-	-	43	33	-	-	-	-

* Chicken broiler and layer flocks were vaccinated once with H5 inactivated vaccine.
** This chicken layer flock was vaccinated two times with H5 inactivated vaccine.
Backyard ducks were not vaccinated.
N/A: Not applied
+ve: Positive

[illegible]

Nine- to11-day-old chicken embryonated eggs were inoculated with samples from ground pulmonary, tracheal, and testicular tissues of dying or dead chickens or ducks. Embryos with extensive hemorrhage died within 48 hrs post inoculation. Severely congested embryos were observed in eggs inoculated with testicular tissues after the first passage (Fig 1E). Allantoic fluids were tested for hemagglutination (HA) reactivity with a routine HA assay and positive titers were detected. Further viral RNA was prepared from the allantoic fluids, which was reverse transcribed to cDNA for amplification of viral HA and NA fragments with polymerase chain reaction (PCR) using primers specific for theH5N1 HA and NA genes (Table 1). Results indicated that the isolates wereHPAIVH5N1 positive. The PCR results showed specific bands in 1.5% agarose gel at 317(Fig 1F) and 245 base pairs in size (data not shown) for HA and NA, respectively. HPAIV subtype H5N1 was detected in34 of 46 birds including both ducks and chickens (Table 2) with a detection rate of73.9%, including 30 of 42 (71.4%) chickens and 4 of 4 (100%) ducks, respectively (Table 2). Further nucleotide sequencing of the purified PCR products confirmed the isolates to be of the HPAIVH5N1 subtypes, and three viral isolates were designated as A/chicken/Egypt/IT-1/2013, A/chicken/Egypt/IT-2/2013, and A/duck/Egypt/IT-3/2013. The relevant nucleotide sequences were deposited at the NCBI GenBank database with deposition numbersKJ192204, KJ192205, KJ192206,KP311329, and KP311330 for the three viral strains, respectively.

Viral RNA in chicken and duck tissues

Chicken and duck tissues including trachea, lung, liver, spleen, intestine, brain, testis, and serum were taken from sick or dead birds for total RNA preparation. After reverse transcription, cDNA of the samples were subjected to TaqMan-based semi-quantitative realtime RT-PCR (qRT-PCR) [22]with primers specific to the M gene to examine viral RNA in each organ type.

As shown in Fig 2, viral RNA of the HPAIV H5N1 M gene was detected in all tissues tested both in chickens and ducks with the exception of testis, which was only positive for chicken layers. Higher levels of viral RNA were in general detected in tissues of broiler and layer chickens, including trachea, lung, spleen, intestines, brain, and serum, than in those of ducks (Fig 2). However, these samples from different birds cannot be compared because they came from natural outbreaks with uncertain timing of the course of infection. In broiler chickens, however, higher viral RNA levels appeared in brain, trachea, and serum samples. No significant differences in viral RNA levels were observed in various tissues of ducks, except for higher levels detected in trachea, lung, and liver tissues (Fig 2).

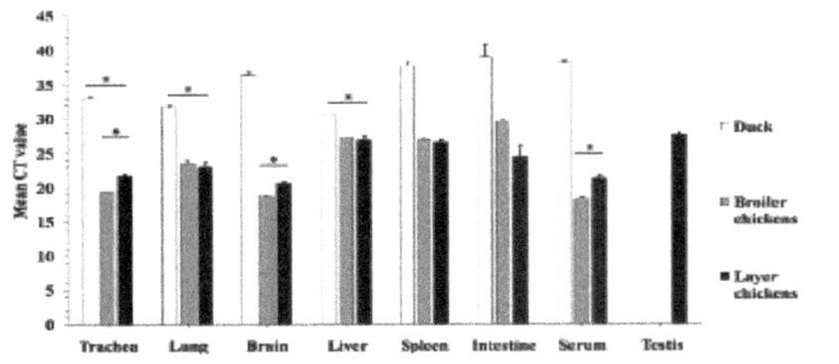

Figure 2: Detection of M gene transcripts by RT-PCR.

Results were expressed as *Ct* values; *Ct* values lower than (35) were considered positive; *Ct* values between 15 and 25 were considered strong positive, while those between 25 and 30 were considered moderate positive; *Ct* values between 30 and 35 were considered weak positive. The tests were performed in triplicates for each sample and the *Ct* numbers are average with 3xSD (* $P<0.05$).

Viral nucleoprotein detected in organs of chickens

Organs and tissues from sick or dead chickens from farms where outbreaks of HPAIV H5N1 occurred were prepared for cross-section slides with routine paraformaldehyde fixation, and subjected to IHC. An antibody to HPAI H5N1 nucleoprotein (NP) was used to stain the samples for detection of viral NP in tissues of infected birds.

As shown in Table 3 and Figs 3 through 7, viral NP was detected in all tested tissues including brain (Fig 4), pancreas and spleen (Fig 5), proventriculus and bursa of Fabricius (Fig 6), and lung and liver (Fig 7). Remarkably, the viral antigen was also detected in testicular tissue in between seminephrous tubules, even sticking to heads of sperm inside them (Fig 7E). The viral antigen was often associated with histologic lesions, although it was also observed in areas without detectable lesions.

Table 3: Summary of Virus Distribution in Tissues of the HPAIV H5N1-Infected Chickens IHC scoring system. (-) no viral antigen detected; (+) sporadic; (++) common; (+++) widespread

Tissue	IHC Score	Type of Cells Expressing Virus Antigen
Trachea	+++	Endothelial cells and epithelial cells
Lung	+	Macrophages, Lymphocytes
Brain	+++	Endothelial cells, neurons and glial cells especially in perkinji cell layer
Spleen	+	Lymphocytes, Endothelial mononuclear cells
Bursa	+	Lymphocytes inside Follicular layer, endothelial cells
Pancreas	+++	Pancreatic acinar epithelium, macrophages and endothelial cells
Proventriculus	+	Glandular epithelium
Testis	++	Inter seminephrous space, intra seminephrous tubules sticking to sperms

IHC scoring system: (-) no viral antigen detected; (+) sporadic; (++) common; (+++) widespread.

doi:10.1371/journal.pone.0120061.t003

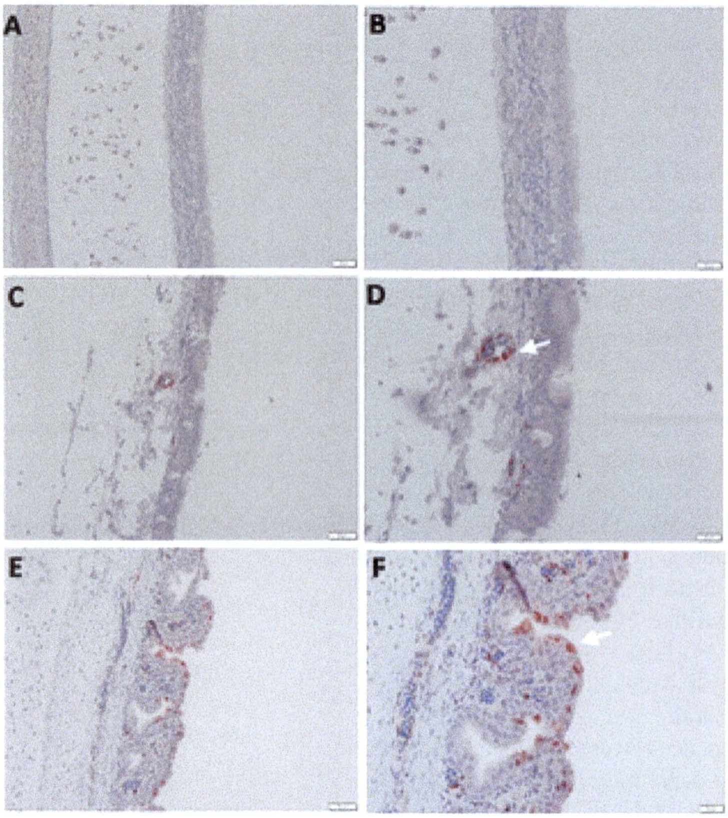

Figure 3: Detection of viral NP antigen in trachea by IHC.

(**A** and **B**) Trachea of non-infected birds (X = 50 and 20μm, respectively). (**C** and **D**) Endothelial cells of trachea of infected birds (X = 50 and 20μm, respectively). (**E** and **F**)Epithelial cells of trachea of infected birds (X = 50 and 20μm, respectively).

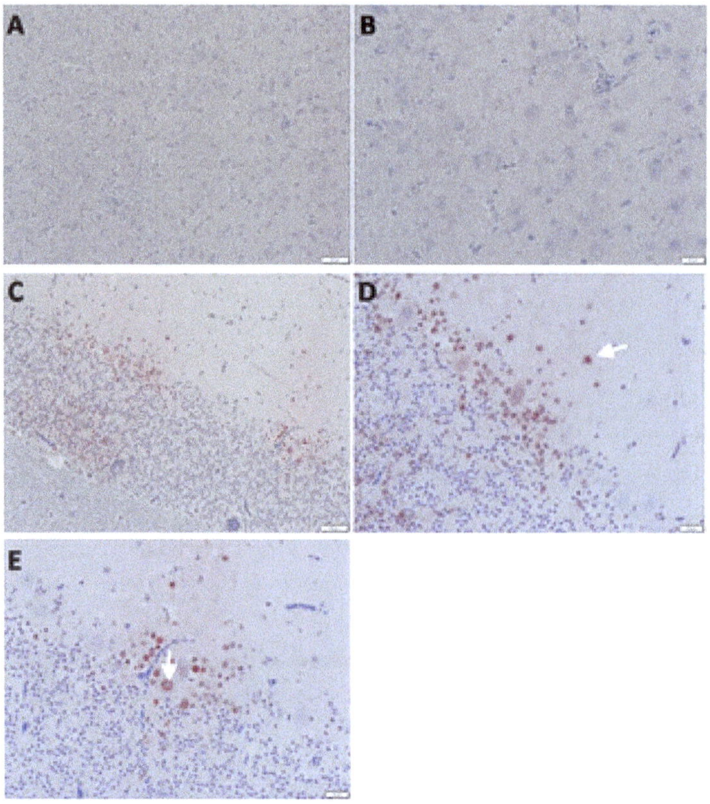

Figure 4: Detection of viral NP antigen in brain by IHC.

(**A** and **B**) Brain of non-infected birds (X = 50 and 20μm, respectively). (**C**) Perkinji cell layer of cerebellum of infected birds (X = 50μm). (**D**) Neurons and glial cells of perkinji cell layer of cerebellum of infected birds (arrow) (X = 20μm). (**E**) Endothelial cells of perkinji cell layer of cerebellum of infected birds (arrow) (X = 20μm).

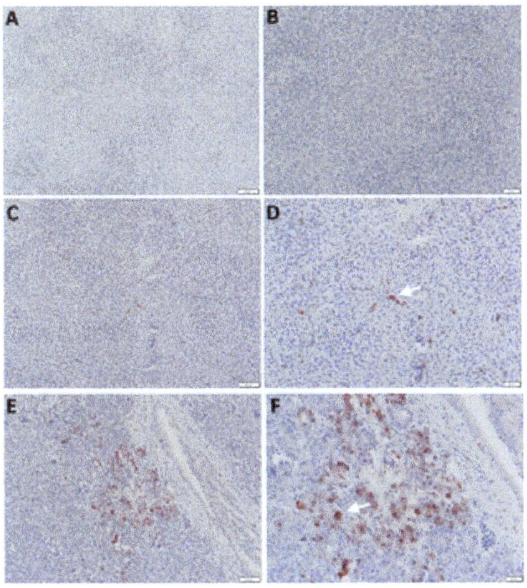

Figure 5: Detection of viral NP antigen in spleen and pancreas by IHC.

(**A** and **B**) Spleen of non-infected birds (X = 50 and 20μm, respectively). (**C**) Lymphocytes in spleen of infected birds (X = 50μm). (**D**) Lymphocytes and mononuclear cells in spleen of infected birds (arrow) (X = 20μm). (**E** and **F)** Acinar epithelium of pancreas of infected birds (X = 50 and 20μm, respectively).

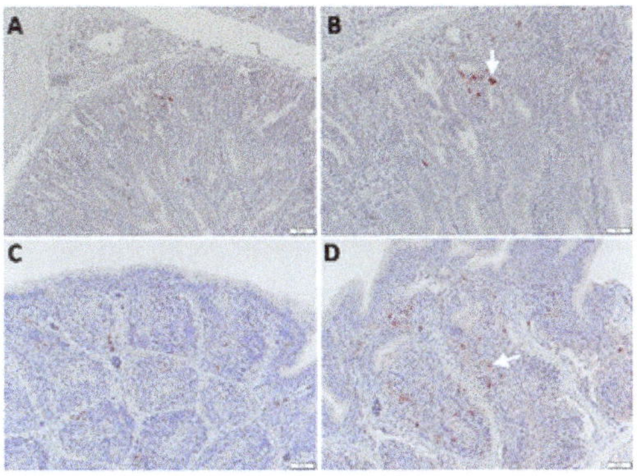

Figure 6: Detection of viral NP antigen in proventriculus and bursa of Fabricius by IHC.

(**A**) Proventriculus of infected birds (X = 50μm). (**B**) Glandular epithelium of proventriculus (arrow) (X = 20μm). (**C** and **D**) Lymphocytes in follicular layer of bursa of Fabricius of infected birds (arrow) (X = 50 and 20μm, respectively).

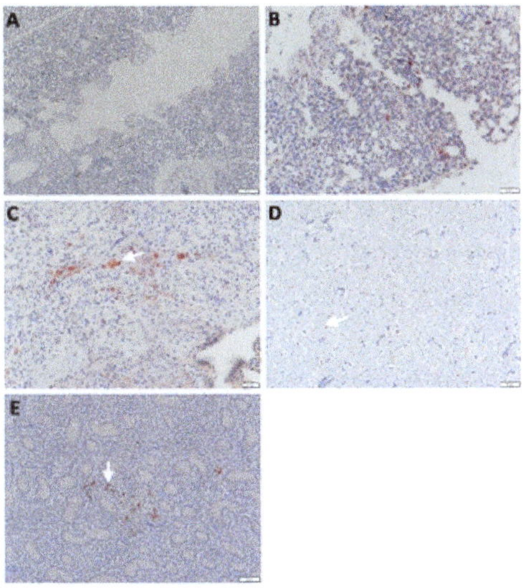

Figure 7: Detection of viral NP antigen in lung, liver and testisby IHC.

(**A**) Lung of non-infected birds (X = 50μm). (**B** and **C**) Macrophages and mononuclear cells in lungs of infected birds (arrow) (X = 50 and 20μm, respectively). (**D**) Liver sinusoids of infected birds (inside van Kuppfer cells) (arrow) (X = 50μm). (**E**) Testis of infected birds (between seminephrous tubules of testicular tissue) (arrow) (X = 50μm).

Staining of most organs revealed a common feature characteristic of the viral antigen detected in their endothelial and mononuclear cells, which suggests that viral pathogenesis of the HPAIV H5N1 may be associated with endothelial invasion, and that the virus could be carried by infected monocytes. We identified viral NP in endothelial (Fig 3D) and epithelial (Fig 3F) cells of the trachea, neurons, glial cells of Perkinji cell layer (Fig 4C and 4D) and endothelial cells of brain (Fig 4E), lymphocytes and mononuclear cells of spleen (Fig 5D), acinar epithelium of pancreas (Fig 5F), glandular epithelium of proventriculus (Fig 6B), and lymphocytes of the follicular layer of the bursa (Fig 6D). A summary of viral antigen staining in various tissues examined is shown in Table 3.

We prepared samples from dead ducks and performed the same IHC staining on duck tissues as chicken tissues with the anti NP antibody. However, we failed to detect viral NP in all tissues examined (data not shown). Our failure could be attributed to the preparation of the samples, since they were collected from dead ducks in the field. Although viral RNA was still present and live virus isolated successfully (Figs 1 and 2), no sufficient viral antigens existed in the tissues due to prolonged exposure at ambient temperature.

Sequence characterization of the HPAIV H5N1 HA and NS genes

Genomic sequences of the HA genes from the isolated viruses were sequenced and the cleavage sites were compared with those of known H5N1 viruses. We found that the HA of our isolates encodes a multibasic amino acid motif, 321-PQGERRRK/KR*GLF-333, at the HA cleavage site, which is a characteristic feature of all HPAIV H5N1 strains. Interestingly, we found that one of our isolates has a substitution of amino acid (R325K) at this cleavage site, to make it PQGEKRRK/KR*GLF. A phylogenetic tree was constructed, indicating that the HA gene belongs to (5J) genotype (Fig 8A). Our isolates formed a uniform cluster, together with the HPAIVH5N1 viruses from Egypt isolated in 2009, 2010, 2011, 2012, and 2013; however, this cluster was not identical to the HPAIV H5 strains used for commercial vaccine development in Egypt, and was also phylogenetically distant from the viruses isolated from Egypt in 2006, 2007, and 2008.

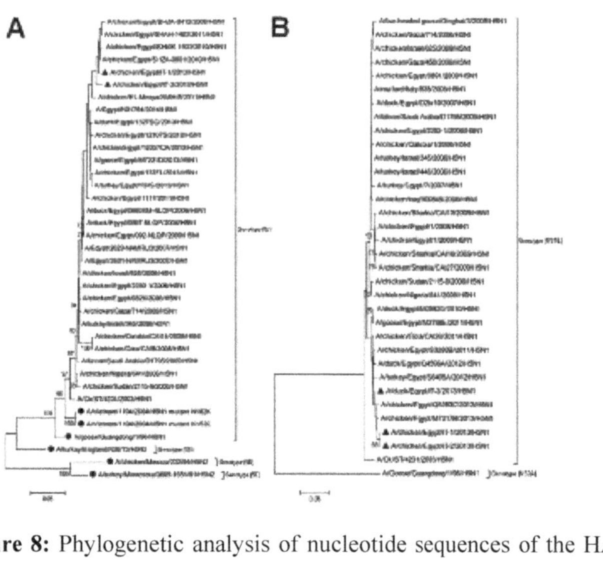

Figure 8: Phylogenetic analysis of nucleotide sequences of the HA and NS genes.

(**A**) Phylogenetic analysis of HA gene nucleotide sequences at the cleavage site. The sequences of known HPAIV HA genes were obtained from GenBank. Vaccine H5 strains were included in the tree and marked with solid circles. The tree was constructed with multiple alignment of a 309 base-nucleotide sequence of HA genes using the Neighborhood-joining method in MEGA5. The tree topology was evaluated by 1,000 bootstrap analyses. The viruses isolated in this study are marked with solid triangle. (**B**) Phylogenetic analysis of NS gene on the basis of nucleotide sequences of the complete coding region (822 bases). The tree was constructed using Neighborhood joining method with bootstrap values calculated for 1,000 replicates and cut off value of 50%. Sequences of the isolates from this study are marked with solid triangles.

We also sequenced the NS genomic segments, which are 822 nucleotides in length and encode for NS1 and NS2/NEP proteins. A phylogenetic tree was constructed indicating that the NS1 gene of our isolates belongs to the NS1EQinghai Lake-like genotype (Fig 8B). Our isolates also formed a uniform cluster, together with the HPAIVH5N1 viruses from Egypt isolated in 2010, 2011, 2012, and 2013; however, this cluster was phylogenetically distant from other HPAIV H5N1 isolated from Egypt in 2006, 2007, 2008, and 2009.

We found that the NS1 protein of our H5N1 viruses had a deletion of the ^{80}TMASV^{84}motif and was 225 amino acids in length. The NS1 had a glutamate at position 92 (92E) and its carboxyl terminus harbored the E-S-E-V motif, both of which have been identified as pathogenic determinants of highly pathogenic viruses [23].

DISCUSSION

In this report we demonstrated that the HPAIV H5N1 is still circulating in commercial poultry farms and backyards and causing outbreaks with significant mortality to both chickens and domestic ducks in Egypt. Our data showed that vaccination with H5N1 and H5N2vaccines may provide significant protection, especially to layers which were vaccinated twice. For both broilers and layers in commercial farms, there appears to be protection with even one-time vaccination when compared to a mortality of over 70% in non-vaccinated chickens [24]. Unfortunately, we did not perform serological test to evaluate the immunological status or vaccine efficacy in chickens of the commercial flocks, and therefore are unable to assess how well the mortality is correlated to the vaccination. Therefore, we cannot conclude emphatically that the much lower mortality in the commercial layers, which were vaccinated twice, was absolutely attributed to the boosted immunity.

Vaccine efficacy may best be assessed in the setting of natural outbreaks, which apparently differs from that designed experimentally. In naturally infected free-living birds, the clinical and pathologic manifestations of an HPAIV infection may be influenced by multiple factors including the age of the bird, the dosage of virus and routes of viral exposure, the presence of concomitant infections, and the levels of immunity acquired from vaccination or during previous exposure to influenza viruses [25, 26], which could be significantly different from trials with experimental challenges. Data about vaccine protection and efficacy from natural outbreaks may be more valuable when case studies are carefully planned and serological survey is thoroughly performed and assessed.

Even though the mortalities were lowered, the pathogenicity of the infection appeared to be severe, and the virus was highly virulent in sick chickens as shown in Fig 1 and Table 2.

Pathogenicity of infection by HPAIV H5N1 has been studied experimentally in chickens and domestic ducks. Vietnam HPAIV H5N1 caused high mortality in two- and four-week-old SPF White Leghorn chickens (*G. gallusdomesticus*) (100%, 48/48) with mean death times (MDT) from 36 to 48 hrs, and two- and five-week-old Pekinwhite ducks (*Anasplatyrhynchus*) (98.4%, 63/64) with MDTs from 2.7 to 4.4 days [27]. Pathogenicity of the Egyptian HPAIV H5N1 have been tested experimentally only in domestic ducks [28]. While A/ck/Egypt/08 killed 8/8 (100%) with an MDT of 4.1 days, A/ck/Egypt/07 killed 4/8 (50%) with an MDT of 7 days, indicating that HPAIV H5N1 isolates differ in their virulence. Although these two isolates are considered to have evolved from the same origin [28], they are far apart within the clade 2.2 in the phylogenetic tree and have evolved different pathogenicity since the HPAIV H5N1 of clade 2.2 was introduced into Egypt. On the other hand, pathogenicity observed in these experimental challenges cannot be directly compared with that in natural outbreaks. Apparent differences exist between SPF birds with a certain age group infected experimentally by the intranasal route (IN) and poultry of various ages in commercial farms by natural exposure. The mortality rates in our report were lower in duck and even much lower in once- and twice-vaccinated chickens during the outbreaks. However, for sick birds the symptoms were severe. Systemic infection was observed and nervous disorders were obvious in both chickens and ducks, and infection was confirmed by viral antigen detection.

The current H5N1 viruses, A/chicken/Egypt/IT-1/2013 and A/chicken/Egypt/IT-2/2013, clearly demonstrate their pantropism in tissues and organs as virulent HPAIV strains. The viral RNA and NP antigen were detected in multiple tissues, including trachea, lung, brain, liver, spleen, pancreas, intestines, serum, proventriculus, bursa of Fabricius, and testis in infected chickens, similar to those observed in chickens infected with the Vietnamese H5N1 virus [28]. Neurotropism of the HPAI H5N1 virus has been previously described [29–32]. Our study shows that high levels of viral RNA were detected in the brains of infected chickens (Fig 2) and that viral NP antigen was observed in the nuclei of neurons and glial cells of the brain, clear signs that the virus replicates in brains. We could also conclude that even though vaccination may lower mortality rates, it does not change pantropism of HPAIV H5N1 in sick birds.

Different pathways have been proposed by which the HPAI H5N1 virus infects the central nervous system (CNS) in chickens. It has been hypothesized that the virus could reach the CNS through the olfactory nerves [33], the peripheral nervous system [34, 35], or even the bloodstream [36]. Interestingly, we observed the viral NP antigen in endothelial cells of brain, which provides direct evidence that the HPAIV H5N1 likely invades the CNS by replicating in blood vessels in the brain, and contributes to the development of severe nervous symptoms. Based on our evidence, we consider this to be one of the routes for HPAIV H5N1 to invade CNS. Severe CNS disorders in birds are probably one of the main causes for mortality when neurons are infected; massive edema due to virus infection-induced altered vascular permeability and multi-organ failure are commonly blamed for high mortality in HPAIV infected birds.

Mechanisms for viral penetration of the blood-brain barrier in the brain have been investigated previously. The virus may invade neurons through the opening of endothelial cell junctional complexes (para-cellular route) [37] or through vesiculo-tubular structures (trans-cellular route) [38]. It could reach the vessels in the brain through the bloodstream, or via a "Trojan horse mechanism" where viral particles are transported through infection of leukocytes and/or mononuclear cells [39]. In our study, viral RNA or antigen was easily detected in blood or sera and infected macrophages and monocytes, which suggests that the endothelial cells may play a crucial role in viral penetration of the blood-brain barrier, leading to severe necrotizing encephalopathy and death. Our finding that endothelial cells of the cerebellum were also strongly positive in viral NP antigen supports this hypothesis (Fig 4).

In this report, the viral antigen was strongly expressed in the acinar epithelium of pancreas, giving rise to the possibility of a potential role of the pancreas in viral pathogenesis. Evidence showed that the virus also replicated in lymphocytes of follicular layer of the bursa, which may be significant in inducing immunity against the virus, a key process for recovery of sick birds from infection. A remarkable finding in our study is the isolation of virus from testicular tissue samples; infection at this site resulted in embryos with severe hemorrhages and congestion (Fig 1E) leading to death within 48hrs post-infection. Moreover, high viral RNA levels were detected from testicular tissue (Fig 2), with viral NP antigen expressed in between seminephrous tubules (Fig 7E). Strikingly, the viral antigen was also detected inside these seminephrous tubules sticking to sperm. However, sexual transmission for apparently healthy cocks to spread HPAIV H5N1 during the incubation period is probably a scenario of low or unlikely probability. It is likely that sperm collected from infected cocks with healthy appearance could disseminate disease to both uninfected birds and farm handlers and workers either via natural insemination or during application of artificial insemination. Thus, the findings in this report not only provide insights on HPAI H5N1 viral pathogenicity and pathogenesis in natural infection, but also emphasize the importance of biosecurity and proper handling in poultry agriculture.

ACKNOWLEDGMENTS

The authors thank Mohamed Azawy for kindly providing clinical samples, Jan Shivers for helping with immunohistochemistry staining, M. Afifi for statistical analysis, and Dr. Rob Porter of Veterinary Diagnostic Laboratory for photographing of slides.

AUTHOR CONTRIBUTIONS

Conceived and designed the experiments: IH SM CJC ZX. Performed the experiments: IH SM AA EBI AS. Analyzed the data: IH ZRZ CJC JC ZX. Contributed reagents/materials/ analysis tools: IH ZRZ CJC JC ZX. Wrote the paper: IH ZX.

REFERENCES

1. Xu X, Subbarao K, Cox NJ, Guo Y. Genetic characterization of the pathogenic influenza A/Goose/Guangdong/1/96 (H5N1) virus: similarity of its hemagglutinin gene to

those of H5N1 viruses from the 1997 outbreaks in Hong Kong. Virology. 1999;261(1):15–9. pmid:10484749 doi: 10.1006/viro.1999.9820

2. Sims L, Ellis T, Liu K, Dyrting K, Wong H, Peiris M, et al. Avian influenza in Hong Kong 1997–2002. Avian diseases. 2003;47(s3):832–8. doi: 10.1637/0005-2086-47.s3.832
3. Sims L, Domenech J, Benigno C, Kahn S, Kamata A, Lubroth J, et al. Origin and evolution of highly pathogenic H5N1 avian influenza in Asia. Veterinary Record. 2005;157(6):159. pmid:16085721 doi: 10.1136/vr.157.6.159
4. Chen H, Smith G, Zhang S, Qin K, Wang J, Li K, et al. Avian flu: H5N1 virus outbreak in migratory waterfowl. Nature. 2005;436(7048):191–2. pmid:16007072 doi: 10.1038/nature03974
5. Liu J, Xiao H, Lei F, Zhu Q, Qin K, Zhang X-w, et al. Highly pathogenic H5N1 influenza virus infection in migratory birds. Science. 2005;309(5738):1206-. pmid:16000410 doi: 10.1126/science.1115273
6. Claas EC, Osterhaus AD, van Beek R, De Jong JC, Rimmelzwaan GF, Senne DA, et al. Human influenza A H5N1 virus related to a highly pathogenic avian influenza virus. The Lancet. 1998;351(9101):472–7. pmid:9482438 doi: 10.1016/s0140-6736(97)11212-0
7. WHO. Cumulative number of confirmed human cases for avian influenza A(H5N1); 2003–2014.
8. Enserink M. H5N1 moves into Africa, European Union, deepening global crisis. Science. 2006;311(5763):932-. pmid:16484460 doi: 10.1126/science.311.5763.932a
9. Freiji M. The poultry industry in the Arab world—present and future. Lohmann Information. 2008:43: 4–52.
10. WHO. H5N1 avian influenza: Timeline of major events.; 2011.
11. Abdelwhab E, Hafez H. An overview of the epidemic of highly pathogenic H5N1 avian influenza virus in Egypt: epidemiology and control challenges. Epidemiology and infection. 2011;139(05):647–57. doi: 10.1017/s0950268810003122
12. Aly M, Arafa A, Hassan M. Epidemiological findings of outbreaks of disease caused by highly pathogenic H5N1 avian influenza virus in poultry in Egypt during 2006. Avian diseases. 2008;52(2):269–77. pmid:18646456 doi: 10.1637/8166-103007-reg.1
13. Hafez M, Arafa A, Abdelwhab E, Selim A, Khoulosy S, Hassan M, et al. Avian influenza H5N1 virus infections in vaccinated commercial and backyard poultry in Egypt. Poultry science. 2010;89(8):1609–13. doi: 10.3382/ps.2010-00708. pmid:20634514
14. Abdelwhab E, Selim A, Arafa A, Galal S, Kilany W, Hassan M, et al. Circulation of avian influenza H5N1 in live bird markets in Egypt. Avian diseases. 2010;54(2):911–4. pmid:20608538 doi: 10.1637/9099-100809-resnote.1
15. Herfst S, Schrauwen EJ, Linster M, Chutinimitkul S, de Wit E, Munster VJ, et al. Airborne transmission of influenza A/H5N1 virus between ferrets. Science. 2012;336(6088):1534–41. doi: 10.1126/science.1213362. pmid:22723413
16. Imai M, Watanabe T, Hatta M, Das SC, Ozawa M, Shinya K, et al. Experimental adaptation of an influenza H5 HA confers respiratory droplet transmission to a reassortant H5 HA/H1N1 virus in ferrets. Nature. 2012;486(7403):420–8. doi: 10.1038/nature10831. pmid:22722205
17. Neumann G, Macken CA, Karasin AI, Fouchier RA, Kawaoka Y. Egyptian H5N1 Influenza Viruses—Cause for Concern? PLoS pathogens. 2012;8(11):e1002932. doi: 10.1371/journal.ppat.1002932. pmid:23166487
18. Njouom R, Aubin JT, Bella AL, Demsa BM, Rouquet P, Gake B, et al. Highly pathogenic avian influenza virus subtype H5N1 in ducks in the Northern part of Cameroon. Vet Microbiol. 2008 Aug 25;130(3–4):380–4. doi: 10.1016/j.vetmic.2008.02.012. pmid:18417301
19. Tsukamoto K, Ashizawa T, Nakanishi K, Kaji N, Suzuki K, Shishido M, et al. Use of reverse transcriptase PCR to subtype N1 to N9 neuraminidase genes of avian influenza viruses. J Clin Microbiol. 2009 Jul;47(7):2301–3. doi: 10.1128/JCM.02366-08. pmid:19403772
20. Hoffmann E, Stech J, Guan Y, Webster R, Perez D. Universal primer set for the full-length amplification of all influenza A viruses. Archives of virology. 2001;146(12):2275–89. pmid:11811679 doi: 10.1007/s007050170002
21. Lu G, Rowley T, Garten R, Donis RO. FluGenome: a web tool for genotyping influenza A virus. Nucleic acids research. 2007;35(suppl 2):W275–W9. doi: 10.1093/nar/gkm365
22. Spackman E, Senne DA, Myers T, Bulaga LL, Garber LP, Perdue ML, et al. Development of a real-time reverse transcriptase PCR assay for type A influenza virus and the avian H5 and H7 hemagglutinin subtypes. Journal of clinical microbiology. 2002;40(9):3256–60. pmid:12202562 doi: 10.1128/jcm.40.9.3256-3260.2002
23. Jackson D, Hossain MJ, Hickman D, Perez DR, Lamb RA. A new influenza virus virulence determinant: the NS1 protein four C-terminal residues modulate pathogenicity. Proceedings of the National Academy of Sciences. 2008;105(11):4381–6. doi: 10.1073/pnas.0800482105. pmid:18334632
24. Grund C, Abdelwhab E-SM, Arafa A-S, Ziller M, Hassan MK, Aly MM, et al. Highly pathogenic avian influenza virus H5N1 from Egypt escapes vaccine-induced immunity but confers clinical protection against a heterologous clade 2.2. 1 Egyptian isolate. Vaccine. 2011;29(33):5567–73. doi: 10.1016/j.vaccine.2011.01.006. pmid:21244859
25. Keawcharoen J, Van Riel D, van Amerongen G, Bestebroer T, Beyer WE, Van Lavieren R, et al. Wild ducks as long-distance vectors of highly pathogenic avian influenza virus (H5N1). Emerging infectious diseases. 2008;14(4):600. doi: 10.3201/eid1404.071016. pmid:18394278
26. Bröjer C, Ågren EO, Uhlhorn H, Bernodt K, Mörner T, Jansson S, et al. Pathology of natural highly pathogenic avian influenza H5N1 infection in wild tufted ducks (Aythya fuligula). Journal of veterinary diagnostic

investigation. 2009;21(5):579–87. pmid:19737752 doi: 10.1177/104063870902100501

27. Pfeiffer J, Pantin-Jackwood M, To T, Nguyen T, Suarez D. Phylogenetic and biological characterization of highly pathogenic H5N1 avian influenza viruses (Vietnam 2005) in chickens and ducks. Virus research. 2009;142(1):108–20. doi: 10.1016/j.virusres.2009.01.019
28. Wasilenko J, Arafa A, Selim A, Hassan M, Aly M, Ali A, et al. Pathogenicity of two Egyptian H5N1 highly pathogenic avian influenza viruses in domestic ducks. Archives of virology. 2011;156(1):37–51. doi: 10.1007/s00705-010-0813-y. pmid:20882306
29. Brown JD, Stallknecht DE, Berghaus RD, Swayne DE. Infectious and lethal doses of H5N1 highly pathogenic avian influenza virus for house sparrows (Passer domesticus) and rock pigeons (Columbia livia). Journal of veterinary diagnostic investigation. 2009;21(4):437–45. pmid:19564491 doi: 10.1177/104063870902100404
30. Pantin-Jackwood M, Swayne D. Pathogenesis and pathobiology of avian influenza virus infection in birds. Revue scientifique et technique (International Office of Epizootics). 2009;28(1):113–36.
31. Tang Y, Wu P, Peng D, Wang X, Wan H, Zhang P, et al. Characterization of duck H5N1 influenza viruses with differing pathogenicity in mallard (Anas platyrhynchos) ducks. Avian Pathology. 2009;38(6):457–67. doi: 10.1080/03079450903349147. pmid:19937535
32. Goletic T, Gagic A, Rešidbegovic E, Kustura A, Kavazovic A, Savic V, et al. Highly pathogenic avian influenza virus subtype H5N1 in mute swans (Cygnus olor) in central Bosnia. Avian diseases. 2010;54(s1):496–501. doi: 10.1637/8705-031609-resnote.1
33. Majde JA, Bohnet SG, Ellis GA, Churchill L, Leyva-Grado V, Wu M, et al. Detection of mouse-adapted human influenza virus in the olfactory bulbs of mice within hours after intranasal infection. Journal of neurovirology. 2007;13(5):399–409. pmid:17994424 doi: 10.1080/13550280701427069
34. Tanaka H, Park C-H, Ninomiya A, Ozaki H, Takada A, Umemura T, et al. Neurotropism of the 1997 Hong Kong H5N1 influenza virus in mice. Veterinary microbiology. 2003;95(1):1–13. doi: 10.1016/s0378-1135(03)00132-9
35. Matsuda K, Park C, Sunden Y, Kimura T, Ochiai K, Kida H, et al. The vagus nerve is one route of transneural invasion for intranasally inoculated influenza A virus in mice. Veterinary Pathology Online. 2004;41(2):101–7. pmid:15017022 doi: 10.1354/vp.41-2-101
36. Mori I, Komatsu T, Takeuchi K, Nakakuki K, Sudo M, Kimura Y. Viremia induced by influenza virus. Microbial pathogenesis. 1995;19(4):237–44. pmid:8825911 doi: 10.1016/s0882-4010(95)90290-2
37. Lossinsky A, Shivers R. Structural pathways for macromolecular and cellular transport across the blood-brain barrier during inflammatory conditions. Review. Histology and histopathology. 2004;19(2):535–64. pmid:15024715
38. Liu NQ, Lossinsky AS, Popik W, Li X, Gujuluva C, Kriederman B, et al. Human immunodeficiency virus type 1 enters brain microvascular endothelia by macropinocytosis dependent on lipid rafts and the mitogen-activated protein kinase signaling pathway. Journal of virology. 2002;76(13):6689–700. pmid:12050382 doi: 10.1128/jvi.76.13.6689-6700.2002
39. Verma S, Lo Y, Chapagain M, Lum S, Kumar M, Gurjav U, et al. West Nile virus infection modulates human brain microvascular endothelial cells tight junction proteins and cell adhesion molecules: Transmigration across the *in vitro* blood-brain barrier. Virology. 2009;385(2):425–33. doi: 10.1016/j.virol.2008.11.047. pmid:19135695

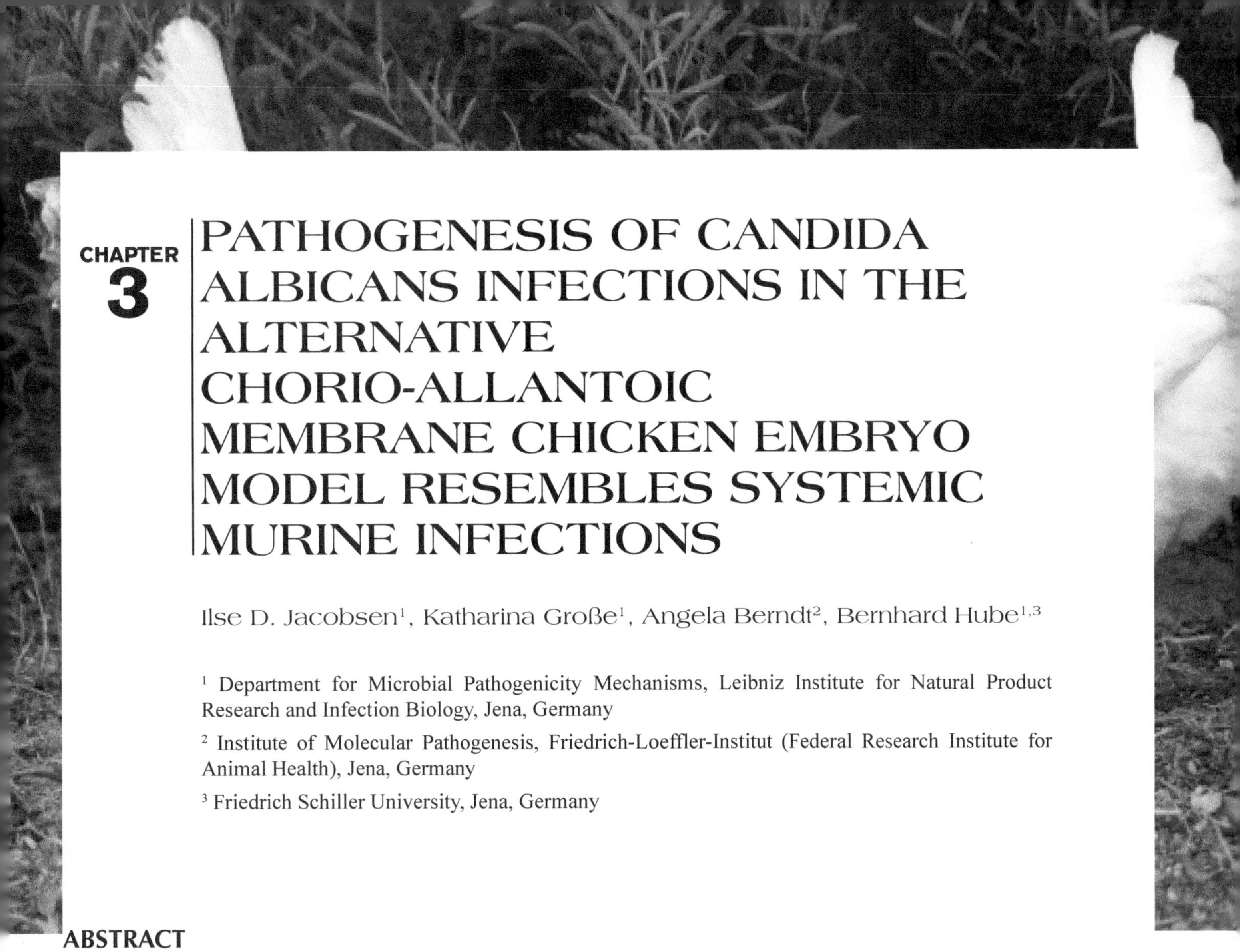

CHAPTER 3

PATHOGENESIS OF CANDIDA ALBICANS INFECTIONS IN THE ALTERNATIVE CHORIO-ALLANTOIC MEMBRANE CHICKEN EMBRYO MODEL RESEMBLES SYSTEMIC MURINE INFECTIONS

Ilse D. Jacobsen[1], Katharina Große[1], Angela Berndt[2], Bernhard Hube[1,3]

[1] Department for Microbial Pathogenicity Mechanisms, Leibniz Institute for Natural Product Research and Infection Biology, Jena, Germany

[2] Institute of Molecular Pathogenesis, Friedrich-Loeffler-Institut (Federal Research Institute for Animal Health), Jena, Germany

[3] Friedrich Schiller University, Jena, Germany

ABSTRACT

Alternative models of microbial infections are increasingly used to screen virulence determinants of pathogens. In this study, we investigated the pathogenesis of Candida albicans and C. glabrata infections in chicken embryos infected via the chorio-allantoic membrane (CAM) and analyzed the virulence of deletion mutants. The developing immune system of the host significantly influenced susceptibility: With increasing age, embryos became more resistant and mounted a more balanced immune response, characterized by lower induction of proinflammatory cytokines and increased transcription of regulatory cytokines, suggesting that immunopathology contributes to pathogenesis. While many aspects of the chicken embryo response resembled murine infections, we also observed significant differences: In contrast to systemic infections in mice, IL-10 had a beneficial effect in chicken embryos. IL-22 and IL-17A were only upregulated after the peak mortality in the chicken embryo model occurred; thus, the role of the Th17 response in this model remains unclear. Abscess formation occurs frequently in murine models, whereas the avian response was dominated by granuloma formation. Pathogenicity of the majority of 15 tested C. albicans deletion strains was comparable to the virulence in mouse models and reduced virulence was associated with significantly lower transcription of proinflammatory cytokines. However, fungal burden did not correlate with virulence and for few mutants like bcr1Δ and tec1Δ different outcomes in survival compared to murine infections were observed. C. albicans strains locked in the yeast stage disseminated significantly more often from the CAM into the embryo, supporting the hypothesis that the yeast morphology is responsible for dissemination in systemic infections. These data suggest that the pathogenesis of C. albicans infections in the chicken embryo model resembles systemic murine infections but also differs in some aspects. Despite its limitations, it presents a useful alternative tool to pre-screen C. albicans strains to select strains for subsequent testing in murine models.

INTRODUCTION

Candida albicans is both a commensal on human mucosal surfaces and one of the most important human fungal pathogens [1]. Disease caused by *C. albicans* ranges from relatively benign infections of skin to oral and vaginal thrush, deep-seated mycoses and life-threatening sepsis [1]. The incidence of *Candida* sepsis has steadily risen over the last two decades and recent studies have identified *Candida* spp. as the fourth most common cause of sepsis in hospital settings [2]. Despite the availability of modern antimycotics, systemic candidiasis is still associated with high mortality rates [3].

To better understand pathogenesis and to identify fungal virulence-associated factors, complex infection models

Citation: Jacobsen ID, Große K, Berndt A, Hube B (2011) Pathogenesis of Candida albicans Infections in the Alternative Chorio-Allantoic Membrane Chicken Embryo Model Resembles Systemic Murine Infections. PLoS ONE 6(5): e19741. doi:10.1371/journal.pone.0019741.

are indispensable. Murine models for both superficial and systemic *C. albicans* infections have been developed and are widely used to study pathogenesis and determine the virulence of defined *C. albicans*mutants [4], [5]. However, the use of murine models is restricted by costs, the requirement of specialized facilities and personnel, legal requirements and ethical considerations. Therefore, infection models using invertebrates, e. g. *Galleria mellonella* larvae and Toll-deficient *Drosophila melanogaster*, as alternative hosts have been developed. These alternative hosts are suitable to determine the virulence of different *C. albicans* strains and to evaluate the efficacy of antifungal compounds [6], [7], [8], [9].

Systemic infections in mice lead to a rapid induction of various cytokines, neutrophil infiltration of affected organs and finally progressive septic shock [10], [11]. This immunopathology is a major difference between murine and insect models, since insect hosts mount a defensive immune response to *C. albicans* infections based on phagocytic cells and the upregulation of antimicrobial peptides but do not develop septic shock[12], [13]. In contrast, the avian immune response to infection resembles the mammalian one to a large extend, including the production of both proinflammatory and regulatory cytokines [14] and development of a systemic response to LPS application [15].

Chicken embryos as alternative model host for fungal pathogens were already described in 1939 by Moore[16]. Until the late 1970s embryonated eggs were frequently used for research in immunology, virology, bacteriology but also mycology [17], [18], [19]. More recently, this alternative model host has also been used to investigate the virulence of *C. albicans* deletion mutants and to investigate efficacy of antimycotics [20],[21]. Infection of the chorio-allantoic membrane within embryonated chicken eggs is technically easy and thus suitable for screening purposes. However, possible pathogenesis mechanisms, the role of the host›s immune system, a comparison with murine models and the potential use of this alternative host for virulence screens have not been addressed in detail. Therefore, we aimed to elucidate the pathogenesis of *C. albicans*infections and the role of the immune system in this alternative host. Furthermore, we analyzed *C. glabrata*and 15 defined *C. albicans* mutants with known virulence potential in mice with regard to virulence, fungal burden and induction of cytokines to determine whether this model is suitable for virulence screening of *C. albicans* mutants.

RESULTS

Establishment and characterization of the infection model

Both preculture conditions and the host have been shown to have a significant influence on survival in systemic *C. albicans* infections in mice [22]. Previous studies using chicken embryos as alternative hosts vary in several technical aspects, thus hampering direct comparison of obtained results. Therefore, we initially thoroughly characterized the model using *C. albicans* SC5314 for infection of the chorio-allantoic membrane (CAM). Mortality was confirmed to be dose-dependent in our model in embryos infected on developmental day 10: Infection with 10^7 cfu/egg led consistently to 75–100% mortality within 7 days. Gradual reduction of mortality was observed with log-fold dilutions of the infectious dose (data not shown). Infection with 10^5cfu/egg resulted in 40–60% final mortality and doses below 10^4 cfu/egg led to no significant mortality (data not shown). Inactivation of *C. albicans* by heat-treatment or thimerosal led to survival rates similar to the PBS control (80–100%). Therefore, the LD_{100} of 10^7 cfu/egg was used for subsequent survival comparisons. Analyses requiring a higher number of surviving embryos throughout a time course were performed using the LD_{50} of 10^5 cfu/egg.

The outcome of infection with various pathogens, including *C. albicans*, in chick embryos has been described to depend on the developmental stage (age) at infection [17], [23]. In agreement with these observations, we found a clear correlation of age at infection and survival. At both high (10^7 cfu, data not shown) and low infectious doses (Fig. 1A), infection on developmental day 8 led to rapid mortality significantly higher than in embryos infected on developmental day 10 (P<0.001), while embryos infected on developmental day 12 were highly resistant and showed survival rates undistinguishable from the PBS control. It has been suggested that the increased resistance of older embryos to infection with pathogens might reflect maturation and increasing competence of the embryonic immune system [17]. Increased immune competence could enable the host to limit fungal burden and prevent dissemination of the pathogen, thus increasing survival of the host. To test this hypothesis, we determined fungal burden in the CAM and dissemination into the liver during the course of infection (day 1–5 post infection (p.i.)) in embryos infected on developmental day 8, 10 and 12 (n=10 per day and age). *C. albicans* could be isolated from the CAM of all infected embryos (Fig. 1B). However, isolation from the liver, indicating systemic dissemination of *C. albicans*, was only sporadically successful. Although we observed a tendency towards lower dissemination rates in oldest embryos, this trend was not statistically significant (Fig. 1C). To determine whether dissemination might be an event associated with imminent death of an embryo, we additionally performed isolation from livers and complete abdomens of freshly deceased embryos. Similarly to living embryos, however, isolation was only infrequently positive (data not shown). Surprisingly, the embryonic age at infection did not have a significant impact on the number of cfu isolated from the CAM (Fig. 1B). Furthermore, cfu did not change over the course of the experiment (Fig. 1B). Neither fungi nor bacteria could be cultured from CAM and embryonic tissue of PBS-mock infected controls (n=15), confirming the absence of contaminations.

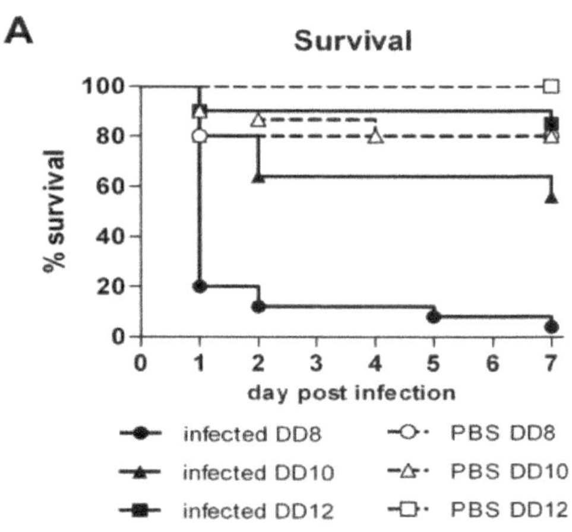

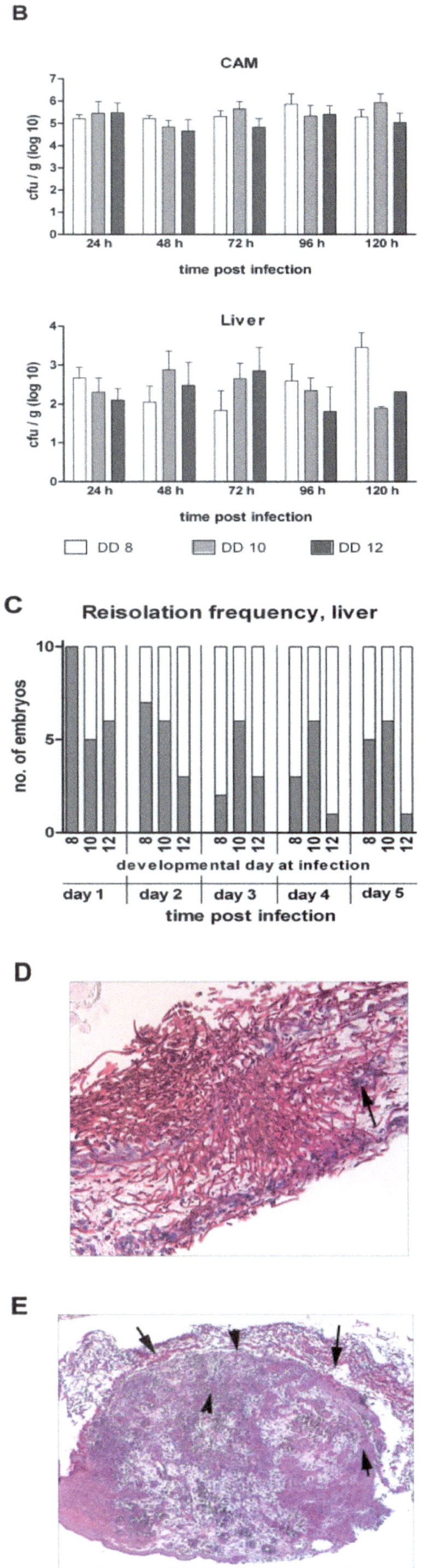

Figure 1: Characterization of the course of infection in chicken embryos infected with *C. albicans* **SC5314 at different developmental days.**

Independent of the fungal burden and dissemination, maturation of the embryo and its organs might lead to increased resistance of tissues to damage. Therefore, we analyzed pathological alterations in embryos infected at different age macroscopically and histologically. Briefly, macroscopically visible white to grayish nodules as well as edematous areas appeared on the CAM 24–48 h p.i. Histological analysis of these alterations revealed focal, invasive, filamentous growth of *C. albicans*, often accompanied with complete destruction of the CAM and angioinvasion (Fig. 1D). In areas were hyphae had not penetrated the whole thickness of the CAM, epithelial hyperplasia, proliferation of fibroblasts and cellular infiltration of the mesoderm was observed. Infiltrates became more prominent at 72 h p.i. as yellowish plaques (Fig. 1E). The majority of examined embryos showed no pathological alterations in internal organs; necrotic lesions containing small numbers of hyphae were observed only sporadically (<10%). These findings were consistent with previous observations by others [19], [21], [24]. Importantly, quality and quantity of the observed alterations were comparable between embryos infected at different developmental stages.

Embryonic maturation influences cytokine production after *C. albicans* infection and susceptibility to endotoxins

In mice, systemic infection with *C. albicans* leads to progressive sepsis [10]. Using *E. coli* LPS applied onto the CAM, we confirmed previous observations by Smith and Thomas [25] that chicken embryos are susceptible to lethal septic shock and that this susceptibility is age-dependent (Fig. 2). Therefore, we hypothesized that an age-dependent sepsis-like response might contribute to the age-dependency of mortality in embryos infected with *C. albicans*. To test this hypothesis, we determined the transcription levels of cytokines, which have been implicated in pathogenesis in mice [11], [26], in the CAM of embryos challenged either with LPS or *C. albicans*. Cytokines function as mediators for immune cell recruitment, activation and immune modulation during infection and are involved in the development of sepsis [27].

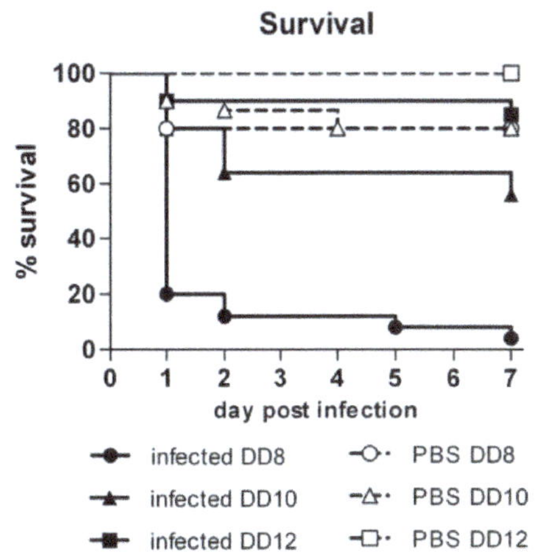

Figure 2: Age-dependent mortality after application of 100 µg LPS on the CAM.

Because mortality after LPS application occurred predominantly within the first 24 h and no deaths were observed after 48 h (Fig. 2), the expression of cytokine genes was analyzed 24 h and 48 h p.i. (Fig. 3A). Upregulation of the proinflammatory cytokines IL-8 (attracting mainly monocytes in chickens), IL-1β, IL-6, IL-12β p40 (note that the subunit p40 is shared with IL-23), the TNFα homologue LITAF (LPS-induced tumor necrosis factor) and K60 (functional orthologue of murine KC; K60 attracts mainly heterophils, the avian homologue of neutrophils) was significantly higher 24 h p.i. in embryos challenged on developmental day 8 compared to older embryos. Similarly, these cytokines (with the exception of LITAF) were upregulated to a greater extend in embryos challenged on day 10 compared to day 12. However, the difference between these two age groups was only significant for IL-8. The kinetics of proinflammatory cytokine gene transcription also differed depending on age: In youngest embryos, transcription levels were consistently highest 24 h p.i. In contrast, transcription of IL-12β p40 and LITAF increased from 24 h to 48 h in embryos challenged on day 10 or 12 and transcription of K60 in oldest embryos was highest 48 h after challenge. IL-6 was only moderately induced at both time points in embryos challenged on day 10 whereas older embryos showed a strong upregulation after 48 h. Age-dependent differences were also observed for IL-10 and IL-4, which exhibit regulatory rather than proinflammatory functions: IL-10 was already upregulated after 24 h in older embryos while the youngest embryos showed upregulation only after 48 h. IL-4 transcripts were upregulated in embryos challenged on developmental day 12 whereas embryos challenged on developmental day 10 transcribed only basal levels of IL-4. In the youngest embryos IL-4 transcripts could not be detected. IL-17A, IL-22 and MIP-1β were not significantly upregulated in any embryo (Fig. 3A). Transcription of IFN-γ was unaltered in all groups at all time points. IL-2 transcripts could not be detected in any group (data not shown). Application of zymosan (consisting of fungal glucan) likewise resulted in age-dependent survival and similar cytokine transcription patterns. However, large doses of zymosan (1 mg/egg) were needed to induce mortality and the transcription level of proinflammatory cytokines was lower than with LPS (data not shown). While fungal glucan can stimulate a proinflammatory response, we cannot exclude that low-level contamination with endotoxins contributed to the observed effects.

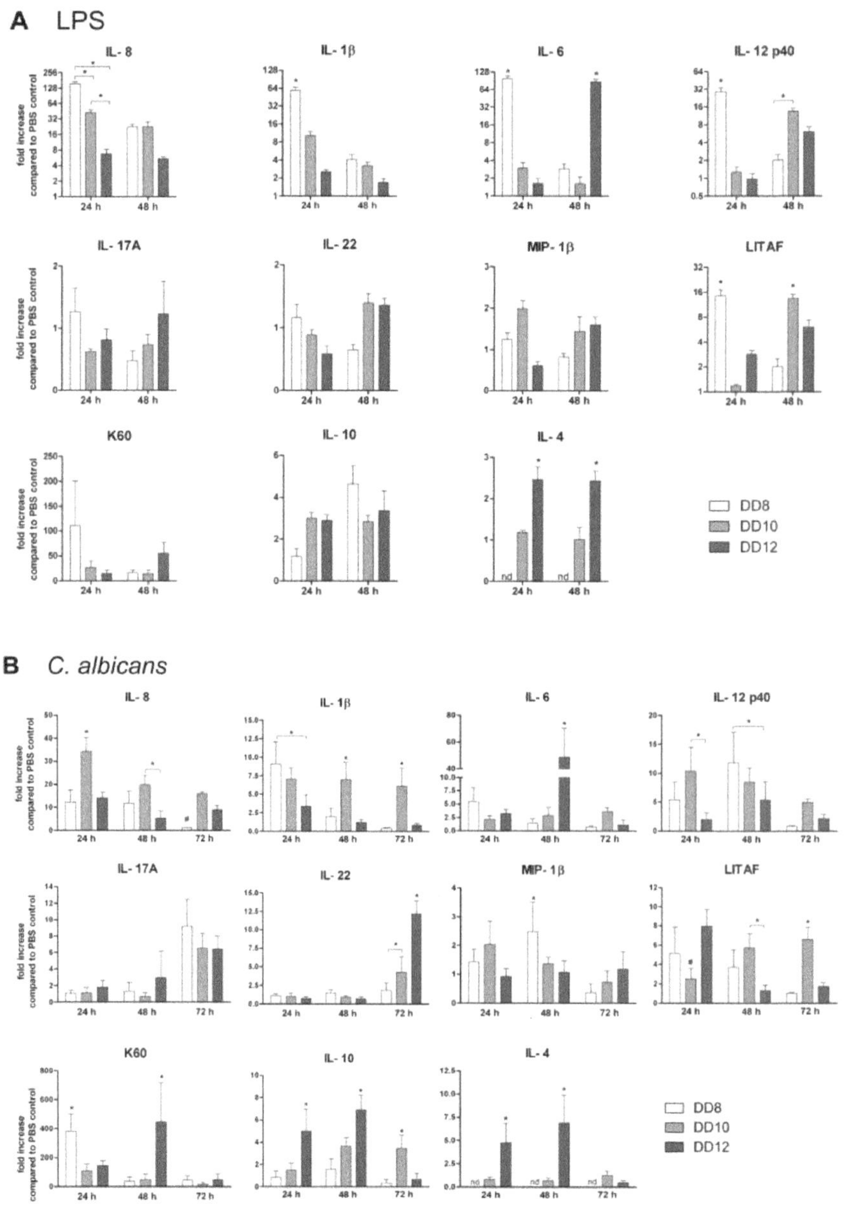

Figure 3: Influence of embryonic age on the transcriptional levels of cytokines after LPS application and infection with *C. albicans*SC5314.

Similarly, the cytokine transcription profiles upon infection with *C. albicans* differed depending on the age of embryos at infection (Fig. 3B). In contrast to LPS, however, only IL-1β and K60 showed highest transcription in youngest embryos 24 h p.i. IL-1β transcription levels declined in embryos infected on developmental day 8 and 12 from 24 h to 48 h whereas embryos infected on developmental day 10 showed continuous high transcription levels throughout 24 h to 72 h p.i. K60 displayed different induction kinetics in oldest embryos where strongest transcription was observed 48 h p.i. IL-8 was most strongly transcribed in embryos infected on day 10. The age groups did not differ in IL-6 induction 24 h p.i., but IL-6 transcription 48 h p.i. was significantly increased in the oldest embryos. Differences to LPS challenge were also observed for IL-12β p40 transcription: Strongest transcription in embryos infected on day 8 was only seen after 48 h, while embryos infected on day 10 responded more rapidly. IL-12β p40 transcription in embryos infected on day 12 was overall lower than in the other age groups. LITAF transcription increased over time in embryos infected on day 10 whereas older embryos showed highest induction 24 h p.i. Comparable to challenge with LPS, transcription of IFN-γ was unaltered in all groups and IL-2 transcripts were not detectable (data not shown). MIP-1β was only moderately (maximum two-fold) upregulated without significant differences between age groups. Transcription of IL-17A and IL-22 increased only 72 h p.i. While this upregulation was comparable amongst age groups for IL-17A, IL-22 transcripts were significantly more abundant in older embryos. Transcription of the regulatory cytokine IL-10 24 h and 48 h p.i. was significantly higher in embryos infected on day 12 compared to day 10. Consistent with the results of LPS challenge, IL-4 transcription only increased in embryos infected on day 12 and transcripts were not detectable in embryos infected on day 8.

This data demonstrate that the age of the host at challenge or infection has a significant influence on the transcriptional cytokine response. The proinflammatory response to LPS declines with increasing age. The response to *C. albicans* infection shows some similarities to LPS challenges, but also displays different kinetics which partially depend on the developmental stage of the embryo. In both LPS challenge and infection with *C. albicans*, increasing age led to stronger transcription of regulatory cytokines.

Modulation of inflammation by IL-10 enhances survival of embryos after infection

Age-dependent resistance of chicken embryos challenged with LPS or infected with *C. albicans* correlated with the transcription levels of IL-10 and IL-4. In mice, the role of IL-10 is not fully clear. While MacCallum et al. showed an inverse correlation of IL-10 with kidney lesion severity and suggested that IL-10 might exert a defensive role [11], Vazquez-Torres et al. demonstrated increased susceptibility of IL-10 knock out mice to systemic candidiasis [28]. To clarify the role of IL-10 in infected chicken embryos, we applied 100 ng recombinant chicken IL-10 onto the CAM of 10 days old eggs 15 min prior to infection. Controls were treated with carrier solution only. IL-10 application alone had no influence on survival of non-infected control embryos. In infected embryos, IL-10 treatment had a minor but reproducible and significant positive effect on survival ($P<0.05$) (Fig. 4).

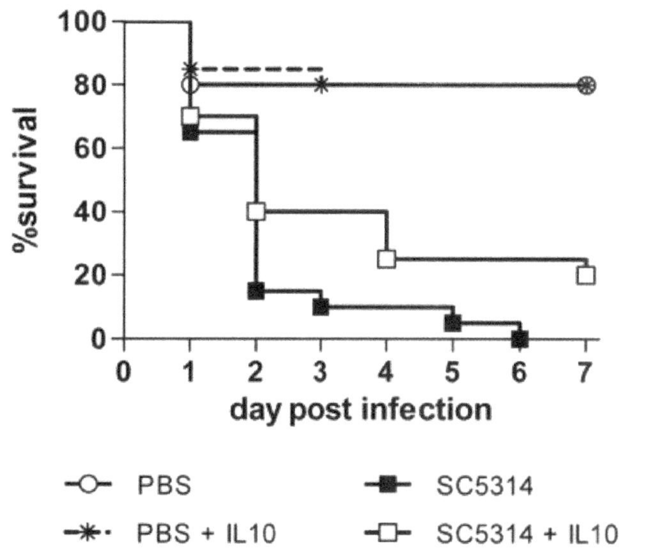

Figure 4: Addition of IL10 reduces mortality after *C. albicans* **infection.**

Candida glabrata survives and disseminates in infected embryos but does not cause mortality

In contrast to *C. albicans*, systemic *C. glabrata* infections in mice do not lead to mortality although the fungus is able to persist within the host [29]. To determine whether chicken embryos as alternative hosts are comparable to mice in this respect, we analyzed the outcome of infection with *C. glabrata* in the egg model.

Independent of the developmental stage at infection, *C. glabrata* infected embryos showed survival almost identical to PBS mock-infected controls (Fig. 5A). However, *C. glabrata* was able to survive and replicate in association with the CAM (Fig. 5B) without significant differences between the age groups. Dissemination occurred frequently in all age groups (Fig. 5C) and *C. glabrata* was isolated from 90–100% of livers 48 h p.i. Histologically, *C. glabrata* was found on and within the CAM (Fig. 5D). Plaque formation occurred earliest 72 h p.i. These plaques were characterized by cellular infiltrations into the mesoderm (Fig. 5D). Thus, although lacking hyphae-dependent penetration mechanisms, *C. glabrata* was able to enter deeper tissues and, similar to mice, *C. glabrata* persisted within infected embryos without gross pathological alterations and mortality.

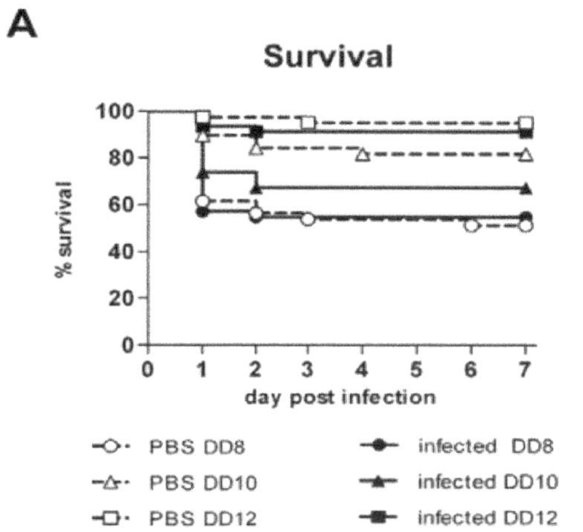

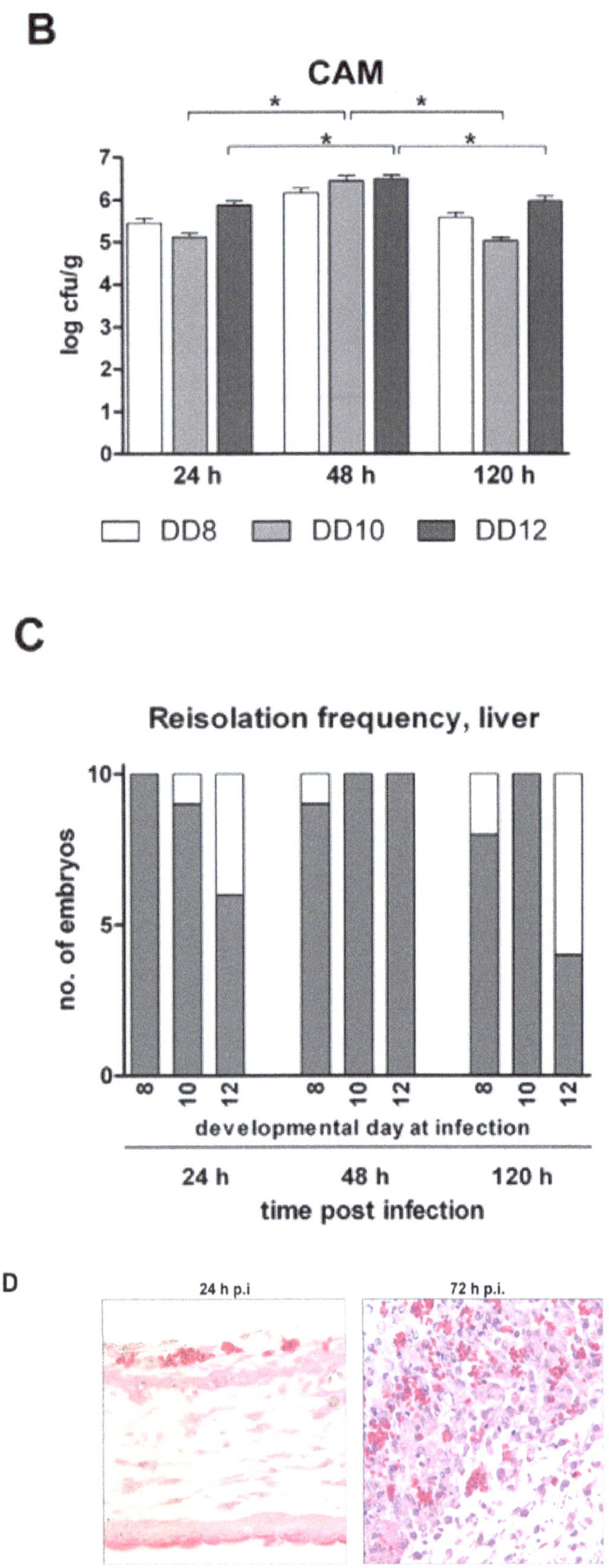

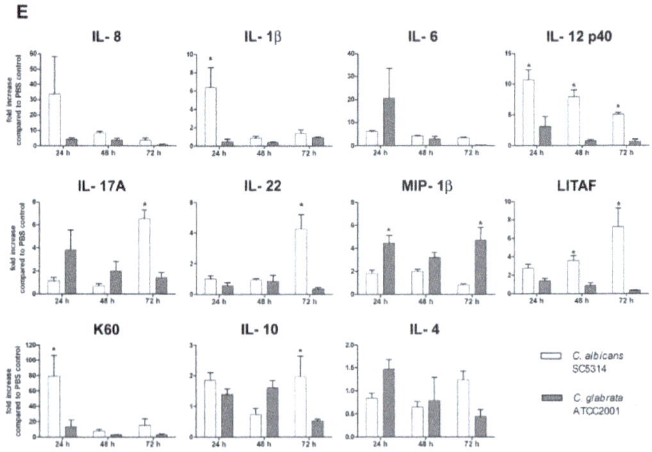

Figure 5: Characterization of the course of infection in chicken embryos infected with *C. glabrata* **ATCC2001.**

In contrast to *C. albicans*, *C. glabrata* infections in mice induce only a transient increase in proinflammatory cytokines and very moderate influx of immune cells [29], [30]. To determine whether similar differences in the host response to *C. albicans* and *C. glabrata* occur in infected chicken embryos, we compared transcription levels of various cytokines and chemokines after infection with either *C. albicans* or *C. glabratain* embryos infected on developmental day 10.

The expression levels of IL-8, IL-1β, IL12 p40 and K60 in *C. glabrata* infected embryos 24 p.i. were only moderately upregulated and lower than in *C. albicans* infected embryos (Fig. 5E). LITAF transcripts were moderately induced both in *C. albicans* and *C. glabrata* infected embryos 24 h p.i. However, while LITAF transcription decreased over time to PBS control levels in *C. glabrata* infected embryos, an increase was observed after infection with *C. albicans* (Fig. 5E). Surprisingly, IL-6, IL-17A and MIP-1β transcripts were higher in *C. glabrata* infected embryos 24 h p.i. (Fig. 5E). However, IL-17A decreased over time in embryos infected with *C. glabrata* while an increase was observed in embryos infected with *C. albicans*. IL-2 transcripts were not detectable in either group. IFN-γ transcription levels in both groups were comparable to PBS controls. IL-10 was upregulated in both groups without quantitative difference (data not shown). Thus, comparable to murine hosts and epithelial models, *C. glabrata* induces overall less proinflammatory cytokines than *C. albicans*.

Embryonated eggs as alternative hosts to determine virulence of *C. albicans* gene deletion mutants

One of the most commonly used applications of alternative model hosts is virulence screening of strains or mutants to select strains of interest for subsequent infection experiments using mammalian hosts. It was shown that chicken embryos are generally suitable for virulence determination of different *Candida* species and *C. albicans* gene deletion mutants [18], [21]. However, only few *C. albicans* mutants with known virulence potential in mice were tested. To gain more comprehensive information on the suitability of the model as a screening tool and possible mechanisms which influence virulence of strains in the chicken embryo model, we analyzed 15 known *C. albicans* gene deletion mutants for their ability to kill chicken embryos. The mutants were selected because of described defects in damaging epithelial cells and/or attenuation in murine infection models. Virulence of the two relevant parental strains, CAI4+pCIp10 and BWP17+pCIp30, was comparable to SC5314 in the embryo model (analyzed by Kaplan-Meyer curves and log rank test, data not shown). Additionally, for mutants, which showed significant attenuation, the complemented mutant, as far as available, was tested.

In survival comparison over a 7 day observation period, ten out of 15 mutants tested showed significantly ($P<0.05$) attenuated virulence in the chicken embryo model. All tested complemented strains led to lower survival rates than infection with the corresponding homozygous deletion mutant, but 3 out of 9 tested complemented strains were significantly reduced in virulence in comparison to the parental strain. Notably, kinetics of mortality onset differed between the mutants: Within the first 24 h, most mutants (*mnt1*Δ, *sap1–3*Δ, *rim101*Δ, *dfg16*Δ, *als3*Δ, *bcr1*Δ, *eed1*Δ) caused similar mortality as the respective parental strain but very few or no deaths in the following days. In contrast, only few embryos died within 24 h after infection with *efg1*Δ and *efg1*Δ*cph1*Δ. Within the first 24 h, *tpk2*Δ caused mortality comparable to the wild type, followed by a delay in killing. However, final mortality rates at the end of the observation period were comparable between *tpk2*Δ and the parental strain CAI4+pCIp10, emphasizing the necessity of a sufficiently long observation period.

To determine whether reduced virulence of mutants was associated with reduced fungal survival in infected eggs, fungal burden was determined as colony forming units (cfu) in the CAM and dissemination into the liver was analyzed 24 h, 48 h and 120 h after infection with *als3*Δ, *bcr1*Δ, *dfg16*Δ, *eed1*Δ, *efg1*Δ*cph1*Δ,*mnt1*Δ, *rim101*Δ, *tec1*Δ, *sap1–3*Δ and the parental strains CAI4+pCIP10 (CAI4) and BWP17+pCIp30 (BWP17). Similar cfu of SC5314 and the parental strains CAI4 and BWP17 could be isolated from the CAM 24 h and 48 h p.i. However, the burden of BWP17 was significantly lower than of SC5314 120 h p.i (Fig. 6A). Dissemination of these strains occurred infrequently without significant differences between the strains (Fig. 6D).

A

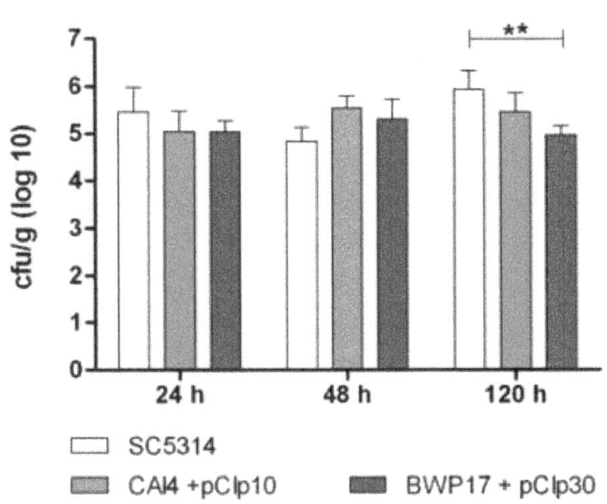

B

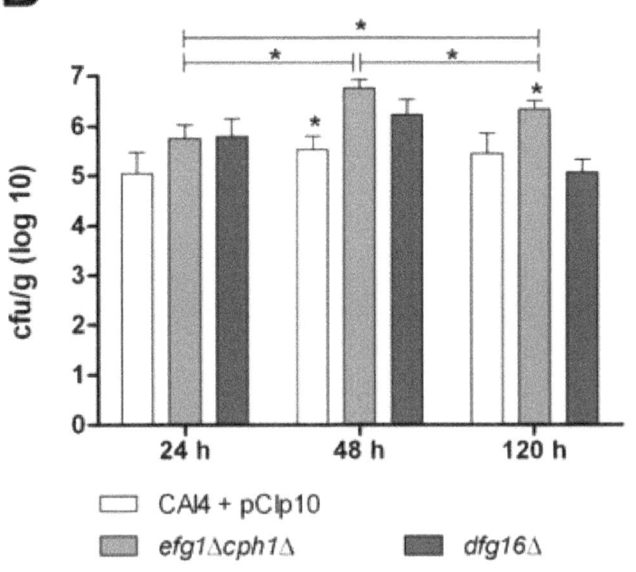

C

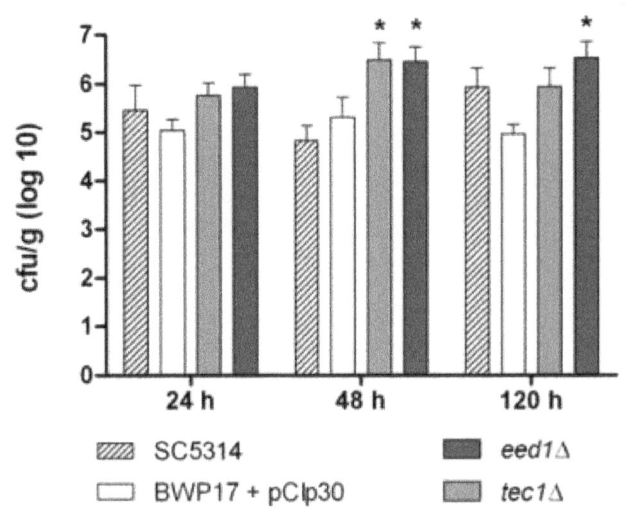

D

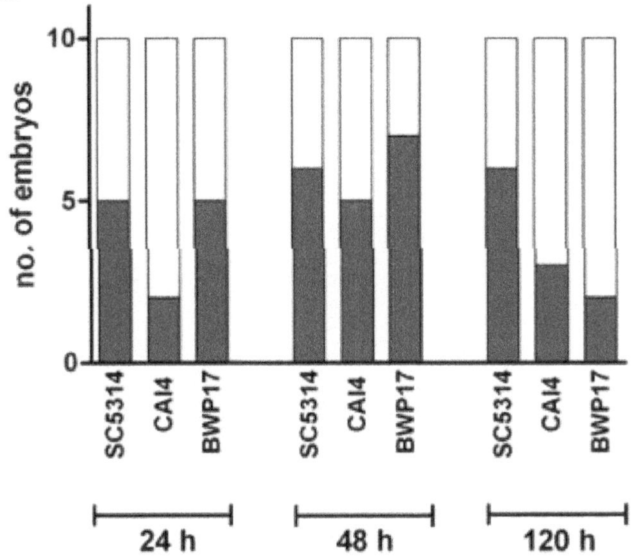

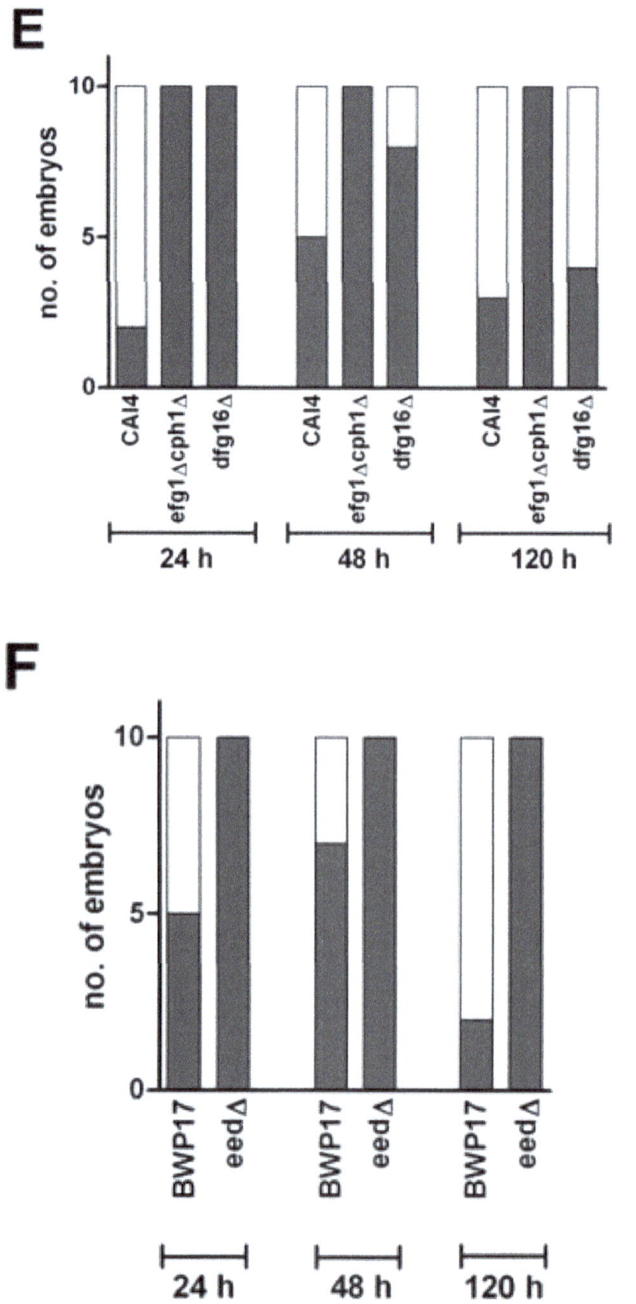

Figure 6: Fungal burden and dissemination frequencies of *C. albicans*mutants in infected embryos.

All mutants could be readily isolated from the CAM and no mutant showed reduced fungal burden within the CAM. In comparison to their respective parental strains, significantly higher cfu of *efg1Δcph1Δ*, *dfg16Δ*,*tec1Δ* and *eed1Δ* were recovered from the CAM of infected eggs (Fig. 6B and C). Dissemination frequencies were similar for most mutants and their parental strain except for *efg1Δcph1Δ*, *eed1Δ* and *dfg16Δ*. *efg1Δcph1Δ* and *eed1Δ* could be isolated from all cultured livers, while dissemination of *dfg16Δ* occurred more frequently within the first 24 h p.i. only (Fig. 6E and F). In summary, these results suggested that (i) increased clearance is unlikely to be the cause of reduced virulence, (ii) dissemination does not necessarily lead to embryonic death and (iii) reduced ability to form hyphae increases likelihood of dissemination.

Hyphae formation is an important virulence factor of *C. albicans* [31]. Consistently, mutants with defects in hyphae formation (*efg1Δcph1Δ*, *eed1Δ*, *dfg16Δ*, *rim101Δ*, *ras1Δ*) were attenuated in the chicken embryo model. However, filament formation depends on various stimuli and defects in hyphae formation can be overcome by appropriate stimuli. This has been shown for *tec1Δ*, which is deficient in hyphae formation *in vitro* but forms wild type-like filaments *in vivo* in the murine kidney after intravenous infection[32]. To confirm known morphology defects of mutants, we analyzed the fungal morphology in the CAM by histology 24 h, 48 h, and 72 h p.i. As described previously [21], wild type and parental strains formed hyphae invading into the CAM within the first 24 h (Fig. 7B–D). Yeast cells were rarely observed in these strains. In contrast, *efg1Δcph1Δ* grew as yeast only (Fig. 7E). Only few, short filaments were observed in*eed1Δ* (Fig. 7F). Interestingly, despite the obvious defect in hyphae formation and similar to *C. glabrata*, both strains were regularly located within the mesoderm of the CAM, supporting that a hyphae-independent invasion mechanism exists in this model. In contrast, *rim101Δ* was found predominantly as yeast cells on the surface of the CAM (Fig. 7G) and invasion was observed only infrequently 72 h p.i. in association with sparse hyphae development (Fig. 7H). Consistent with *in vitro* results [33], *dfg16Δ* produced only short hyphae and showed reduced invasion into the CAM (Fig. 7I). Both *als3Δ* and *bcr1Δ* were able to produce filaments and invade the CAM (Fig. 7K and L). However, compared to the parental strains, more yeast cells were present in these strains and invasion occurred less frequently. *tec1Δ*, *sap1–3Δ* and *mnt1Δ* all formed filaments but showed differences in frequency and depth of invasion: While *mnt1Δ* and *tec1Δ* (Fig. 7M and N) frequently penetrated the full width of the CAM, *sap1–3Δ* was predominantly found on the surface of the CAM and invading filaments were only occasionally and in few numbers observed within the mesoderm (Fig. 7O).

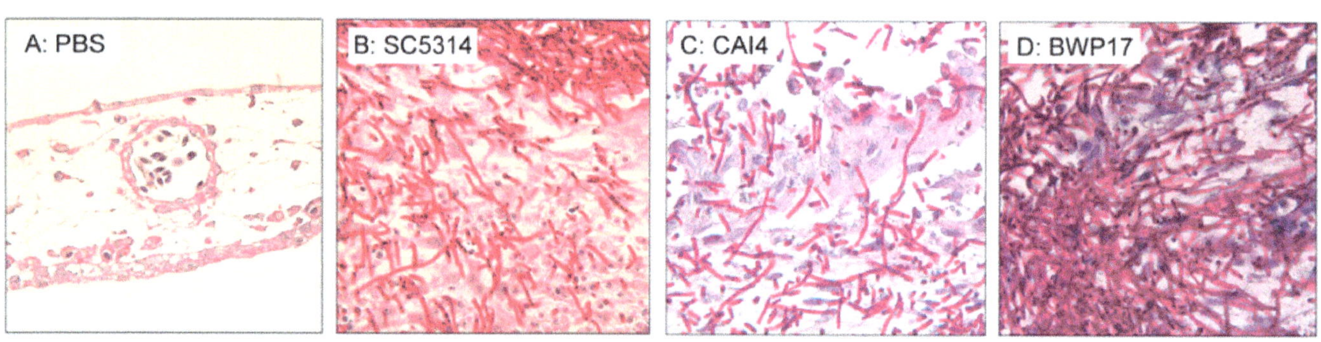

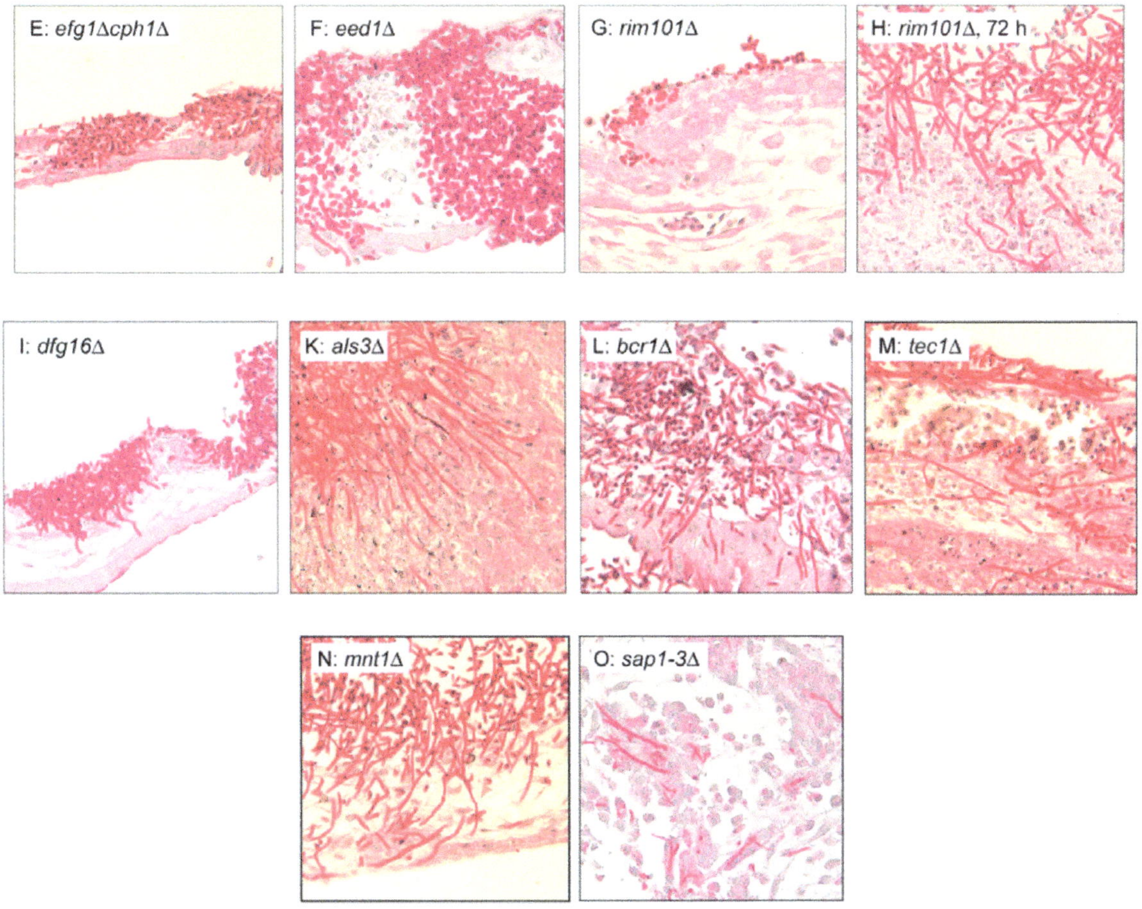

Figure 7: Fungal morphology during infection of the CAM.

In intravenously challenged mice, induction of proinflammatory cytokines in kidneys is directly correlated with the virulence of *C. albicans* strains [11], [26]. To assess whether a similar correlation exists in chicken embryo infection, we determined K60, IL-8, IL-1β and IL-10 transcription in the CAM of embryos infected with *C. albicans* deletion mutants in comparison to their parental strain. Attenuated *C. albicans* mutants generally induced less proinflammatory cytokine transcripts 24 p.i. (Fig. 8), but specific differences were observed between mutants: Only *efg1*Δ*cph1*Δ and *sap1–3*Δ showed reduced transcription levels of all three proinflammatory cytokines (Fig. 8A). *mnt1*Δ and *rim101*Δ induced significantly less IL-8 and IL-1β but levels of K60 were not or only moderately reduced, respectively (Fig. 8A). A similar induction pattern was observed for *bcr1*Δ (Fig. 8B). *dfg16*Δ and *eed1*Δ induced high levels of IL-8 but reduced levels of K60 and IL-1β (Fig. 8A and B). Wildtype-like IL-1β induction but less K60 and IL-8 transcripts were observed with*als3*Δ. Finally, *tec1*Δ differed in transcription kinetics from both the parental strain and the other mutants by showing a reduced induction 24 h p.i. but a strong late induction of IL-1β (48 h p.i., Fig. 8B) and K60 (72 h p.i., Fig. 8B). IL-10 was only moderately induced by CAI4 and BWP and most mutants showed no increase compared to the PBS control (Fig. 8).

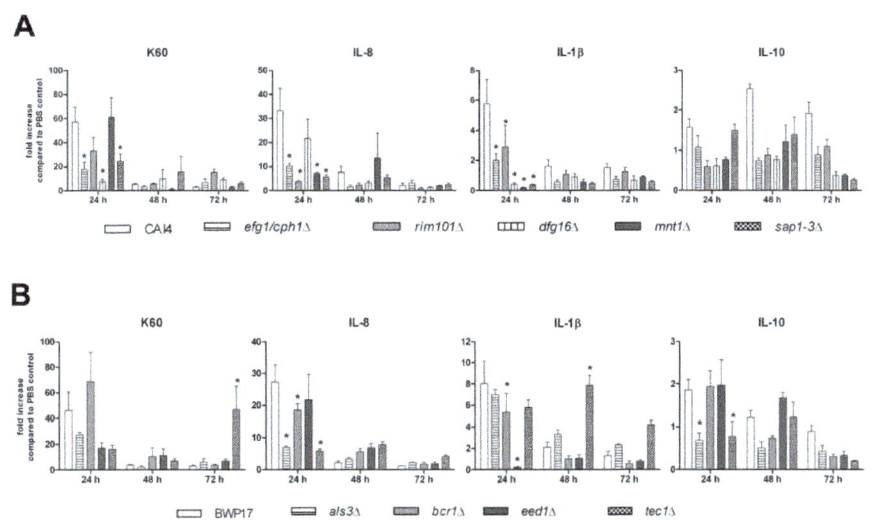

Figure 8: Cytokine transcription in the CAM after infection with *C. albicans*mutants.

DISCUSSION

Mammalian infection models, in particular mouse models, are commonly considered the gold standard to study host-pathogen interactions of human pathogens. However, the use of mammalian models is limited by several factors, including ethical considerations, costs and requirement of specialized facilities. Under these conditions, alternative model hosts of a lower phylogenetic or ontogenetic stage, like invertebrates or avian embryos, can provide an important and alternative tool to study virulence. Chicken embryos have been used previously to investigate *C. albicans* virulence and morphological alterations during infection have been described [20], [21], [23], [24]. Nonetheless, it is of yet unclear which alterations lead to mortality, how the host responds and to which extend interaction of *C. albicans* with the embryo reflects the well studied murine models.

It should be noted that we did not screen buffers and chemicals used in our study for potential endotoxin contamination. Therefore, we cannot completely exclude that endotoxin contaminations might have influenced results obtained in this study. However, all buffers used were tested in a control group of chicken embryos (PBS control) in each individual experiment. The survival of PBS controls was comparable with sham operated embryos (data not shown). The low mortality observed in PBS controls thus appears to be attributable to the necessary mechanical manipulations. All cytokine data were calculated as fold increase to the above mentioned PBS controls within the same experiment to obviate buffer-mediated changes in cytokine transcription.

We aimed at characterizing the host-pathogen interaction during *C. albicans* infection in embryonated eggs to elucidate the potential use of this model as a screening tool for virulence of *C. albicans*. We confirmed previous observations by others that *C. albicans* readily colonizes and invades the CAM, including blood vessels. While Gow et al. [21] could not detect dissemination of SC5314 into the embryo, we observed infrequent dissemination. Given the small size of the liver in young embryos and the low fungal burdens, methodological differences can easily influence detection of dissemination and might therefore explain the differing results. Using a different wild type *C. albicans* strain, Fox et al. [23] observed an age-dependent decrease in fungal burden in the liver, whereas we observed a trend but no significant age-dependency. Our observation that *C. glabrata* and some hyphae-deficient *C. albicans* mutants (*efg1Δcph1Δ*, *eed1Δ*, *dfg16Δ*) disseminate at high frequency suggests that strain specific differences in dissemination exist and supports the hypothesis that yeast cells are the morphological form responsible for dissemination. Additionally, our results confirm the conclusion of Gow et al. [21] that dissemination is no necessary prerequisite for lethal outcome after infection of the CAM.

While dissemination frequencies and the fungal burden in the liver and CAM per weight did not change significantly with increasing age, we observed a strong decrease in mortality in older embryos. Thus, age-dependent susceptibility is unlikely to be an effect of changes in the ratio of infectious dose to embryonic body weight. Likewise, the fungal burden per weight in the CAM did not change depending on embryonic age and during the course of infection, suggesting that (i) at an early stage, the embryonic immune system is able to control fungal proliferation but incapable of clearing infection and (ii) that other mechanisms than clearance of fungi mediate resistance.

In systemically infected mice, the local proinflammatory cytokine response in the kidneys correlates with kidney lesions and lethality [11], [26]. Similarly, we observed higher proinflammatory cytokine production in younger, more susceptible chicken embryos, suggesting that immunopathology in the chicken embryo model contributes to pathogenesis. This hypothesis is further supported by our finding that *C. glabrata*, which does not cause significant mortality in infected chicken embryos, and attenuated *C. albicans* mutants induce significantly less proinflammatory cytokines than *C. albicans* wild type strains, consistent with reports from systemic murine candidiasis [11], [29]. Moreover, the age-dependent susceptibility to LPS-induced septic shock in chicken embryos mirrors susceptibility to *C. albicans* infection. Although a Th2 response is generally considered detrimental in systemic candidiasis, IL-4 deficiency in mice enhances susceptibility to systemic murine *C. albicans* infection [28]. Thus, the age-dependent ability of chicken embryos to increase IL-4 transcription upon infection might contribute to age-dependent resistance. However, whether IL-4 directly influences susceptibility in chicken embryos or if the embryo›s ability to produce IL-4 is only an indicator of a more complex response involving other effectors, remains to be determined. In contrast to the role of IL-10 in mice, where deletion of IL-10 is protective against systemic candidiasis [28], we observed a protective effect of addition of IL-10 to chicken embryos at a susceptible age. Since the general function of IL-10 is modulation and downregulation of proinflammatory responses, the protective effect of IL-10 in chicken embryos could be mediated by an immune-modulatory function which downregulates an otherwise destructive proinflammatory response, thus differing from its role in candidiasis in mice. We suggest that the key to protection is the appropriate balance of the immune response: The proinflammatory response must be sufficient to control the fungus but inflammation needs to be restricted to avoid excessive inflammation-mediated damage.

In addition to Th1, a Th17 response is essential for a protective immune response against disseminated candidiasis in mice [34]. While one study showed increased IL-17A levels in mice 24 h p.i. [34], IL-17 could not be detected within the first 48 h in another study [11]. In chicken embryos, we only observed transcriptional upregulation of IL-17A at 72 h p.i. Similarly, IL-22, another cytokine which has been implicated in Th17 responses, was only upregulated after 72 h. Thus, even though chicken embryos mount a measurable Th17 response on the transcriptional level, it occurs only after main mortality occurred. Furthermore, only IL-22 showed transcriptional differences depending on embryonic age at the time of infection. Therefore, in contrast to mice, IL-17A and IL-22 may not directly contribute to the reduced susceptibility of older chicken embryos.

Macroscopically, *C. albicans* infections lead to the formation of plaques on the CAM. These plaques are granuloma-like structures [24], which are typical for an avian immune response. In contrast to neutrophil infiltration in mammals, which often leads to the formation of abscesses and tissue destruction, heterophil infiltration in birds is resolved by demarcation of necrotic heterophils (and pathogens) by epithelioid macrophages and fibroblasts. The resulting granuloma-like structure isolates pathogens and potential harmful heterophil components from the surrounding tissue [35]. Formation of granuloma-like structures in the *C. albicans* chicken embryo model is likely triggered by the early increase in chemoattractant cytokines, especially IL-8 and K60, which recruit macrophages and heterophils to the site of infection. Visible plaque formation coincides with the decline in cytokine transcription, suggesting that successful demarcation of the pathogen removes the immune stimulus. Moreover, the majority of deaths in the chicken embryo model occur before mature granuloma are formed. Thus, we suggest that while a proinflammatory response in the CAM is necessary to demarcate infected areas, an imbalanced, excessive cytokine response contributes to deaths of young embryos after *C. albicans* infection. In older embryos, the mounted immune response appears to be more balanced and sufficiently induces granuloma formation without causing additional harm.

As cytokines function as signal molecules in infection, the defensive efficacy of the immune response is mediated by immune cells, antibacterial peptides and the complement system. Although we did not analyze effector functions in this study, others have shown that antibacterial peptides are differentially expressed during ontogenesis and that the phagocytic capacity increases during embryonic development [23], [36]. Therefore, it appears likely that functional maturation of immune effector mechanisms additionally contributes to increasing resistance. Furthermore, we cannot exclude that younger embryos are more sensitive to damage of the CAM. Although the quality and quantity of lesions within the CAM was comparable between embryos of different age, higher sensibility of younger embryos could additionally contribute to the influence of embryonic age on the outcome of infection.

To gain further insights into the host-pathogen interaction and to determine the value of chicken embryos as alternative hosts for virulence determination, we analyzed several *C. albicans* deletion mutants for their ability to kill chicken embryos, invade the CAM and induce proinflammatory cytokine transcription. Interestingly, all mutants were isolated in similar or higher cfu compared to the parental strain, suggesting that observed virulence defects are due to altered pathogenesis rather than decreased fitness. In accordance with the role of hyphae and hyphae-associated gene expression in other infection models [31], hyphae-deficient mutants were attenuated in the chicken embryo model. Furthermore, these mutants induced less proinflammatory cytokine transcripts in the chicken embryo model, consistent with the observations of Moyes et al., that hyphae formation and invasion are necessary to trigger cytokine production in cell culture models [37].

Different murine models mimicking different manifestations of human candidiasis are used to investigate the role of putative virulence factors, but only few *C. albicans* mutants have been tested in several murine models. For *TPK2* and *CKA2*, the role in virulence appears to depend on the murine infection model used, as the respective deletion mutants are fully virulent in murine systemic candidiasis, but attenuated in oropharyngeal candidiasis and epithelial cell models [38], [39], [40]. In chicken embryos, *tpk2*Δ led to delayed mortality, but showed no significant attenuation and *cka2*Δ was fully virulent. Thus, virulence of these two mutants in chicken embryos grossly resembled systemic but not mucosal infection in mice. In contrast, *tec1*Δ is attenuated in the systemic mouse model [32], but fully virulent in the chicken embryo model. It has been suggested that the attenuation in the systemic mouse model is due to the decreased ability to evade macrophages after phagocytosis [32]. However, in contrast to intravenous infection which directly exposes the fungus to phagocytic cells, there are no residential macrophages within the CAM, thus delaying the exposure of fungal cells to phagocytes until these cells immigrate from the blood. Thus, a disadvantage of the CAM infection model is that it might not appropriately mimic initial survival in the blood stream after systemic infection. While intravenous infection of chicken embryos is possible [24], it is technically more challenging than infection of the CAM and therefore not suitable for screening purposes. Interestingly, *tec1*Δ induced a delayed increase in proinflammatory cytokines compared to the parental strain. The cause for this delay is not clear, but since Tec1 acts as a transcriptional regulator, deletion of *TEC1* might influence the stimulation of host cells via altered expression of surface-associated molecules. For example, Tec1 indirectly influences transcriptional activation of *ALS3* via Bcr1 [41].

The transcription factor Bcr1 is important for biofilm formation *in vitro* and *in vivo* [42]. Part of these biofilm defects are mediated by Bcr1-dependent regulation of Als3, a well studied adhesin, invasin and ferritin receptor [42], [43], [44]. Despite its role for biofilm formation *in vivo*, *bcr1*Δ is not essential for virulence in a systemic mouse model [42]. In contrast, we observed significant attenuation of both *bcr1*Δ and *als3*Δ in the chicken embryo model. These differences could be explained by the different inoculation routes: Application onto the CAM requires adhesion of fungal cells to the CAM and the typical growth of *C. albicans* in foci on the CAM suggests that aggregation of fungal cells is involved in establishment of infection. Biofilm-related mechanisms might be involved in this step. Furthermore, reduced induction of proinflammatory cytokines by both *bcr1*Δ and *als3*Δ might also contribute to attenuation.

Glycosylation of secreted and surface proteins influences filamentation, adhesion, cell wall stability, and interaction with host cells [45], [46]. In contrast to Gow et al. [21], we found the o-mannosyltransferase mutant *mnt1*Δ to be attenuated in chicken embryos. These discrepancies might be due to differences in methodology, like the age of embryos at infection, since glycosylation is involved in the interaction of *C. albicans* with macrophages [45] and the ability of embryonic macrophages to kill *C. albicans* increases with age [23]. Furthermore, attenuation of *mnt1*Δ only became evident after a prolonged observation period while mortality rates after 24 h were indistinguishable between *mnt1*Δ and its parental strain. Thus, rating mortality over several days is necessary to determine the virulence potential of strains.

Conflicting results have also been published regarding the role of secreted aspartic proteases (Saps) for virulence of *C. albicans* in chicken embryos. Saps are expressed during infection of chicken embryos [21]and protease-deficient *C. albicans* strains were found to be attenuated in virulence and unable to invade the CAM [47]. Furthermore, Kobayashi et al. [48] described that a purified *Candida* protease disrupts intercellular junctions of the CAM and protease-treatment as well as damage to the CAM allowed a protease-deficient *C. albicans* strain to invade. However, differences in virulence were found amongst protease-producing strains [47] and Gow et al. [21] found *SAP* deletion mutants to be fully virulent in chicken embryos. In our hands, a *sap1–3Δ* mutant was significantly attenuated while a *sap4–6Δ* mutant was fully virulent. Histology revealed normal hyphae formation of *sap1–3Δ* but reduced numbers of hyphae invading into deeper layers of the CAM and reduced induction of proinflammatory cytokines. While methodological differences might account for some of the variation we also cannot exclude polar effects in the *sap1–3Δ* mutant due to the use of the *URA*-blaster method in mutant generation. However, it also appears plausible that proteases might aid *C. albicans* in initial invasion into the CAM but that other factors determine the final outcome of infection.

Complex genetic effects might likewise contribute to the observation that some of the complemented mutants tested showed only incomplete recovery of the wild type virulence phenotype. Commonly, only a single copy of the deleted gene is reintroduced into a mutant. Thus, gene dosage effects might influence virulence of a complemented strain. The locus at which the wild type gene is reintroduced and unspecific effects due to more rounds of genetic manipulation performed to construct complemented strains might also affect virulence in this model. While incomplete rescue of virulence has also been described for some strains in murine models [49], it appears to be more common in the chicken embryos model. This should be taken into consideration when evaluating results obtained with the chicken embryo model.

C. glabrata lacks virulence in moderately immunosuppressed mice [29] and chicken embryos although it›s ability to cause lethal infections in humans is well documented [2]. Therefore, both murine models and chicken embryos as alternative hosts are obviously not ideal systems to study pathogenesis of human candidiasis caused by *C. glabrata*.

While it is apparent that we do not fully understand pathogenesis in chicken embryos infected with *C. albicans* on the CAM yet, based on our data and previous work published by others, we propose the following model: The initial phase after application of *C. albicans* is determined by the fungal ability to adhere and form microcolonies on the CAM. In the second phase, rapid hyphae formation and invasion into the CAM triggers a strong proinflammatory host response. An imbalanced, sepsis-like immune response in combination with immature effector functions of the embryonic immune system and damage of the CAM putatively contribute to mortality. Invasion of blood vessels is frequently observed in this stage but dissemination into internal organs of the embryo occurs only infrequently and does not contribute significantly to pathogenesis. If the embryo survives the second phase, foci of fungal invasion are demarcated by immune cells and fibroblasts, visible as plaques, thus limiting further expansion of invasive fungal growth without eliminating the pathogen. Therefore, fungal burden remains stable over time and does not correlate with survival. This demarcation phase coincides with a decline of the proinflammatory response and decrease of mortality frequency in surviving embryos.

In summary, infection of the CAM combines aspects of invasion assays and murine systemic infection in a complex *in vivo* model using an alternative vertebrate host. The advantages of the CAM model lie in comparatively low costs and the technical simplicity with no need for specialized facilities and expertise. The main differences between the chicken embryo model and systemic murine models lie in the application route and the immune status of the host. Systemic infections in mice are predominantly performed in immunocompetent animals, whereas chicken embryos should be considered naturally immunocompromised. Although the immune response of chicken embryos and mice are similar with regard to the induction of proinflammatory cytokines, the effect of IL-10 clearly differs in the two models. Furthermore, the role of IL17A, and a Th17 response in general, remain unclear in the chicken embryo model. In addition, candidiasis in mice generally leads to abscess formation while chicken embryos demarcate infected areas by granuloma. This difference might explain why attenuation of strains in the chicken embryo model was not accompanied by reduction of fungal burden. As the age of chicken embryos at infection has a major influence on the outcome, preincubation and infection procedures need to be standardized to gain comparable results. Our results indicate that attenuation of mutants might be less pronounced in the embryo model compared to systemic murine infections and that complementation might not sufficiently rescue virulence phenotypes in all cases. Thus, the chicken model might yield false-negative results. However, the model still provides a suitable screening tool to determine the virulence of large numbers of mutants strains to identify attenuated strains for subsequent testing in murine models. Furthermore, if specialized animal facilities are not available, the chicken embryo model can be employed as alternative *in vivo* system. In combination with survival analysis, histology and determination of the cytokine response, the CAM chicken model provides insights into pathogenesis. If applied to testing *C. albicans* mutants, this information aids in formulating hypotheses for subsequent refined testing in appropriate mammalian models.

MATERIALS AND METHODS

Ethics statement

All experiments were performed in compliance with the German animal protection law. According to this, no specific approval is needed for work performed in avian embryos before the time of hatching. Experiments were terminated latest on developmental day 18, three days before hatching, by chilling the eggs on ice for 30–60 min.

Candida strains and preparation for infection

The *Candida* strains used in this study have been described. For infection experiments, strains were subcultured once on YPD agar plates for 24 h at 37°C. A single colony was then inoculated into 20 ml liquid YPD and cultured for 12–14 h at 30°C with 200 rpm. Cells were harvested by centrifugation (3,000× g, 5 min, 4°C) and washed twice with cold sterile phosphate buffered saline (PBS), pH 7.4. After determining the cell number with a Cellometer™ Auto T4 (Nexcelom Bioscience, Lawrence, MA, U.S.A.), the suspensions were adjusted to the desired concentration with cold, sterile PBS. Inocula were maintained on ice and used within 1–2 h. The cell numbers in inocula were confirmed by plating serial dilutions on YPD agar plates. Colony forming units (cfu) were determined after 36 h incubation at 30°C. Experiments were only considered valid if the difference between calculated cell number and counted cfu was <20%.

Inactivation of *C. albicans*

For heat inactivation, *C. albicans* suspension adjusted to the appropriate concentration were incubated for 15 min at 80°C. Alternatively, diluted fungal suspensions were inactivated by adding 100 mM thimerosal (Sigma, Steinheim, Germany) and incubating for 45 min at 37°C. Following thimerosal treatment, fungal cells were washed 3× with sterile PBS. Inactivation was confirmed by plating serial dilutions on YPD agar plates.

Preparation of embryonated eggs and inoculation on the chorio-allantoic membrane (CAM)

Fertilized chicken eggs of the breed "weiße Leghorn" were obtained from a local producer. The eggs were stored at 8°C for a maximum of seven days prior to incubation at 37.6°C and 50–60% relative humidity in a specialized incubator (BSS 300, Grumbach, Germany). Eggs were turned four times a day starting on the fourth day of incubation until infection. Prior to infection, vitality of the embryo was assessed by candling. For survival experiments and determination of fungal burden, inoculation on the CAM was performed as described previously [50]. Twenty eggs were infected per group and survival was monitored for up to 7 days by candling. Experiments were repeated at least two times. Survival data were plotted as Kaplan-Meyer curves and statistically analyzed by log rank test using Graph Pad Prism Version 5.00 for Windows (GraphPad Software, San Diego California USA).

For determination of the immune response and histological analyses, the technique was modified to allow easier localizing of the site of infection: 50 µl *Candida* inoculum containing 1×10^5 cells was placed onto sterile nylon membrane filters (0.45 µm pore size, 13 mm in diameter, cut in half; Carl Roth GmbH, Karlsruhe, Germany) on sterile Whatman® blotting paper (GE Healthcare, München, Germany). After excessive liquid had soaked through the membranes, the wet membranes were placed onto YPD agar plates until inoculation. Embryonated eggs were prepared as described above but the hole at the longitudinal side was elongated to a 5 mm slit. The inoculated membrane was carefully inserted through the slit with the inoculated site facing the CAM. Survival curves obtained using the membrane method were comparable to survival after inoculation of suspensions containing the same number of fungal cells.

Age-matched PBS mock-infected embryos were used as negative controls in all experiments.

Application of lipopolysaccharides, zymosan and IL-10

Lipopolysaccharides (LPS, prepared by phenol extraction from *Escherichia coli* O55:B5, Sigma) and zymosan (prepared from *Saccharomyces cerevisiae*, Sigma) were solved in sterile PBS. Chicken recombinant IL-10 (Kingfisher Biotech Inc., St. Paul, MN, U.S.A.) was solved in sterile PBS containing 0.2% BSA (Serva, Heidelberg, Germany) as carrier protein. Both LPS, zymosan and IL-10 were applied onto the CAM as described above for survival experiments.

Determination of fungal burden

Embryonated eggs were infected with 10^5 cfu/egg as described above for survival experiments. At given time points, viable embryos (defined by embryonic movement at candling) were humanely sacrificed by chilling the eggs on ice for 30–60 min. The eggs› surface was then disinfected with 70% ethanol. The shell was cut in half with sterile scissors. Approximately 0.5–1 g CAM (comprising 1/3 to 1/2 of total CAM), were removed. The embryo was then carefully removed from its surrounding membranes and placed in 70% ethanol for 2–3 min. Using a sterile set of scissors and forceps, the abdominal cavity was opened to remove the liver. Samples were homogenized in 2 ml sterile, cold PBS using an Ultra-Turrax® T10 basic (IKA® GmbH, Staufenberg, Germany). Undiluted homogenate (liver: 4×500 µl; CAM: 100 µl) and serial dilutions were plated onto YPD agar plates and incubated for 36 h prior to colony counting. Fungal burden of CAM and liver were determined for at least ten embryos per fungal strain and time point. Statistical analysis was performed by 2-way ANOVA and Bonferroni post test using GraphPad Prism® Version 5.00 for Windows. Dissemination frequencies were compared by chi-square test.

Histological analysis

For histological analysis, embryonated eggs were infected with the nylon membrane method and dissected as described above 24 h, 48 h and 72 h post infection (p.i.). The CAM underneath and beside the membrane was removed *in toto* with the nylon membrane, placed into biopsy bags and fixed in neutral formalin (Histofix®, Roth). Paraffin-embedded specimens were cut into 5 µm sections, stained with periodic acid-Schiff (PAS) stain according to standard protocols and examined using bright field microscopy at the indicated magnification.

Determination of cytokine and chemokine transcription levels

For analysis of cytokine and chemokine transcription levels, embryonated eggs were infected with *C. albicans* by the nylon membrane method and dissected as described above at the indicated time points. Samples were taken and processed as previously described [50]. Quantitative real time RT-PCR reactions were set up with the One step RT qPCR MasterMix Plus for SYBR® GreenI kit (Eurogentec, Seraing, Belgium) according to the manufacturer›s instructions using 100 ng total RNA as template. Primers and temperature protocols used have been published previously [50], [51], [52] with the exception of IL-10. For IL-10 the following primers were used with an annealing temperature of 56°C: forward 5-*AGGAGACGTTCGAGAAGATGGAT -3*; reverse 5-*TCACTTCCTCCTCCTCATCAGC-3*. The amplification and detection of specific products was performed on a 7300 Real Time PCR System (Applied Biosystems, Foster City, USA) using the dissociation curve mode to check the specificity of amplification products. Specific mRNA levels were quantified using the threshold method [53] and normalized to GAPDH (ΔC_T values). The results are expressed as n-fold change to age-matched PBS control embryos by calculating $2^{(-\Delta\Delta CT)}$. The groups at a given time point were compared by 1-way ANOVA followed by Bonferroni post test (for three groups) or unpaired, two-tailed *t* test (for two groups) using Graph Pad Prism Version 5.00 for Windows.

ACKNOWLEDGMENTS

We thank J. F. Fink, J. Ernst, N. A. R. Gow, W. A. Fonzi, K. Schroeppel, A. P. Mitchell, S. G. Filler, K. Haynes, and F. Muehlschlegel for kindly providing wild type and mutant strains and A. J. Brown for providing pCIP10 and pCIP30; Birgit Weber and Ursula Stöckel for excellent technical help and Betty Wächtler for helpful discussions.

REFERENCES

1. Odds FC. *Candida* and Candidosis. London: Baillière Tindall; 1988.
2. Pfaller MA, Diekema DJ. Epidemiology of invasive candidiasis: a persistent public health problem. Clin Microbiol Rev. 2007;20:133–163.
3. Pappas PG, Rex JH, Lee J, Hamill RJ, Larsen RA, et al. A prospective observational study of candidemia: epidemiology, therapy, and influences on mortality in hospitalized adult and pediatric patients. Clin Infect Dis. 2003;37:634–643.
4. Naglik JR, Fidel PL, Jr, Odds FC. Animal models of mucosal *Candida* infection. FEMS Microbiol Lett.2008;283:129–139.
5. de Repentigny L. Animal models in the analysis of *Candida* host-pathogen interactions. Curr Opin Microbiol. 2004;7:324–329.
6. Brennan M, Thomas DY, Whiteway M, Kavanagh K. Correlationbetweenvirulenceof*Candidaalbicans*mutants in mice and *Galleria mellonella* larvae. FEMS Immunol Med Microbiol. 2002;34:153–157.
7. Rowan R, Moran C, McCann M, Kavanagh K. Use of *Galleria mellonella* larvae to evaluate the in vivo anti-fungal activity of [Ag2(mal)(phen)3]. Biometals. 2009;22:461–467.
8. Chamilos G, Lionakis MS, Lewis RE, Lopez-Ribot JL, Saville SP, et al. *Drosophila melanogaster* as a facile model for large-scale studies of virulence mechanisms and antifungal drug efficacy in *Candida* species.J Infect Dis. 2006;193:1014–1022.
9. Alarco AM, Marcil A, Chen J, Suter B, Thomas D, et al. Immune-deficient *Drosophila melanogaster*: a model for the innate immune response to human fungal pathogens. J Immunol. 2004;172:5622–5628.
10. Spellberg B, Ibrahim AS, Edwards JE, Jr, Filler SG. Mice with disseminated candidiasis die of progressive sepsis. J Infect Dis. 2005;192:336–343.
11. MacCallum DM, Castillo L, Brown AJ, Gow NA, Odds FC. Early-expressed chemokines predict kidney immunopathology in experimental disseminated *Candida albicans* infections. PLoS One. 2009;4:e6420.
12. Bergin D, Murphy L, Keenan J, Clynes M, Kavanagh K. Pre-exposure to yeast protects larvae of*Galleria mellonella* from a subsequent lethal infection by *Candida albicans* and is mediated by the increased expression of antimicrobial peptides. Microbes Infect. 2006;8:2105–2112.
13. Hoffmann JA, Reichhart JM. *Drosophila* innate immunity: an evolutionary perspective. Nat Immunol.2002;3:121–126.
14. Beeckman DS, Rothwell L, Kaiser P, Vanrompay DC. Differential cytokine expression in*Chlamydophila psittaci* genotype A-, B- or D-infected chicken macrophages after exposure to *Escherichia coli* O2:K1 LPS. Dev Comp Immunol. 2010;34:812–820.
15. De Boever S, Beyaert R, Vandemaele F, Baert K, Duchateau L, et al. The influence of age and repeated lipopolysaccharide administration on body temperature and the concentration of interleukin-6 and IgM antibodies against lipopolysaccharide in broiler chickens. Avian Pathol. 2008;37:39–44.
16. Moore M. The Chorio-Allantoic Membrane of the Developing Chick as a Medium for the Cultivation and Histopathologic Study of Pathogenic Fungi. Science. 1939;89:514–515.
17. Buddingh GJ. The chick embryo for the study of infection and immunity. J Infect Dis. 1970;121:660–663.
18. Partridge BM, Athar MA, Winner HI. Chick embryo inoculation as a pathogenicity test for *Candida*species. J Clin Pathol. 1971;24:645–648.
19. Cawson RA. Induction of epithelial hyperplasia by *Candida albicans*. Br J Dermatol. 1973;89:497–503.
20. Härtl A, Hillesheim HG, Kunkel W, Schrinner EJ. [The *Candida* infected hen's egg. An alternative test system for systemic anticandida activity]. Arzneimittelforschung. 1995;45:926–928.
21. Gow NA, Knox Y, Munro CA, Thompson WD. Infection of chick chorioallantoic membrane (CAM) as a model for invasive hyphal growth and pathogenesis of *Candida albicans*. Med Mycol. 2003;41:331–338.
22. Odds FC, Van Nuffel L, Gow NA. Survival in experimental *Candida albicans* infections depends on inoculum growth conditions as well as animal host. Microbiology. 2000;146(Pt 8):1881–1889.
23. Fox AJ, Reid TMS, Solomon JB. J. B. Solomon ISoDaCI, editor. 1980; Aberdeen. Pergamon Press; Development of resistance to invading *Candida albicans* in the chicken embryo. pp. 295–300.
24. Norris RF, Shorey WK, Bongiovanni AM. Lesions produced in chick embryos by *Candida* (*Monilia*) *albicans*. Arch Pathol (Chic) 1948;45:506–512.
25. Smith RT, Thomas L. The lethal effect of endotoxins on the chick embryo. J Exp Med. 1956;104:217–231.
26. MacCallum DM. Massive induction of innate immune response to *Candida albicans* in the kidney in a murine intravenous challenge model. FEMS Yeast Res. 2009;9:1111–1122.
27. Sriskandan S, Altmann DM. The immunology of sepsis. J Pathol. 2008;214:211–223.
28. Vazquez-Torres A, Jones-Carson J, Wagner RD, Warner T, Balish E. Early resistance of interleukin-10 knockout mice to acute systemic candidiasis. Infect Immun. 1999;67:670–674.
29. Jacobsen ID, Brunke S, Seider K, Schwarzmuller T, Firon A, et al. *Candida glabrata* persistence in mice does not depend on host immunosuppression and is unaffected by fungal amino acid auxotrophy. Infect Immun. 2010;78:1066–1077.

30. Brieland J, Essig D, Jackson C, Frank D, Loebenberg D, et al. Comparison of pathogenesis and host immune responses to *Candida glabrata* and *Candida albicans* in systemically infected immunocompetent mice. Infect Immun. 2001;69:5046–5055.

31. Kumamoto CA, Vinces MD. Contributions of hyphae and hypha-co-regulated genes to *Candida albicans* virulence. Cell Microbiol. 2005;7:1546–1554.

32. Schweizer A, Rupp S, Taylor BN, Rollinghoff M, Schroppel K. The TEA/ATTS transcription factor CaTec1p regulates hyphal development and virulence in *Candida albicans*. Mol Microbiol. 2000;38:435–445.

33. Thewes S, Kretschmar M, Park H, Schaller M, Filler SG, et al. *In vivo* and *ex vivo* comparative transcriptional profiling of invasive and non-invasive *Candida albicans* isolates identifies genes associated with tissue invasion. Mol Microbiol. 2007;63:1606–1628.

34. Huang W, Na L, Fidel PL, Schwarzenberger P. Requirement of interleukin-17A for systemic anti-Candida albicans host defense in mice. J Infect Dis. 2004;190:624–631.

35. Harmon BG. Avian heterophils in inflammation and disease resistance. Poult Sci. 1998;77:972–977.

36. Meade KG, Higgs R, Lloyd AT, Giles S, O›Farrelly C. Differential antimicrobial peptide gene expression patterns during early chicken embryological development. Dev Comp Immunol. 2009;33:516–524.

37. Moyes DL, Runglall M, Murciano C, Shen C, Nayar D, et al. A biphasic innate immune MAPK response discriminates between the yeast and hyphal forms of *Candida albicans* in epithelial cells. Cell Host Microbe. 2010;8:225–235.

38. Park H, Myers CL, Sheppard DC, Phan QT, Sanchez AA, et al. Role of the fungal Ras-protein kinase A pathway in governing epithelial cell interactions during oropharyngeal candidiasis. Cell Microbiol.2005;7:499–510.

39. Sonneborn A, Bockmuhl DP, Gerads M, Kurpanek K, Sanglard D, et al. Protein kinase A encoded by TPK2 regulates dimorphism of *Candida albicans*. Mol Microbiol. 2000;35:386–396.

40. Chiang LY, Sheppard DC, Bruno VM, Mitchell AP, Edwards JE, Jr, et al. *Candida albicans* protein kinase *CK2* governs virulence during oropharyngeal candidiasis. Cell Microbiol. 2007;9:233–245.

41. Argimon S, Wishart JA, Leng R, Macaskill S, Mavor A, et al. Developmental regulation of an adhesin gene during cellular morphogenesis in the fungal pathogen *Candida albicans*. Eukaryot Cell 2007

42. Nobile CJ, Andes DR, Nett JE, Smith FJ, Yue F, et al. Critical role of Bcr1-dependent adhesins in *C. albicans* biofilm formation in vitro and in vivo. PLoS Pathog. 2006;2:e63.

43. Phan QT, Myers CL, Fu Y, Sheppard DC, Yeaman MR, et al. Als3 Is a *Candida albicans* Invasin That Binds to Cadherins and Induces Endocytosis by Host Cells. PLoS Biol. 2007;5:e64.

44. Almeida RS, Brunke S, Albrecht A, Thewes S, Laue M, et al. The hyphal-associated adhesin and invasin Als3 of *Candida albicans* mediates iron acquisition from host ferritin. PLoS Pathog.2008;4:e1000217.

45. McKenzie CG, Koser U, Lewis LE, Bain JM, Mora-Montes HM, et al. Contribution of Candida albicans cell wall components to recognition by and escape from murine macrophages. Infect Immun. 78:1650–1658.

46. Munro CA, Bates S, Buurman ET, Hughes HB, Maccallum DM, et al. Mnt1p and Mnt2p of *Candida albicans* are partially redundant alpha-1,2-mannosyltransferases that participate in O-linked mannosylation and are required for adhesion and virulence. J Biol Chem. 2005;280:1051–1060.

47. Shimizu K, Kondoh Y, Tanaka K. Proteinase production and pathogenicity of Candida albicans. I. Invasion into chorioallantoic membrane by *C. albicans* strains of different proteinase activity. Microbiol Immunol. 1987;31:1045–1060.

48. Kobayashi I, Kondoh Y, Shimizu K, Tanaka K. A role of secreted proteinase of *Candida albicans* for the invasion of chick chorio-allantoic membrane. Microbiol Immunol. 1989;33:709–719.

49. Lo HJ, Kohler JR, DiDomenico B, Loebenberg D, Cacciapuoti A, et al. Nonfilamentous *C. albicans*mutants are avirulent. Cell. 1997;90:939–949.

50. Jacobsen ID, Grosse K, Slesiona S, Hube B, Berndt A, et al. Embryonated eggs as an alternative infection model to investigate *Aspergillus fumigatus* virulence. Infect Immun. 2010;78:2995–3006.

51. Pieper J, Methner U, Berndt A. Heterogeneity of avian gammadelta T cells. Vet Immunol Immunopathol.2008;124:241–252.

52. Carvajal BG, Methner U, Pieper J, Berndt A. Effects of *Salmonella enterica* serovar Enteritidis on cellular recruitment and cytokine gene expression in caecum of vaccinated chickens. Vaccine. 2008;26:5423–5433.

53. Pfaffl MW. A new mathematical model for relative quantification in real-time RT-PCR. Nucleic Acids Res. 2001;29:e45.

CHAPTER 4

AVIAN COLIBACILLOSIS AND SALMONELLOSIS: A CLOSER LOOK AT EPIDEMIOLOGY, PATHOGENESIS, DIAGNOSIS, CONTROL AND PUBLIC HEALTH CONCERNS

S. M. Lutful Kabir[1, 2]

[1] Graduate School of Life and Environmental Sciences, Osaka Prefecture University, Osaka, Japan

[2] Department of Microbiology and Hygiene, Faculty of Veterinary Science, Bangladesh Agricultural University, Mymensingh-2202, Bangladesh

ABSTRACT

Avian colibacillosis and salmonellosis are considered to be the major bacterial diseases in the poultry industry world-wide. Colibacillosis and salmonellosis are the most common avian diseases that are communicable to humans. This article provides the vital information on the epidemiology, pathogenesis, diagnosis, control and public health concerns of avian colibacillosis and salmonellosis. A better understanding of the information addressed in this review article will assist the poultry researchers and the poultry industry in continuing to make progress in reducing and eliminating avian colibacillosis and salmonellosis from the poultry flocks, thereby reducing potential hazards to the public health posed by these bacterial diseases.

INTRODUCTION

Avian colibacillosis is an infectious disease of birds caused by *Escherichia coli*, which is considered as one of the principal causes of morbidity and mortality, associated with heavy economic losses to the poultry industry by its association with various disease conditions, either as primary pathogen or as a secondary pathogen. It causes a variety of disease manifestations in poultry including yolk sac infection, omphalitis, respiratory tract infection, swollen head syndrome, septicemia, polyserositis, coligranuloma, enteritis, cellulitis and salpingitis. Colibacillosis of poultry is characterized in its acute form by septicemia resulting in death and in its subacute form by peri-carditis, airsacculitis and peri-hepatitis [1]. On the other hand, *Salmonella* infection caused by a variety of *Salmonella* species is one of the most important bacterial diseases in poultry causing heavy economic losses through mortality and reduced production [2]. Avian salmonella infection may occur in poultry either acute or chronic form by one or more member of genus *Salmonella*, under the family Enterobacteriaceae [3]. Besides, motile Salmonellae (paratyphoid group) infection cause salmonellosis in chickens and have zoonotic significance.

Avian colibacillosis has been noticed to be a major infectious disease in birds of all ages. This disease has an important economic impact on poultry production worldwide. The majority of economic losses results from mortality and decrease in productivity of the affected birds [4]. Infectious bursal disease (IBD), mycoplasmosis, coccidiosis, Newcastle disease or infectious bronchitis, as well as nutritional deficiencies all predispose the birds to this disease [5]. However, faecal contamination of egg may result in the penetration of*E. coli* through the shell and may spread to the chickens during hatching and is often associated with high mortality rates,

Citation: S. M. Lutful Kabir, Avian Colibacillosis and Salmonellosis: A Closer Look at Epidemiology, Pathogenesis, Diagnosis, Control and Public Health Concerns, doi: 10.3390/ijerph7010089.

or it may give rise to yolk sac infection. On the other hand, with the great expansion of poultry rearing and farming, avian salmonellosis is the most devastating disease worldwide. The epidemiology of fowl typhoid and pullorum disease in poultry, particularly with regard to transmission from one generation to the next is known to be closely associated with infected eggs [6]. The birds that survive from clinical disease when infected at a young stage may show few signs of infection but can become carriers [7].

At slaughter, resistant strains from the gut readily soil poultry carcasses and as a result poultry meats are often contaminated with multiresistant *E. coli* [8–14]; likewise eggs become contaminated during laying [15]. Hence, resistant faecal *E. coli* from poultry can infect humans both directly and via food. These resistant bacteria may colonize the human intestinal tract and may also contribute resistance genes to human endogenous flora [16]. Similarly, the emergence of multidrug resistance among *Salmonella* spp. is an increasing concern. *Salmonella* serovar Hadar has been reported as one of the most resistant *Salmonella*serotypes [17–19].

Microbial food safety is an increasing public health concern worldwide. Epidemiological reports suggest that poultry meat is still the primary cause of human food poisoning [20]. Poultry meat is more popular in the consumer market because of advantages such as easy digestibility and acceptance by the majority of people [21]. However, the presence of pathogenic and spoilage microorganisms in poultry meat and its by-products remains a significant concern for suppliers, consumers and public health officials worldwide. *E. coli* and*Salmonella* has been consistently associated with foodborne illnesses in most countries of the world.

There are many poultry diseases transmissible to human, among them avian colibacillosis and avian salmonellosis are the prime concerns. But the detailed information about avian colibacillosis and avian salmonellosis in connection to the public health concerns are not available yet in one place. So, I intend to write this review article focusing on the various aspects of avian colibacillosis and avain salmonellosis in connection to the public health concerns.

PIDEMIOLOGY OF AVIAN COLIBACILLOSIS AND AVIAN SALMONELLOSIS

Epidemiology of Avian Colibacillosis

E. coli is a gram-negative, non-acid-fast, uniform staining, non-spore-forming bacillus that grows both aerobically and anaerobically and may be variable in size and shape. Many strains are motile and have peritrichous flagella. *E. coli* is considered as a member of the normal microflora of the poultry intestine, but certain strains, such as those designated as avian pathogenic *E. coli* (APEC), spread into various internal organs and cause colibacillosis characterized by systemic fatal disease [22,23]. *E. coli* isolates pathogenic for poultry commonly belong to certain serogroups, particularly the serogroups O78, O1, and O2, and to some extent O15 and O55 [24,25]. In domestic poultry, avian colibacillosis is frequently associated with *E. coli*strains of serotypes O78:K80, O1:K1 and O2:K1 (2-Filali E). The avian colibacillosis was found widely prevalent in all age group of chickens (9.52 to 36.73%) with specially high prevalence rate in adult layer birds (36.73%) [26].

The most important reservoir of *E. coli* is the intestinal tract of animals, including poultry. In chickens, there are about 10^9 colony forming units (CFU) of bacteria per gram of feces and of these, 10^6 CFU are *E. coli*. *E. coli* has also been commonly isolated from the upper respiratory tract. In addition, it is present on the bird's skin and feathers. These strains always belong to both pathogenic and non-pathogenic types [27]. In the caecal flora of healthy chickens, 10 to 15% of the *E. coli* strains may belong to an O-serotype that can also be isolated from colibacillosis lesions [28]. As soon as the first hours after hatching, the birds start building up their *E. coli* flora. The bacteria drastically increase their numbers in the gut. In a single bird a large number of different *E. coli* types is present, obtained via horizontal contamination from the environment, more specifically from other birds, faeces, water and feed [29]. Moreover, rodents may be carriers of APEC and hence a source of contamination for the birds [22].

The risk for colibacillosis increases with increasing infection pressure in the environment. A good housing hygiene and avoiding overcrowding are very important. Other principal risk factors are the duration of exposure, virulence of the strain, breed, and immune status of the bird [30–34]. Every damage to the respiratory system favours infection with APEC. Several pathogens, like NDV, IBV and MG, both wildtype and vaccine strains, may play a part in this process. An unfavourable housing climate, like an excess of ammonia or dust, renders the respiratory system more susceptible to APEC infections through deciliation of the upper respiratory tract [22].

Pulsed field gel electrophoresis (PFGE) is considered to be the most reliable molecular finger-printing technique to differentiate organisms but restriction fragment length polymorphism (RFLP) is the one that is used most frequently. However, both techniques require large quantities of DNA, are time consuming, and require expensive equipment [35]. Other techniques such as ERIC–PCR and REP–PCR [36,37] and random amplification of polymorphic DNA (RAPD)–PCR [38] have been proposed as alternatives and used to characterize *Escherichia coli* isolates of avian origin [39,40]. Other molecular techniques such as ribotyping and isoenzyme profile have also been used to evaluate the clonality of avian *E. coli* [41]. Some clones are specific to APEC and a small-scale comparison of commensal and pathogenic isolates revealed that 83% of pathogenic strains belong to only five clones, whereas each of the 10 non-pathogenic strains belong to different clones [42]. On the other hand, clonal relationships were found for O2:K1 isolates from humans and chickens [43] and for O78 isolates from humans, cattle, sheep, pigs and chickens [44], indicating that these species too might act as a source of infection for chickens.

Even though certain O-types are more frequently detected in APEC than in commensal *E. coli* [45], the isolates are very heterogenous, both in their pheno- and genotype [43,45–47]. On the other hand, the prevalence of certain serotypes is linked with the geographical localisation of a flock [48].

Since avian pathogenic *E. coli* (APEC) and human uropathogenic *E. coli* (UPEC) may encounter similar challenges when establishing infection in extraintestinal locations, they may share a similar content of virulence genes and capacity to cause disease. In this regard, Rodriguez-Siek *et al.* [49] compared 200 human uropathogenic *E. coli* (UPEC) and 524 avian pathogenic *E. coli* (APEC) isolates for their content of virulence genes (Table 1), including many implicated in extraintestinal pathogenic *E. coli* (ExPEC) virulence as well as those associated with APEC plasmids for assessing the potential of APEC to cause human extraintestinal diseases and a well-documented ability of avian *E. coli* to spread to human beings, the potential for APEC to act as human UPEC or as a reservoir of virulence genes for UPEC should be considered.

Table 1: ExPEC/APEC genes used in virulence genotyping*

Gene	Description	Reference
pTJ100-related genes		
cvaC+	Structural gene for the colicin V operon	[50]
iroN±	Catecholate siderophore receptor gene	[51]
iss+	Increased serum survival gene	[52,53]
iucC±	Involved in aerobactin synthesis	[54,55]
iutA±	Ferric aerobactin receptor gene; iron transport	[55]
sitA±	Putative iron transport gene	[56]
traT+	Outer membrane protein gene; surface exclusion; serum resistance	[57,58]
tsh≠	Temperature-sensitive hemagglutinin gene	[59]
Iron-Related		
feoB	Gene which mediates ferric iron uptake	[56]
ireA	Encodes an iron-responsive element; putative sideropohore receptor gene	[60]
irp-2	Iron repressible gene associated with yersiniabactin synthesis	[61]
Toxins		
hlyD	Transport gene of the hemolysin operon	[62]
Miscellaneous		
fliC (H7)	Produces flagellin protein associated with the H7 antigen group	[63]

* Descriptions of genes encoding components of certain adhesins (i.e., genes encoding parts of the P pilus, papA; papC; papEF; papG, including papG alleles I, II, and III; the S pilus, sfa and the gene encoding the S fimbrial tip, sfaS; the Type 1 fimbrial adhesin, fimH; the F1C fimbrial tip, focG; and other genes encoding portions of miscellaneous adhesins, iha; afa; gafD; and bmaE); toxins (cnf-1 and cdtB); protectins (kpsMT K1; kpsMT II; kpsMT III; and rfc); siderophores (fyuA); and other miscellaneous structures (ibeA; ompT; and PAI(CFT073), a fragment from archetypal UPEC strain CFT073) can be found in Johnson and co-workers [64]. Also, the description of papG allele I' can be found in Johnson and Stell [65].

+ These genes are listed as pTJ100-related, but they could also be listed as protectins.

± These genes are listed as pTJ100-related, but they could also be listed with the iron-related genes.

≠ These genes are listed as pTJ100-related, but they also could be listed in the miscellaneous group.

Avian pathogenic *E. coli* strains are often resistant to antimicrobials approved for poultry including cephradine [66], tetracyclines [66–70], chloramphenicol [66], sulfonamides [67,69–71], amino-glycosides [68–70,72,73] and β-lactam antibiotics [66,67,69,71]. Resistance to fluoroquinolones was reported within several years of the approval of this class of drugs for use in poultry [45,71,74,75]. There is reason for concern that genes conferring resistance to extended-spectrum beta-lactams will emerge in avian pathogenic*E. coli* strains [76] and reduce the efficacy of ceftiofur, which is currently used on a limited basis in poultry breeding flocks and hatcheries. In one study, conducted at the University of Georgia, 97 of 100 avian pathogenic *E. coli* isolates were resistant to streptomycin and sulfonamide and 87% of these multiple antimicrobial resistant strains contained a class 1 integron, intI1, which carried multiple antibiotic resistance genes [70]. Multiple antimicrobial resistance traits of avian pathogenic *E. coli* have also been associated with transmissible R-plasmids [77].

Epidemiology of Avian Salmonellosis

Avian *Salmonella* infections are important as both a cause of clinical disease in poultry and as a source of food-borne transmission of disease to humans. Under the family of

Enterobacteriaceae, the genus *Salmonella*is a facultative intracellular pathogen causing localized or systemic infections; as well as a chronic asymptomatic carrier state [78]. The etiological agent of fowl typhoid and pullorum disease is *Salmonella enterica* subsp. *enterica* serovar Gallinarum, which is divided into two distinct biovars under the serogroup D1, Gallinarum and Pullorum, which are denoted as *S. gallinarum* and *S. pullorum,* respectively [78,79]. In addition to *S. gallinarum-pullorum*, other salmonellae such as *S. enteritidis, S. panama* and *S. dublin* also belong to the serogroup D1 [79]. The various motile and non-host adapted highly invasive serotypes such as*Salmonella enteritidis* and *Salmonella typhimurium* are commonly referred to as paratyphoid salmonellae [80]. Age wise prevalence of avian salmonellosis showed highest infection rate in adult layers (53.25%) in comparison to brooding (14.55%), growing (16.10%) and pullet (16.10%) chickens [26].

Various routes of infection have been described. Oral route of infection represents the normal route of infection [81]. Although infection in newly hatched chicks by nasal and cloacal route are also considered as the important route of transmission. Chicks may be infected early by vertical transmission either from an infected ovary, oviduct or from the infected eggs during the passage through the cloacal faeces from infected or carrier hens. The birds survive from clinical disease when infected in young stage may show few signs of infection but they become carriers [82]. In adult carriers the reproductive organs are the predilection sites that often lead to the infection of ovarian follicles and as a result transovarian transmission of the disease occurs. The bacteria are passed out through the faeces and lateral spread takes place through the fecal contaminated feeds, water and litter [78].

Although more than 2,300 serotypes of *Salmonella* have been identified, only about 10% of these have been isolated from poultry [80]. Chickens are the natural hosts for the highly host adapted biovar *S. gallinarum*and *S. pullorum*, but natural outbreaks have also been reported in turkeys, guinea fowl, quail and pheasants [83]. Fowl typhoid is a peracute, acute or chronic form of disease affecting mostly adult chickens, whereas pullorum disease affects the very young chickens, mostly 2–3 weeks of age. In the adult it tends to be chronic [78,84]. Fowl typhoid is frequently referred to as a disease of adult birds; still, there are also reports of high morbidity and mortality in young chickens [85]. *S. gallinarum* can produce lesions in chicks, which are indistinguishable from those associated with pullorum disease [78]. A certain percentage of chickens that survive from the initial infection become carriers with or without presence of clinical signs and pathological lesions [83]. Crowding, malnutrition, and other stressful conditions as well as unsanitary surroundings can exacerbate mortality and performance losses due to salmonellosis, especially in young birds [86]. The potential risk factors responsible for *Salmonella* contamination of broiler-chicken flocks are summarized in Table 2.

Table 2: A list of risk factors responsible for *Salmonella* contamination of broiler-chicken flocks

Risk factors	Reference
Inadequate level of hygiene	[87,88]
Salmonella contamination of the previous flock with a persistence inside the house	[89,90] [91]
Contaminated day-old chicks and feed	[89,92-94]
The farm structure (>3 houses on the farm)	[89]
Wet and cold season	[89]
Litter-beetle infestation of the house	[91]

In more recent years, the use of DNA-related techniques such as plasmid analysis [95,96], ribotyping [97–100], and PFGE [101,102] have proved to be useful in discriminating isolates of *Salmonella* species. Lapuz *et al.* [103] investigated the prevalence of *Salmonella* in four layer farms in eastern Japan between 2004 and 2006 to determine the role of roof rats (*Rattus rattus*) in the epizootology of *Salmonella enterica*subsp. *enterica* serovar Enteritidis (*S. enteritidis*) and they suggested that roof rats were carriers of *S. enteritidis* and *S. infantis* and that persistent *S. enteritidis* and *S. infantis* infections in a rat population might play an important role in the spread and maintenance of these pathogens inside the layer premises.

Fowl typhoid and pullorum disease are distributed in many countries of the world, and have economic significance [104]. They are mainly distributed in Latin America, the Middle East, the Indian subcontinent, Africa and perhaps other parts of the world [78,105]. Salmonellosis has also been reported in many countries of South-East Asia including Bangladesh [106,107], India [108,109], Pakistan [110,111] and Nepal [112]. Fowl typhoid is common in both backyard chickens and in commercial poultry [113].

Salmonella and other food borne pathogens acquire antibiotic resistance by random chromosomal mutations, mutation of existing genes, and through specific mechanisms such as transduction, tranformation, and conjugation [114]. These mechanisms involve transfer of drug resistant genes by means of circular DNA plasmids such as R-factor, conjugative plasmid, or chromosomal elements [115–122]. The occurrence and proliferation of antibiotic-resistant *Salmonella* in environmental samples, poultry, and other animals and humans may be due to the use of medicated feeds [123–125], the practice of dipping hatching eggs in solutions containing antimicrobial agents [126–128], routine inoculation of day-old poults with antibiotics [126–128] and treatment of other animals [129] and humans [117] with antibiotics. *Salmonella* strains of avian origin are also often resistant to variety of antimicrobials approved for poultry including tetracycline [130–133], oxytetracycline [134], penicillin [66,130–134], aminoglycosides [130,132,133], sulfisoxazole [133] and fluoroquinolones [135]. On the other hand, Manie *et al.* [136] found several strains of multiple antibiotic-resistant *Salmonella* strains in chicken.

PATHOGENESIS AND DISEASE SYNDROMES OF AVIAN COLIBACILLOSIS AND AVIAN SALMONELLOSIS

Pathogenesis and Disease Syndromes of Avian Colibacillosis

The mechanisms by which avian pathogenic *E. coli* cause infection are largely unknown. The virulence factors contributing to the pathogenesis of avian colibacillosis are summarized in Table 3.

Table 3: A list of virulence factors contributing to the pathogenesis of avian colibacillosis

Virulence facors	Reference
F (type 1) and P fimbrial adhesins	[137-140]
Curli	[141,142]
Factors contributing to adhesion, resistance to immunologic defense, survival in physiologic fluids, and cytotoxic effects	[143]
Factors conferring resistance to serum and phagocytosis	[138,140,144,145]
Aerobactin siderophores	[138,146]
*hyl*E, a hemolysin gene	[147]
The *tsh* gene encoding temperature sensitive hemagglutinin	[141,148]
K1 Capsular antigen	[149]
Cytotoxins	[150-152]
Outer membrane proteins	[153]
Coligenicity	[151]
The heat-labile chick lethal toxin (CLT)	[154]
Verotoxin-2 like toxin	[152]

Recently, Hughes *et al.* [155] described a cross-sectional study of wild birds in northern England to determine the prevalence of *E. coli*-containing genes that encoded Shiga toxins (*stx1* and *stx2*) and intimin (*eae*), important virulence determinants of STEC associated with human disease and they stated that while wild birds were unlikely to be direct sources of STEC infections, they did represent a potential reservoir of virulence genes.

APEC are responsible for a considerable number of various diseases at different ages. Neonatal infection of chicks can occur horizontally, from the environment, or vertically, from the hen. A laying hen suffering from*E. coli*-induced oophoritis or salpingitis may infect the internal egg before shell formation. Faecal contamination of the eggshell is possible during the passage of the egg through the cloaca and after laying. The latter possibility is considered as the main route of infection for the egg [22]. Before hatching, APEC causes yolk sac infections and embryo mortality. The chick can also be infected during or shortly after hatching. In these cases, retained infected yolk, omphalitis, septicemia and mortality of the young chicks up to an age of three weeks is seen [22]. Broilers may be affected by necrotic dermatitis, also known as cellulitis, characterized by a chronic inflammation of the subcutis on abdomen and thighs [22].

Swollen head syndrome (SHS), mainly a problem in broilers, causes oedema of the cranial and periorbital skin. SHS can cause a reduction in egg production of 2 to 3%, and a mortality of 3 to 4% [156]. Data on this disease are contradictory. Picault *et al.* [157] and Hafez & Löhren [158] considered SHS as a disease caused by avian pneumovirus (APV), usually followed by an opportunistic *E. coli* infection. Nakamura *et al.* [159] however reported that APEC were probably playing a significant part in the disease, but that the role of APV was not at all clear. This had been confirmed by Georgiades *et al.* [160], who did not detect APV in any of the flocks affected by SHS during a field study, but instead detected infectious bronchitis virus (IBV), avian adenovirus, avian reovirus, and Newcastle disease virus (NDV), as well as *Mycoplasma synoviae* and *M. gallisepticum* (MG).

APEC probably do not cause intestinal diseases. Nevertheless, enterotoxigenic *E. coli* (ETEC) are occasionally isolated from poultry suffering from diarrhoea [161–163] and diarrhoea was experimentally induced after intramuscular inoculation of APEC [164]. On the other hand, enteropathogenic *E. coli* (EPEC) were isolated from clinically healthy chickens [165]. In turkeys, experimentally inoculated EPEC can only cause enteritis in combination with coronavirus [166].

Layers as well as broilers may suffer from acute or chronic salpingitis [167,168]. Salpingitis can be the result of an ascending infection from the cloaca [167,168] or an infection of the left abdominal airsac [22], although Bisgaard and Dam [167] considered the latter possibility less likely than an ascending infection. Salpingitis can lead to the loss of egg-laying capacity [163]. In the case of chronic salpingitis, the oviduct has a yellowish-gray, cheese-like content, with a concentric structure [168]. In layers, salpingitis can cause egg peritonitis if yolk material has been deposited in the peritoneal cavity, characterised by a sero-fibrinous inflammation of the surrounding tissues [22].

Airsacculitis is observed at all ages. The bird is infected by inhalation of dust contaminated with faecal material, which may contain 10^6 CFU of *E. coli* per gram [169]. This aerogenic route of infection is considered as the main origin of systemic colibacillosis or colisepticemia [33,143,170].

Septicemia also affects chickens of all ages, and is mainly described in broilers. It is the most prevalent form of colibacillosis, characterised by polyserositis [143]. It causes depression, fever and often high mortality. Although its pathogenesis has not been elucidated, several routes of infection are possible: neonatal infections [22], infections through skin lesions [171], infection of the reproductive organs [22,167,168], of the respiratory tract [33] and even infection *per os* [172]. When *E. coli* reaches the vascular system, the internal organs and the heart are infected. The infection of the myocard causes heart failure [173]. Septicemia occasionally also leads to synovitis and osteomyelitis [22,174] and on rare occasions to panophthalmia [22]. Coligranuloma or Hjarre's disease is characterised by granulomas in liver, caeca, duodenum and mesenterium, but not in the spleen. It is a rare form of colibacillosis, but in affected flocks it may cause up to 75% mortality [22].

Further studies are needed to determine the role of newly identified putative virulence genes and genes with unknown functions as virulence markers of APEC to strengthen the current understanding of mechanisms underlying the pathogenesis of avian colibacillosis.

Pathogenesis and Disease Syndrome of Avian Salmonellosis

The pathogenicity of *Salmonella* depends on the invasive properties and the ability of the bacteria to survive and multiply within the cells, particularly macrophages [175]. The main site of multiplication of these bacteria is the digestive tract, which may result in widespread contamination of the environment due to bacterial excretion through feces. Following invasion through the intestinal mucosa, cecal tonsils and Peyer's patches, the organisms are engulfed by macrophages, and through the blood stream and/or lymphatic systems, they spread to organs rich in reticuloendothelial tissues (RES), such as liver and spleen, which are the main sites of multiplication [176]. In case of inadequate body defense mechanism, they may lead to second invasion and be localized in other organs, particularly ovary, oviduct, myocardium, pericardium, gizzard, yolk sac and/or lungs [177]. In the bird challenge, *S. typhimurium* rapidly caused inflammation of the intestinal mucosa, but*S. pullorum* preferentially targeted the bursa of Fabricius prior to eliciting intestinal inflammation [178]. Pullorum disease manifests itself predominantly as an enteric disease of chickens, while fowl typhoid shows signs of septicemic disease [78]. Both biovars can cause septicemic infections, which may be acute or chronic, but unlike *S. pullorum*, *S. gallinarum* is capable of producing peracute infection and hemolytic anemia in both young and adults [84]. *S. gallinarum* is extremely pathogenic to young broiler chicks [179].

Fowl typhoid is indistinguishable from pullorum disease unless the etiological agent is isolated and identified [113]. Clinical signs in chicks and poults include anorexia, diarrhea, dehydration, weakness and high mortality [83]. In mature fowls, fowl typhoid and pullorum disease are manifested by anorexia, drop in egg production, increased mortality, reduced fertility and hatchability [83]. *S. pullorum* infected adult birds may or may not exhibit any clinical signs, or they cannot be detected by their physical appearance [78]. Furthermore, the exact mechanisms of getting these poultry diseases are still remained to be obscured.

DIAGNOSIS OF AVIAN COLIBACILLOSIS AND AVIAN SALMONELLOSIS

Colibacillos is suspected based on the clinical features and the typical macroscopic lesions. The diagnosis is obtained by *E. coli* isolation from cardiac blood and affected tissues, like liver, spleen, pericard or bone marrow. Experimentally it was shown that in acute cases, isolation is possible from six hours to three days after infection; in subacute cases, isolation is only possible until seven days after infection [180]. Contamination from the intestines is rarely a problem, if fresh material is used and standard bacteriological procedures are applied [181]. Selective media like McConkey, eosin-methylene blue or drigalki agar are used for isolation. Further identification of the isolated colonies is based on biochemical reactions (indol production, fermentation of glucose with gas production, presence of ß-galactosidase, absence of hydrogen sulphite production and urease, and the inability to use citrate as a carbon source) [29]. O-serotyping is a frequently used typing method. An ELISA, based on sonicated *E. coli*, has been developed for detection of antibodies against two important pathogenic serotypes of *E. coli*: O78:K80 and O2:K1 [182]. Another ELISA was based on fimbrial antigen [183]. Both have limited value because they can only detect homologous APEC types. All currently known virulence-associated factors, detected in strains isolated from colibacillosis lesions, can also be detected in faecal isolates from clinically healthy chickens. For this reason, none of these traits can be used for APEC identification.

Diagnosis of avian salmonellosis should be confirmed by isolation, identification, and serotyping of*Salmonella* strains. Infections in mature birds can be identified by serologic tests, followed by necropsy evaluation complemented by microbiologic culture and typing for confirmation. A serological ELISA test for the diagnosis of avian salmonellosis either with *S. typhimurium* or *S. enteritidis* has been established [184]. Szmolka *et al.* [185] established a diagnostic and a real-time PCR system for rapid and reliable genus- and serovar- (*S. enteritidis* and *S. typhimurium*) specific detection of *Salmonella* for monitoring purposes in the poultry food chain.

PREVENTIVE MEASURES FOR CONTROLLING AVIAN COLIBACILLOSIS AND AVIAN SALMONELLOSIS

Avian Colibacillosis

A first step is the prevention of egg contamination by fumigating them within two hours after lay, and by removing cracked eggs or eggs soiled with faecal material. It is recommended to vent the incubators and hatchers to the outside and to have as few breeder flocks as possible per breeding unit [22]. In chicks, contamination with APEC from the environment must be controlled by reduction and control of intestinal infection. This can be achieved using competitive exclusion (CE) [186–190], *i.e.*, inoculating day-old chicks with normal bacterial flora of healthy adult chickens or a monoculture, for instance of *Bacillus subtilis*. Birds also need to be protected against pathogens that promote infections with APEC. This is possible by using*Mycoplasma*-free birds [22] and protecting the birds against mycoplasmas and viral diseases by vaccinations [170]. Disease introduction must also be avoided [170] by a suitable house infrastructure, the correct use of a transition zone (for changing clothes and shoes, and washing hands), and pest control: rodent faeces are a source of pathogenic *E. coli* [22]. The housing climate must be kept optimal for bird density, humidity, ventilation, dust and ammonia [29,170].

The great diversity among APEC strains limits the possibilities of vaccination, and vaccines are not used on a large scale. Several vaccines based on killed or attenuated strains have been tested experimentally. In general, they give sufficient protection against infection with homologous strains, but protection against heterologous strains is less efficient [29]. However, Melamed *et al.* [191] reported a certain degree of heterologous protection obtained with an inactivated vaccine. Passive immunisation of young birds via the breeder hens is efficient for two weeks [192], if the birds are challenged with homologous strains. Vaccines based on virulence factors like fimbriae, also give a good homologous protection, *i.e.*, against APEC possessing the same fimbriae [193].

Avian Salmonellosis

Although fowl typhoid and pullorum disease are widely distributed in most parts of the world, the diseases have been eradicated from commercial poultry in developed countries such as the United States of America, Canada and most countries of Western Europe [78]. Successful control programs can be achieved by developing good hygiene and management together with routine serological tests and slaughter policy [177]. The principal management procedures should include chicks free from infections, and the chicks should be placed in a cleaned, sanitized and *S. gallinarum* and *S. pullorum* free environment with strict biosecurity measures [194]. The feed and water should be free from *Salmonella* contamination. The dead birds need to be well disposed. Adequate precautions are needed to prevent infections from mechanical carriers like footwear, human clothing, hatchery disciplines, equipments, litters, crates, trucks and processing plants [195]. Wray *et al.* [196] described that the birds need to be tested at the age of 16 weeks due to immunologic maturity, at the point of lay due to stress and two consecutive times one month apart to provide the acceptable evidence that the flock is free from fowl typhoid [177]. Kabir *et al.* [189] and Kabir [190] demonstrated the potential role of probiotics for the controlling of *Salmonella* strains of poultry via the mechanisms of competitive exclusion. Vaccines may be used to control the disease, and antibiotics can be used for the treatment of fowl typhoid and pullorum disease.

PUBLIC HEALTH CONCERNS OF AVIAN COLIBACILLOSIS AND AVIAN SALMONELLOSIS

E. coli of the O2:K1 serotype isolated from human urinary tract infections and from septicemic chickens are phenotypically highly related. A distinction between both groups was only possible by examining their plasmid contents [43]. Cherifi *et al.* [44] obtained similar results for a group of O78 isolates and concluded that chickens might be a source of septicemic human O78 infections. However, contrasting results were obtained in a study by Caya *et al.* [197]. In this study, avian *E. coli* isolates from healthy and diseased birds (airsacculitis and cellulitis) and *E. coli* strains isolated from sick humans during the same period and in the same geographical area as the avian isolates were compared. The study results suggested that these avian isolates possessed very few of the attributes required to cause disease in humans. Reversely, human isolates can be pathogenic to day-old chicks after subcutaneous inoculation. Strains tested were of the serotypes O1, O2, O18 and O78 [198]. Although O157 verotoxigenic *E. coli* (VTEC) had been detected in broilers [158], the chicken was not considered as an important reservoir for this zoonotically often reported serotype. Experimental studies showed that chickens might be functioned as a reservoir: O157 strains easily infected the young birds, even at a low dose, and persisted in the caecum for up to three months [199]. The study by Stavric *et al.* [200] showed that layers were also susceptible to colonisation by O157:H7 and other VTEC after inoculation *per os*. The intestines were increasingly colonised if increasing inoculation doses were used. The older the bird, the more restricted the colonisation and persistence were. All birds involved in the experiment remained clinically healthy. Histologically, attachment and effacement lesions were detected in the proximal caeca. Chapman *et al.* [199] reported that at that time no bacteriologically confirmed human cases of O157 infections had been observed, caused by poultry. Nonetheless, chicken meat was sometimes positive for VTEC [201,202]. In addition, Manges *et al.* [203] conducted a case-control study between April 2003 and June 2004 and they demonstrated that antimicrobial resistant, urinary tract infection (UTI) causing*E. coli* could have a food reservoir, possibly in poultry or pork. Uncontrolled, avian *E. coli* represents a serious animal welfare concern and risk to public health as it is a zoonotic organism with avian *E. coli* species known to adapt to humans.

Salmonellosis is of public health concern because most of the strains of *Salmonella* are potentially pathogenic to humans and animals. Avian salmonellosis can pose a health risk to people if exposed. Symptoms appear similar to food poisoning, such as diarrhea and acute gastroenteritis. However, it appears that birds mainly acquire the disease from the environment and that infected birds play a relatively small role in the transmission of disease to domestic animals and humans. Public health concerns and the potential for foodborne zoonotic transmission have made *Salmonella* the subject of numerous international, national, and local surveillance programs [204].

STRATEGIES FOR REDUCING PUBLIC HEALTH HAZARDS

The risk of colibacillosis can be reduced through simple precautions.

- By thorough cleaning of poultry houses.
- By ensuring proper ventilation of the poultry houses and chlorination of drinking water.
- By washing hands carefully before and after food preparation and after toileting.
- By avoiding eating raw or undercooked poultry.
- By wrapping fresh meats in plastic bags at the market to prevent fluids from dripping on other foods.
- By ensuring the correct internal cooking temperature especially when using a microwave.

The risk of salmonellosis can be also reduced through simple precautions.

- By washing hands carefully before and after food preparation and after toileting or changing diapers.
- By avoiding eating raw or undercooked eggs (or foods made with raw eggs) and poultry.
- By wrapping fresh meats in plastic bags at the market to prevent fluids from dripping on other foods.
- By ensuring the correct internal cooking temperature especially when using a microwave.
- By avoiding chicks and ducklings as pets for small children.

CONCLUSIONS

Avian colibacillosis and salmonellosis are considered to be the major bacterial disease problems in the poultry industry world-wide and these diseases constitute a major public health burden and represent a significant cost in many countries. The economic and public health burden of these diseases have made this topic time demanding. It is suggested from this review article that more effective application of existing control methods would greatly reduce the hazards to public health.

ACKNOWLEDGMENTS

I would like to thank all the reviewers for their constructive suggestions and comments.

REFERENCES

1. Calnek BW, Barnes HJ, Beard CW, McDougald LR, Saif YM. Diseases of Poultry. 10th ed. Iowa State University Press; Ames, IA, USA: 1997.
2. Haider MG, Hossain MG, Hossain MS, Chowdhury EH, Das PM, Hossain MM. Isolation and characterization of enterobacteria associated with health and disease in sonali chickens. Bangl. J. Vet. Med.2004;2:15–21.
3. Hofstad MS, John BH, Calnek BW, Reid WN, Yoder HW., Jr . Diseases of Poultry. 8th ed. Panima Education Book Agency; New Delhi, India: 1992. pp. 65–123.
4. Otaki Y. Poultry disease control programme in Japan. Asian Livestock. 1995;20:65–67.
5. Wray C, Davies RH. Enterobacteriacae. In: Jordan F, Pattison M, Alexander D, Faragher T, editors.Poultry Diseases. 5th ed. W. B. Saunders; Philadelphia, PA, USA: 2001. pp. 95–130.
6. Wigley P, Berchieri A, Jr, Page KL, Smith AL, Barrow PA. *Salmonella enterica* serovar Pullorum persists in splenic macrophages and in the reproductive tract during persistent, disease free carriage in chickens.Infect. Immun. 2001;69:7873–7879.
7. Berchieri A, Jr, Murphy CK, Marston K, Barrow PA. Observations on the persistence and vertical transmission of *Salmonella enterica* serovars Pullorum and Gallinarum in chickens: Effect of bacterial and host genetic background. Avian Pathol. 2001;30:221–231.
8. Caudry SD, Stanisich VA. Incidence of antibiotic resistant *Escherichia coli* associated with frozen chicken carcasses and characterization of conjugative R-plasmids derived from such strains. Antimicrob. Agents Chemother. 1979;16:701–709.
9. Nazer AH. Transmissible drug resistance in *Escherichia coli* isolated from poultry and their carcasses in Iran. Cornell. Vet. 1980;70:365–371.
10. Bensink JC, Botham FP. Antibiotic resistant coliform bacilli, isolated from freshly slaughtered poultry and from chilled poultry at retail outlets. Aust. Vet. J. 1983;60:80–83.
11. Linton AH, Howe K, Hartley CL, Clements HM, Richmond MH, Osborne AD. Antibiotic resistance among *Escherichia coli* O-serotypes from the gut and carcasses of commercially slaughtered broiler chickens: a potential public health hazard. J. Appl. Bacteriol. 1977;42:365–378.
12. Chaslus Dancla E, Lafont JP. IncH plasmids in *Escherichia coli* strains isolated from broiler chicken carcasses. Appl. Environ. Microbiol. 1985;49:1016–1018.
13. Jayaratne A, Collins-Thompson DL, Trevors JT. Occurrence of aminoglycoside phosphotransferase subclassIandIIstructuralgenesamongEnterobacteriaceae spp. isolated from meat samples. Appl. Microbiol. Biotechnol. 1990;33:547–552.
14. Turtura GC, Massa S, Chazvinizadeh H. Antibiotic resistance among coliform bacteria isolated from carcasses of commercially slaughtered chickens. Int. J. Food Microbiol. 1990;11:351–354.
15. Lakhotia RL, Stephens JF. Drug resistance and R factors among enterobacteria isolated from eggs. Poult. Sci. 1973;52:1955–1962.
16. van den Bogaard E, London N, Driessen C, Stobberingh EE. Antibiotic resistance of faecal *Escherichia coli* in poultry, poultry farmers and poultry slaughterers. J. Antimicrob. Chemother. 2001;47:763–771.
17. Cruchaga S, Echeita A, Aladueña A, García-Peña J, Frias N, Usera MA. Antimicrobial resistance in salmonellae from humans, food and animals in Spain in 1998. J. Antimicrob. Chemother. 2001;47:315–321.
18. van Looveren M, Chasseur-Libotte ML, Godard C, Lammens C, Wijdooghe M, Peeters L, Goossens H. Antimicrobial susceptibility of nontyphoidal *Salmonella* isolated from humans in Belgium. Acta Clin. Belg.2001;56:180–186.
19. Wybot I, Wildemauwe C, Godard C, Bertrand S, Collard JM. Antimicrobial drug resistance in nontyphoid human *Salmonella* in Belgium: Trends for the period 2000–2002. Acta Clin. Belg. 2004;59:152–160.
20. Mulder RW. Hygiene during transport, slaughter and processing. In: Richardson RI, Mead GC, editors.Poultry Meat Science Poultry Science Symposium Series. CABI Publishing; Oxford shire, UK: 1999. pp. 277–285.
21. Yashoda KP, Sachindra NM, Sakhare PZ, Rao DN. Microbiological quality of broiler chicken carcasses processed hygienically in a small scale poultry processing unit. J. Food Qual. 2001;24:249–259.
22. Barnes HJ, Gross WB. Colibacillosis. In: Calnek BW, Barnes HJ, Beard CW, McDougald LR, Saif YM, editors. Diseases of Poultry. 10th ed. Iowa State University Press; Ames, IA, USA: 1997. pp. 131–141.
23. La Ragione RM, Woodward MJ. Virulence factors of *Escherichia coli* serotypes associated with avian colisepticemia. Res. Vet. Sci. 2002;73:27–35.
24. Gross WB. Diseases due to *Escherichia coli* in poultry. In: Gyles CL, editor. Escherichia coli in Domestic Animals and Humans. CAB International Library; Wallingford, UK: 1994. pp. 237–260.
25. Chart H, Smith HR, La Ragione RM, Woodward MJ. An investigation into the pathogenic properties of*Escherichia coli* strains BLR, BL21, DH5α, and EQ1. J. Appl. Microbiol. 2000;89:1048–1058.
26. Rahman MA, Samad MA, Rahman MB, Kabir SML. Bacterio-pathological studies on salmonellosis, colibacillosis and pasteurellosis in natural and experimental infections in chickens. Bangl. J. Vet. Med.2004;2:1–8.
27. Harry EG, Hemsley LA. The relationship between

environmental contamination with septicemia strains of *Escherichia coli*. Vet. Rec. 1965;77:241–245.

28. Harry EG, Hemsley LA. The association between the presence of septicemia strains of *Escherichia coli*in the respiratory and intestinal tracts of chickens and the occurrence of coli septicemia. Vet. Rec.1965;77:35–40.
29. Dho-Moulin M, Fairbrother JM. Avian pathogenic *Escherichia coli* (APEC) Vet. Res. 1999;30:299–316.
30. Gross WB, Siegel PB, Hall RW, Domermuth CH, DuBoise RT. Production and persistence of antibodies in chickens to sheep erythrocytes. 2. Resistance to infectious diseases. Poult. Sci. 1980;59:205–210.
31. Rosenberger JK, Fries PA, Cloud SS, Wilson RA. *In vitro* and *in vivo* characterization of avian*Escherichia coli*. II. Factors associated with pathogenicity. Avian Dis. 1985;29:1094–1107.
32. Gross WB. Effect of short-term exposure of chickens to corticosterone on resistance to challenge exposure with *Escherichia coli* and antibody response to sheep erythrocytes. Am. J. Vet. Res. 1992;53:291–293.
33. Pourbakhsh SA, Boulianne M, Martineau-Doizé B, Dozois CM, Desautels C, Fairbrother JM. Dynamics of*Escherichia coli* infection in experimentally inoculated chickens. Avian Dis. 1997;41:221–233.
34. McGruder ED, Moore GM. Use of lipopolysaccharide (LPS) as a positive control for the evaluation of immunopotentiating drug candidates in experimental avian colibacillosis models. Res. Vet. Sci. 1998;66:33–37.
35. da Silveiraa WD, Ferreiraa A, Lancellottia M, Barbosaa AGCD, I, Leitea DS, de Castrob AFP, Brocchi M. Clonal relationships among avian *Escherichia coli* isolates determined by enterobacterial repetitive intergenic consensus (ERIC)–PCR. Vet. Microbiol. 2002;89:323–328.
36. Gilson E, Clément JM, Brutlag D, Hofnung M. A family of dispersed repetitive extragenic palindromic DNA sequences in *Escherichia coli*. EMBO J. 1984;3:1417–1421.
37. Hulton CS, Higgins CF, Sharp PM. ERIC sequences: A novel family of repetitive elements in the genomes of *Escherichia coli*, *Salmonella typhimuirum* and other enterobacteria. Mol. Microbiol.1991;5:825–834.
38. Welsh J, McClelland M. Fingerprinting genomes using PCR with arbitrary primers. Nucleic Acids Res.1990;18:7213–7218.
39. Chansiripornchai N, Ramasoota P, Sasipreyajan J, Svenson SB. Differentiation of avian *Escherichia coli*(APEC) isolates by random amplified polymorphic DNA (RAPD) analysis. Vet. Microbiol. 2001;80:77–83.
40. de Moura AC, Irino K, Vidotto MC. Genetic variability of avian *Escherichia coli* isolates evaluated by enterobacterial reptitive intergenic consensus and repetitive extragenic palindromic polymerase chain reation.Avian Dis. 2001;45:173–181.
41. Silveira WD, Lancellotti M, Ferreira A, Solferini VN, de Castro AFP, Stehling EG, Brocchi M. Determination of the clonal structure of avian *Escherichia coli* strains by isoenzyme and ribotyping analysis.J. Vet. Med. B Infect. Dis. Vet. Public Hlth. 2003;50:63–69.
42. White DG, Dho-moulin M, Wilson RA, Whittam TS. Clonal relationships and variation in virulence among *Escherichia coli* strains of avian origin. Microb. Pathog. 1993;14:399–409.
43. Achtman M, Heuzenroeder M, Kusecek B, Ochman H, Caugant D, Selander RK, Vaïsanen-Rhen V, Korhonen TK, Stuart S, Orskov F, Orskov I. Clonal analysis of *Escherichia coli* O2: K1 isolated from diseased humans and animals. Infect. Immun. 1986;51:268–276.
44. Cherifi A, Contrepois M, Picard B, Goullet P, Orskov I, Orskov F. Clonal relationships among*Escherichia coli* serogroup O78 isolates from human and animal infections. J. Clin. Microbiol.1994;32:1197–1202.
45. Blanco JE, Blanco M, Mora A, Blanco J. Production of toxins (enterotoxins, verotoxins, and necrotoxins) and colicins by *Escherichia coli* strains isolated from septicemic and healthy chickens: relationship with *in vivo* pathogenicity. J. Clin. Microbiol. 1997a;35:2953–2957.
46. de Moura AC, Irino K, Vidotto MC. Genetic variability of avian *Escherichia coli* strains evaluated by enterobacterial repetitive intergenic consensus and repetitive extragenic palindromic polymerase chain reaction. Avian Dis. 2001;45:173–181.
47. Ewers C, Janßen T, Kießling S, Philipp HC, Wieler LH. Molecular epidemiology of avian pathogenic*Escherichia coli* (APEC) isolated from colisepticemia in poultry. Vet. Microbiol. 2004;104:91–101.
48. Blanco JE, Blanco M, Mora A, Jansen WH, Garcia V, Vazquez ML, Blanco J. Serotypes of *Escherichia coli* isolated from septicemic chickens in Galicia (Northwest Spain) Vet. Microbiol. 1998;61:229–235.
49. Rodriguez-Siek KE, Giddings CW, Doetkott C, Johnson TJ, Fakhr MK, Lisa KN. Comparison of*Escherichia coli* isolates implicated in human urinary tract infection and avian colibacillosis. Microbiolo gy.2005;151:2097–2110.
50. Gilson L, Mahanty HK, Kolter R. Four plasmid genes are required for colicin V synthesis, export, and immunity. J. Bacteriol. 1987;169:2466–2470.
51. Russo TA, Carlino UB, Mong A, Jodush ST. Identification of genes in an extraintestinal isolate of*Escherichia coli* with increased expression after exposure to human urine. Infect. Immun. 1999;67:5306–5314.
52. Binns MM, Davies DL, Hardy KG. Cloned fragments of the plasmid ColV, I-K94 specifying virulence and serum resistance. Nature. 1979;279:778–781.
53. Chuba PJ, Leon MA, Banerjee A, Palchaudhuri S. Cloning and DNA sequence of plasmid determinant*iss*, coding for increased serum survival and surface exclusion, which has homology with lambda DNA. Mol. Gen. Genet. 1989;216:287–292.
54. de Lorenzo V, Neilands JB. Characterization of *iucA* and *iucC* genes of the aerobactin system of plasmid ColV-K30 in *Escherichia coli*. J. Bacteriol. 1986;167:350–355.

55. de Lorenzo V, Bindereif A, Paw BH, Neilands JB. Aerobactin biosynthesis and transport genes of plasmid ColV-K30 in *Escherichia coli* K-12. J. Bacteriol. 1986;165:570–578.

56. Runyen-Janecky LJ, Reeves SA, Gonzales EG, Payne SM. Contribution of the *Shigella flexneri* Sit, Iuc, and Feo iron acquisition systems to iron acquisition *in vitro* and in cultured cells. Infect. Immun.2003;71:1919–1928.

57. Achtman M, Kennedy N, Skurray R. Cell–cell interactions in conjugating *Escherichia coli*: Role of TraT protein in surface exclusion. Proc. Natl. Acad. Sci. USA. 1977;74:5104–5108.

58. Moll A, Manning PA, Timmis KN. Plasmid determined resistance to serum bactericidal activity: A major outer membrane protein, the *traT* gene product, is responsible for plasmid-specified serum resistance in*Escherichia coli*. Infect. Immun. 1980;28:359–367.

59. Provence DL, Curtiss R., III Isolation and characterization of a gene involved in hemagglutination by an avian pathogenic *Escherichia coli* strain. Infect. Immun. 1994;62:1369–1380.

60. Russo TA, Carlino UB, Johnson JR. Identification of a new iron-regulated virulence gene, *ireA*, in an extraintestinal pathogenic isolate of *Escherichia coli*. Infect. Immun. 2001;69:6209–6216.

61. Schubert S, Rakin A, Karch H, Carniel E, Heesemann J. Prevalence of the "high-pathogenicity island" of *Yersinia* species among *Escherichia coli* strains that are pathogenic to humans. Infect. Immun.1998;66:480–485.

62. Hacker J, Goebel W, Hof H, Konig W, Konig B, Scheffer J, Hughes C, Marre R. Adhesins, serum resistance and cytolysins of *E coli*-genetic structure and role in pathogenicity. In: Cabello FC, Pruzzo C, editors. Bacteria, Complement and the Phagocytic Cell. Springer-Verlag; New York, NY, USA: 1988. pp. 221–229.

63. Fields PI, Blom K, Hughes HJ, Helsel LO, Feng P, Swaminathan B. Molecular characterization of the gene encoding H antigen in *Escherichia coli* and development of a PCR restriction fragment length polymorphism test for identification of *E. coli* O157:H7 and O157:NM. J. Clin. Microbiol. 1997;35:1066–1070.

64. Johnson JR, Delavari P, Kuskowski M, Stell AL. Phylogenetic distribution of extraintestinal virulence-associated traits in *Escherichia coli*. J. Infect. Dis. 2001;183:78–88.

65. Johnson JR, Stell AL. Extended virulence genotypes of *Escherichia coli* strains from patients with urosepsis in relation to phylogeny and host compromise. J. Infect. Dis. 2000;181:261–272.

66. Rahman MA, Samad MA, Rahman MB, Kabir SML. *In vitro* antibiotic sensitivity and therapeutic efficacy of experimental salmonellosis, colibacillosis and pasteurellosis in broiler chickens. Bangl. J. Vet. Med. 2004;2:99–102.

67. Cloud SS, Rosenberger JK, Fries PA, Wilson RA, Odor EM. *In vitro* and *in vivo* characterization of avian *Escherichia coli*. I. Serotypes, metabolic activity, and antibiotic sensitivity. Avian Dis. 1985;29:1084–1093.

68. Irwin RJ, McEwen SA, Clarke RC, Meek AH. The prevalence of verocytotoxin-producing *Escherichia coli* and antimicrobial resistance patterns of nonverocytotoxin-producing *Escherichia coli* and *Salmonella* in Ontario broiler chickens. Can. J. Vet. Res. 1989;53:411–418.

69. Blanco JE, Blanco M, Mora A, Blanco J. Prevalence of bacterial resistance to quinolones and other antimicrobials among avian *Escherichia coli* strains isolated from septicemic and healthy chickens in Spain.J. Clin. Microbiol. 1997;35:2184–2185.

70. Bass L, Liebert CA, Lee MD, Summers AO, White DG, Thayer SG, Maurer JJ. Incidence and characterization of integrons, genetic elements mediating multiple-drug resistance, in avian *Escherichia coli*.Antimicrob. Agents Chemother. 1999;43:2925–2929.

71. Li XS, Wang GQ, Du XD, Cui BA, Zhang SM, Shen JZ. Antimicrobial susceptibility and molecular detection of chloramphenicol and florfenicol resistance among *Escherichia coli* isolates from diseased chickens. J. Vet. Sci. 2007;8:243–247.

72. Dubel JR, Zink DL, Kelley LM, Naqi SA, Renshaw HW. Bacterial antibiotic resistance: frequency of gentamicin-resistant strains of *Escherichia coli* in the fecal microflora of commercial turkeys. Am. J. Vet. Res. 1982;43:1786–1789.

73. Allan BJ, van den Hurk JV, Potter AA. Characterization of *Escherichia coli* isolated from cases of avian colibacillosis. Can. J. Vet. Res. 1993;57:146–151.

74. White DG, Piddock LJ, Maurer JJ, Zhao S, Ricci V, Thayer SG. Characterization of fluoroquinolone resistance among veterinary isolates of avian *Escherichia coli*. Antimicrob. Agents Chemother.2000;44:2897–2899.

75. van den Bogaard AE, London N, Driessen C, Stobberingh EE. Antibiotic resistance of faecal*Escherichia coli* in poultry, poultry farmers and poultry slaughterers. J. Antimicrob. Chemother.2001;47:763–771.

76. Zhao S, White DG, McDermott PF, Friedman S, English L, Ayers S, Meng J, Maurer JJ, Holland R, Walker RD. Identification and expression of cephamycinase bla*cmy* genes in *Escherichia coli* and*Salmonella* isolated from food animals and ground meats. Antimicrob. Agents Chemother. 2001;45:3647–3650.

77. Wooley RE, Spears KR, Brown J, Nolan LK, Dekich MA. Characteristics of conjugative R plasmids from pathogenic avian *Escherichia coli*. Avian Dis. 1992;36:348–352.

78. Shivaprashad HL. Pullorum disease and fowl typhoid. In: Calnek BW, Barnes HJ, Beard CW, McDoughald LR, Saif YM, editors. Diseases of Poultry. 10th ed. Iowa State University press; Ames, IA, USA: 1997. pp. 82–96.

79. Minor L. In: Bergey's Manual of Systemic Bacteriology. Boone R, Castenholz W, editors. Williams & Wilkins; Philadelphia, PA, USA: 1984. pp. 427–458.

80. Gast RK. Paratyphoid Infections. In: Calnek BW, Barnes HJ, Beard CW, McDoughald LR, Saif YM,

editors. Diseases of Poultry. 10th ed. Iowa State University press; Ames, IA, USA: 1997. pp. 97–121.

81. Brito JR, Xu Y, Hinton M, Pearson GR. Pathological findings in the intestinal tract and liver of chicks after exposure to *Salmonella* serotypes Typhimurium or Kedougou. Br. Vet. J. 1995;151:311–323.

82. Berchieri A, Jr, Murphy CK, Marston K, Barrow PA. Observation on the persistence and vertical transmission *Salmonella enterica* serovars pullorum and gallinarum in chickens: Effect of bacterial and host genetic background. Avian Pathol. 2001;30:221–231.

83. Shivaprasad HL. Fowl typhoid and pullorum disease. Rev. Sci. Tech. 2000;19:405–424.

84. Christensen JP. Phenotypic and genotypic characterization of *Salmonella enterica* serovar Gallinarum biovars gallinarum and pullorum in relation to typing and virulencePh.D. Thesis, Department of Veterinary Microbiology, The Royal Veterinary and Agricultural University; Copenhagen, Denmark: 1996

85. Hall WJ, Legenhausen DH, Macdonald AD. Studies on fowl typhoid. 1. Nature and dissemination.Poult. Sci. 1949;28:344–362.

86. Waltman WD, Gast RK, Mallinson ET. Isolation and Identification of Avian Pathogens. 5th ed. American Association of Avian Pathologists; Jacksonville, FL, USA: 2008. Salmonellosis; pp. 3–9.

87. Henken AM, Frankena K, Goelema JO, Graat EAM, Noordhuizen JPTM. Multivariate epidemiological approach to salmonellosis in broiler breeder flocks. Poult. Sci. 1992;71:838–843.

88. Fris C, van den Bos J. A retrospective case-control study of risk factors associated with *Salmonella enterica* subsp. *enterica* serovar Enteritidis infections on Dutch broiler breeder farms. Avian Pathol.1995;24:255–272.

89. Oystein A, Skov MN, Chriel M, Agger JF, Bisgaard M. A retrospective study on *Salmonella* infection in Danish broiler flocks. Prev. Vet. Med. 1996;26:223–237.

90. Lahellec C, Colin P, Bennejean G, Paquin J, Guillerm A, Debois JC. Influence of resident *Salmonella* on contamination of broiler flocks. Poult. Sci. 1986;65:2034–2039.

91. Baggesen DL, Olsen JE, Bisgaard M. Plasmid profiles and phages types of *Salmonella typhimurium*isolated from successive flocks of chickens on three parent stock farms. Avian Pathol. 1992;21:569–579.

92. Vaughn JB, Williams LP, LeBlanc DR, Helsdon HL, Taylor C. *Salmonella* in a modern broiler operation: a longitudinal study. Am. J. Vet. Res. 1974;35:737–741.

93. Christensen JP, Brown DJ, Madsen M, Olsen JE, Bisgaard M. Hatchery-borne *Salmonella enterica*serovar Tennessee infections in broilers. Avian Pathol. 1997;26:155–168.

94. Davies RH, Nicholas RAJ, Mclaren IM, Corkish JD, Lanning DG, Wray C. Bacteriological and serological investigation of persistent *Salmonella enteritidis* infection in an integrated poultry organisation. Vet. Microbiol. 1997;58:277–293.

95. Martinetti G, Altwegg M. rRNA gene restriction patterns and plasmid analysis as a tool for typing*Salmonella enteritidis*. Res. Microbiol. 1990;141:1151–1162.

96. Stubbs AD, Hickman-Brenner FW, Cameron DN, Farmer JJ., III Differentiation of *Salmonella enteritidis*phage type 8 strains: evaluation of three additional phage typing systems, plasmid profiles, antibiotic susceptibility patterns, and biotyping. J. Clin. Microbiol. 1994;32:199–201.

97. Altwegg M, Hinckman-Brenner FW, Farmer JJ., III Ribosomal RNA gene patterns provide increased sensitivity for typing *Salmonella typhi* strains. J. Infect. Dis. 1989;160:145–149.

98. Esteban E, Snipes K, Hiird D, Kasten R, Kinde H. Use of ribotyping for characterization of *Salmonella*serotypes. J. Clin. Microbiol. 1993;31:233–237.

99. Nastasi A, Mammina C, Villafrate MR. rDNA fingerprinting as a tool in epidemiological analysis of*Salmonella typhi* infections. Epidemiol. Infect. 1991;107:565–576.

100. Usera MA, Popovic T, Bopp CA, Stockbine NA. Molecular subtyping of *Salmonella enteritidis* phage type 8 strain from the United States. J. Clin. Microbiol. 1994;32:194–198.

101. Olsen JE, Skov MN, Threlfall EJ, Brown DJ. Clonal lines of *Salmonella enteritica* serotype enteritidis documented by IS200-, ribo-, pulsed-field gel electrophoresis and RFLP typing. J. Med. Microbiol.1994;40:15–22.

102. Thong KL, Cheong YM, Puthucheary S, Koh CL, Pang T. Epidemiological analysis of sporadic*Salmonella typhi* isolates and those from outbreaks by pulsed-field gel electrophoresis. J. Clin. Microbiol.1994;32:1135–1141.

103. Lapuz R, Tani H, Sasai K, Shirota K, Katoh H, Baba E. The role of roof rats (*Rattus rattus*) in the spread of *Salmonella enteritidis* and *S. infantis* contamination in layer farms in eastern Japan. Epidemiol Infect. 2008;136:1235–1243.

104. Barrow PA, Berchieri A, Jr, Al-Haddad O. Serological response of chickens to infection with*Salmonella gallinarum–Salmonella pullorum* detected by enzyme linked immunosorbent assay. Avian Dis.1992;36:227–236.

105. Bouzoubaa K, Lemainguer K, Bell JG. Village chickens as a reservoir of *Salmonella pullorum* and*Salmonella gallinarum* in Morocco. Prev. Vet. Med. 1992;12:95–100.

106. Bhattacharjee PS, Kundu RL, Mazumder JU, Hossain E, Miah AH. A retrospective analysis of chicken diseases diagnosed at the Central Disease Investigation Laboratory, Dhaka, Bangladesh. Bangladesh Vet. Jr.1996;30:105–113.

107. Begum F, Khan MSR, Choudhury KA, Rahman MM, Amin MM. Studies on immune response of chickens to fowl typhoid vaccines. Bangladesh J. Microbiol. 1993;10:51–56.

108. Ghosh SS. Incidence of pullorum disease in Nagaland. Indian Vet. J. 1988;65:949–951.

109. Kumur A, Kaushik RK. Investigation of fowl typhoid in Haryana State. Indian J. Poult. Sci.1988;23:104–106.

110. Javed T, Hameed A. Prevalence of *Salmonella* carriers among broiler breeders in Pakistan. Veterinarski Arhiv. 1989;59:185–191.

111. Muneer MA, Arshad M, Sheikh MA, Ahmad MD. Identification of pullorum disease carriers using spot agglutination test. Pakistan Vet. J. 1988;8:93–94.

112. Jha VC, Thakur RP, Chand-Thakuri K, Yadav JN. Prevalence of salmonellosis in chickens in the eastern Nepal. Veterinary Review Kathmandu. 1994;9:4–6.

113. Fricker CR. Isolation of *Salmonella* and *Campylobacter*. J. Appl. Bacteriol. 1987;63:99–116.

114. Okolo MI. Bacterial drug resistance in meat animals: A review. Int. J. Zoonoses. 1986;13:143–152.

115. Vidon DJ, Jacob S, Ganzenmuller M. Incidences of simple and transferable drug resistance in*Escherichia coli* and *Salmonella* isolated from various foods: Identification of a R plasmid in *S. Saint-Paul.*Ann. Microbiol. 1978;129:155–159.

116. O'Brien TF, Hopkins JD, Gilleece ES, Mederios AA, Kent RL, lackburn BO, Holmes MB, Reardon JP, Vergeront JM, Schell WL, Christenson E, Bissett ML, Morse EV. Molecular epidemiology of antibiotic resistance in *Salmonella* from animals and human beings in the United States. N. Engl. J. Med. 1982;307:1–6.

117. Holmberg SD, Osterholm MT, Senger KA, Cohen ML. Drug-resistant *Salmonella* from animals fed antimicrobials. N. Engl. J. Med. 1984;311:617–622.

118. Poppe C, Gyles CL. Relation of plasmids to virulence and other properties of salmonellae from avian sources. Avian Dis. 1987;31:844–854.

119. Schuman JD, Zottola EA, Harlander SK. Preliminary characterization of a food-borne multiple antibiotic resistant *Salmonella typhimurium* strain. Appl. Environ. Microbiol. 1989;55:2344–2348.

120. Salyers AA, Whitt DD. Bacterial Pathogenesis: A Molecular Approach. ASM Press; Washington, DC, USA: 1994. Antibiotics: mechanisms of action and mechanisms of bacterial resistance; pp. 97–110.

121. Poppe C, McFadden KA, Demczuk WH. Drug resistance, plasmids, biotypes and susceptibility to bacteriophages of *Salmonella* isolated from poultry in Canada. Int. J. Food Microbiol. 1996;30:325–344.

122. Wagner J, Hahn H. Increase of bacterial resistance in human medicine by resistance genes of bacteria from meat supplying animals. Berl. Munch. Tierarztl. Wochenschr. 1999;112:380–384.

123. Holmberg SD, Osterholm MT, Senger KA, Cohen ML. Drug-resistant *Salmonella* from animals fed antimicrobials. N. Eng. J. Med. 1984;311:617–622.

124. Gast RK, Stephens JF. Effects of kanamycin administration to poultry on the proliferation of drug-resistant *Salmonella*. Poult. Sci. 1988;67:689–698.

125. Gast RK, Stephens JF, Foster DN. Effects of kanamycin administration to poultry on the interspecies transmission of drug-resistant *Salmonella*. Poult. Sci. 1988;67:699–706.

126. Dubel JR, Zink DL, Kelley LM, Naqi SA, Renshaw HW. Bacterial antibiotic resistance: frequency of gentamicin-resistant strains of *Escherichia coli* in the faecal microflora of commercial turkeys. Am. J. Vet. Res. 1982;43:1786–1789.

127. Hirsh DC, Ikeda JS, Martin LD, Kelley BJ, Ghazikhanian GY. R plasmid-mediated gentamicin resistance in salmonellae isolated from turkeys and their environment. Avian Dis. 1983;27:766–772.

128. Ekperigin HE, Jang S, McCapes RH. Effective control of a gentamicin resistant *Salmonella arizonae*infection in turkey poults. Avian Dis. 1983;27:822–829.

129. Pacer RE, Spika JS, Thurmond MC, Hargrett-Bean N, Potter ME. Prevalence of *Salmonella* and multiple antimicrobial-resistant *Salmonella* in California dairies. J. Am. Vet. Med. Assoc. 1989;195:59–63.

130. Poppe C, Kolar JJ, Demczuk WHB, Harris JE. Drug resistance and biochemical characteristics of*Salmonella* from Turkeys. Can. J. Vet. Res. 1995;59:241–248.

131. Oliveira WF, Cardoso WM, Salles RPR, Romão JM, Teixeira RSC, Câmara SR, Siqueira AA, Marques LCL. Initial identification and sensitivity to antimicrobial agents of *Salmonella* sp. isolated from poultry products in the state of Ceara, Brazil. Rev. Bras. Cienc. Avic. 2006;8:193–199.

132. Berrang ME, Ladely SR, Simmons M, Fletcher DL, Fedorka-Cray PJ. Antimicrobial resistance patterns of *Salmonella* from retail chicken. Int. J. Poult. Sci. 2006;5:351–354.

133. Parveen S, Taabodi M, Schwarz JG, Oscar TP, Harter-Dennis J, White DG. Prevalence and antimicrobial resistance of *Salmonella* recovered from processed poultry. J. Food Prot. 2007;70:2466–2472.

134. Sharma M, Katock RC. Deadly outbreak in chicks owing to *Salmonella typhimurium*. Indian J. Poult. Sci. 1996;31:60–62.

135. Herikstad H, Hayes P, Mokhtar M, Fracaro ML, Threlfall EJ, Angulo FJ. Emerging quinolone-resistant*Salmonella* in the United States. Emerg. Infect. Dis. 1997;3:371–372.

136. Manie T, Khan S, Brozel VS, Veith WJ, Gouws PA. Antimicrobial resistance of bacteria isolated from slaughtered and retail chickens in South Africa. Lett. Appl. Microbiol. 1998;26:253–258.

137. Dho-Moulin M, van den Bosch JF, Girardeau JP, Bree A, Barat T, Lafont JP. Surface antigens from*Escherichia coli* O2 and O78 strains of avian origin. Infect. Immun. 1990;58:740–745.

138. Dozois CM, Fairbrother JM, Harel J, Bosse M. Pap- and pil-related DNA sequences and other virulence determinants associated with *Escherichia coli* isolated from septicemic chickens and turkeys. Infect. Immun.1992;60:2648–2656.

139. van den Bosch JF, Hendriks JH, Gladigau I, Willems HM, Storm PK, de Graaf FK. Identification of F11 fimbriae on chicken *Escherichia coli* strains. Infect. Immun. 1993;61:800–806.

140. Pourbakhsh SA, Dho-Moulin M, Bree A, Desautels C, Martineau-Doize B, Fairbrother JM. Localization of the *in vivo* expression of P and F1 fimbriae in chickens experimentally inoculated with pathogenic *Escherichia coli*. Microb. Pathog. 1997;22:331–341.

141. Maurer JJ, Lee MD, Lobsinger C, Brown T, Maier M, Thayer SG. Molecular typing of avian*Escherichia coli* isolates by random amplification of polymorphic DNA. Avian Dis. 1998;42:431–451.

142. Foley SL, Horne SM, Giddings CW, Robinson M, Nolan LK. *Iss* from a virulent avian *Escherichia coli*. Avian Dis. 2000;44:185–191.

143. Dho-Moulin M, Fairbrother JM. Avian pathogenic *Escherichia coli* (APEC) Vet. Res. 1999;30:299–316.

144. Ellis MG, Arp LH, Lamont SJ. Serum resistance and virulence of *Escherichia coli* isolated from turkeys. Am. J. Vet. Res. 1988;49:2034–2037.

145. Pfaff-McDonough SJ, Horne SM, Giddings CW, Ebert JO, Doetkott C, Smith MH, Nolan LK. Complement resistance-related traits among *Escherichia coli* isolates from apparently healthy birds and birds with colibacillosis. Avian Dis. 2000;44:23–33.

146. Lafont JP, Dho M, d›Hauteville HM, Brée A, Sansonetti PJ. Presence and expression of aerobactin genes in virulent avian strains of *Escherichia coli*. Infect. Immun. 1987;55:193–197.

147. Reingold J, Starr N, Maurer J, Lee MD. Identification of a new *Escherichia coli* She haemolysin homolog in avian *E. coli*. Vet. Microbiol. 1999;66:125–134.

148. Provence DL, Curtiss R., III Isolation and characterization of a gene involved in hemagglutination by an avian pathogenic *Escherichia coli* strain. Infect. Immun. 1994;62:1369–1380.

149. Bree A, Dho M, Lafont JP. Comparative infectivity of axenic and specific pathogen free chickens of O2*E. coli* strains with or without virulence factors. Avian Dis. 1989;33:134–139.

150. Emery DA, Nagaraja KV, Shaw DP, Newman JA, White DG. Virulence factors of *Escherichia coli*associated with *coli*septicemia in chickens and turkeys. Avian Dis. 1992;36:504–511.

151. Blanco JE, Blanco M, Mora A, Blanco J. Production of toxins (enterotoxins, verotoxins, and necrotoxins) and colicins by *Escherichia coli* strains isolated from septicemic and healthy chickens: relationship with *in vivo* pathogenicity. J. Clin. Microbiol. 1997;35:2953–2957.

152. Parreira VR, Yano T. Cytotoxin produced by *Escherichia coli* isolated from chickens with swollen head syndrome (SHS) Vet. Microbiol. 1998;62:111–119.

153. Chaffer M, Heller ED, Schwartsburd B. Relationship between resistance to complement, virulence and outer membrane protein patterns in pathogenic *Escherichia coli* O2 isolates. Vet. Microbiol. 1999;64:323–332.

154. Truscott RB, Lopez-Alvarez J, Pettit JR. Studies of *Escherichia coli* infection in chickens. Can. J. comp. Med. 1974;38:160–167.

155. Hughes LA, Bennett M, Coffey P, Elliott J, Jones TR, Jones RC, Lahuerta-Marin A, McNiffe K, Norman D, Williams NJ, Chantrey J. Risk factors for the occurrence of *Escherichia coli* virulence genes *eae,stx1* and *stx2* in wild bird populations. Epidemiol. Infect. 2009;137:1574–82.

156. Morley AJ, Thomson DK. Swollen-head syndrome in broiler chickens. Avian Dis. 1984;28:238–243.

157. Picault JP, Giraud P, Drouin P, Guittet M, Bennejean G, Lamande J, Toquin D, Gueguen C. Isolation of a TRTV-like virus from chickens with swollen-head syndrome. Vet. Rec. 1987;121:135.

158. Hafez HM, Löhren U. Swollen head syndrome: clinical observations and serology in West Germany.Deutsche Tierärztliche Wochenschrift. 1990;97:322–324.

159. Nakamura K, Mase M, Tanimura N, Yamaguchi S, Yuasa N. Attempts to reproduce swollen head syndrome in specific pathogen-free chickens by inoculating with *Escherichia coli* and/or turkey rhinotracheitis virus. Avian Pathol. 1998;27:21–27.

160. Georgiades G, Iordanidis P, Koumbati M. Cases of swollen head syndrome in broiler chickens in Greece. Avian Dis. 2001;45:745–750.

161. Tsuji T, Joya JE, Honda T, Miwatani T. A heat-labile enterotoxin (LT) purified from chicken enterotoxigenic *Escherichia coli* is identical to porcine LT. FEMS Microbiol. Lett. 1990;55:329–332.

162. Akashi N, Hitotsubashi S, Yamanaka H, Fujii Y, Tsuji T, MiyamaA, JoyaJE, OkamotoK. Production ofheat-stable enterotoxin II by chicken clinical isolates of *Escherichia coli*. FEMS Microbiol. Lett.1993;109:311–316.

163. Dho-Moulin M, Fairbrother JM. Avian pathogenic *Escherichia coli* (APEC) Vet. Res. 1999;30:299–316.

164. ZanellaA,AlboraliGL,BardottiM,CandottiP,Guadagnini PF, Anna Martino P, Stonfer M. Severe*Escherichia coli* O111 septicemia and polyserositis in hens at the start of lay. Avian Pathol. 2000;29:311–317.

165. Kariuki S, Gilks C, Kimari J, Muyodi J, Getty B, Hart CA. Carriage of potentially pathogenic*Escherichia coli* in chickens. Avian Dis. 2002;46:721–724.

166. Guy JS, Smith LG, Breslin JJ, Vaillancourt JP, Barnes HJ. High mortality and growth depression experimentally produced in young turkeys by dual infection with enteropathogenic *Escherichia coli* and turkey coronavirus. Avian Dis. 2000;44:105–113.

167. Bisgaard M, Dam A. Salpingitis in poultry. I. Prevalence, bacteriology and possible pathogenesis in broilers. Nordisk Veterinaermedicin. 1980;32:361–368.

168. Bisgaard M, Dam A. Salpingitis in poultry. I. Prevalence, bacteriology and possible pathogenesis in egg-laying chickens. Nordisk Veterina ermedicin. 1981;33:81–89.

169. Harry EG. The survival of *E. coli* in the dust of poultry houses. Vet. Rec. 1964;76:466–470.

170. Goren E. Colibacillose bij pluimvee: etiologie, pathologie en therapie. Tijdschrift voor Diergeneeskunde. 1991;116:1122–1129.

171. Norton RA, Macklin KS, McMurtrey BL. The association of various isolates of *Escherichia coli* from the United States with induced cellulitis and colibacillosis in young broiler chickens. Avian Pathol.2000;29:571–574.

172. Leitner G, Heller ED. Colonization of *Escherichia coli* in young turkeys and chickens. Avian Dis.1992;36:211–220.

173. Gross WB. Electrocardiographic changes in *Escherichia coli* infected birds. Am. J. Vet. Res.1966;27:1427–1436.

174. Dho-Moulin M. Les *Escherichia coli* pathogènes des volailles. Annales de Médecine Vétérinair.1993;137:353–357.

175. Humbert F, Salvat G. The risk of transmission of salmonellae in poultry farming: Detection and prevention in Europe. Rev. Sci. Tech. 1997;16:83–90.

176. Barrow PA, Huggins MB, Lovell MA. Host specificity of *Salmonella* infection in chickens and mice is expressed *in vivo* primarily at the level of the reticuloendothelial system. Infect. Immun. 1994;62:4602–4610.

177. Barrow PA. *Salmonella* control- past, present and future. Avian Pathol. 1993;22:651–669.

178. Henderson SC, Bounous DI, Lee MD. Early events in the pathogenesis of avian salmonellosis. Infect. Immun. 1999;67:3580–3586.

179. Lowry VK, Tellez GI, Nisbet DJ, Garcia G, Urquiza O, Stanker LH, Kogut MH. Efficacy of *Salmonella enteritidis*-immune lymphokines on horizontal transmission of *S. arizonae* in turkeys and *S. gallinarum* in chickens. Int. J. Food Microbiol. 1999;48:139–148.

180. Gomis SM, Watts T, Riddell C, Potter AA, Allan BJ. Experimental reproduction of *Escherichia coli* cellulitis and septicemia in broiler chickens. Avian Dis. 1997;41:234–240.

181. Gross WB, Domermuth CH. Colibacillosis. In: Hitchner SB, Domermuth CH, Purchase HG, Williams JE, editors. Isolation and Identification of Avian Pathogens. Arnold Printing Corporation; New York, NY, USA: 1975. pp. 34–37.

182. Leitner G, Melamed D, Drabkin N, Heller ED. An enzyme-linked immunosorbent assay for detection of antibodies against *Escherichia coli*: association between indirect hemagglutination test and survival. Avian Dis. 1990;34:58–62.

183. Bell CJ, Finlay DA, Clarke HJ, Taylor MJ, Ball HJ. Development of a sandwich ELISA and comparison with PCR for the detection of F11 and F165 fimbriated *Escherichia coli* isolates from septicemic disease in farm animals. Vet. Microbiol. 2002;85:251–257.

184. Kles V, Morin M, Humbert F, Lalande F, Guittet M, Bennejean G. Serologic diagnosis of avian salmonelloses: Adjustment of an ELISA test using antigens adsorbed with the aid of anti-colibacillary sera. Zentralbl Veterinarmed B. 1993;40:305–325.

185. Szmolka A, Kaszanyitzky E, Nagy B. Improved diagnostic and real-time PCR in rapid screening for *Salmonella* in the poultry food chain. Acta. Vet. Hung. 2006;54:297–312.

186. Weinack OM, Snoeyenbos GH, Smyser CF, Soerjadi AS. Competitive exclusion intestinal colonization of *Escherichia coli* in chicks. Avian Dis. 1981;25:696–705.

187. La Ragione RM, Casula G, Cutting SM, Woodward MJ. *Bacillus subtilis* spores competitively exclude *Escherichia coli* O78:K80 in poultry. Vet. Microbiol. 2001;79:133–142.

188. Hofacre CL, Johnson AC, Kelly BJ, Froyman R. Effect of a commercial competitive exclusion culture on reduction of colonization of an antibiotic-resistant pathogenic *Escherichia coli* in day-old broiler chickens. Avian Dis. 2002;46:198–202.

189. Kabir SML, Rahman MM, Rahman MB, Hosain MZ, Akand MSI, Das SK. Viability of probiotics in balancing intestinal flora and effecting histological changes of crop and caecal tissues of broilers. Biotechnology. 2005;4:325–330.

190. Kabir SML. The Role of probiotics in the poultry industry. Int. J. Mol. Sci. 2009;10:3531–3546.

191. Melamed D, Leitner G, Heller ED. A vaccine against avian colibacillosis based on ultrasonic inactivation of *Escherichia coli*. Avian Dis. 1991;35:17–22.

192. Heller ED, Leitner G, Drabkin N, Melamed D. Passive immunisation of chicks against *Escherichia coli*.Avian Pathol. 1990;19:345–354.

193. Gyimah JE, Panigrahy B, Williams JD. Immunogenicity of an *Escherichia coli* multivalent pilus vaccine in chickens. Avian Dis. 1986;30:687–689.

194. Pomery BS, Nagaraja KV. Fowl typhoid. In: Calnek BW, Barnes HJ, Beard CW, Reid WM, Yoder HW Jr, editors. Diseases of Poultry. 9th ed. Wolfe publishing Ltd; London, UK: 1991. pp. 87–99.

195. Christensen JP, Skov MN, Hinz KH, Bisgaard M. *Salmonella enterica* serovar Gallinarum biovar gallinarum in layers: epidemiological investigations of a recent outbreak in Denmark. Avian Pathol.1994;23:489–501.

196. Wray C, Davies RH, Corkish JD. Enterobacteriaceae. In: Jordan TW, Pattison M, editors. Poultry Diseases. 4th ed. W. B. Saunders; Philadelphia, PA, USA: 1996. pp. 9–43.

197. Caya F, Fairbrother JM, Lessard L, Quessy S. Characterization of the risk to human health of pathogenic *Escherichia coli* isolates from chicken carcasses. J. Food Prot. 1999;62:741–746.

198. Czirók E, Dho M, Herpay M, Gadó I, Milch H. Association of virulence markers with animal pathogenicity of *Escherichia coli* in different models. Acta Microbiol. Hungarica. 1990;37:207–217.

199. Chapman PA, Siddons CA, Gerdan Malo AT, Harkin MA. A 1-year study of *Escherichia coli* O157 in cattle, sheep, pigs and poultry. Epidemiol. Infect. 1997;119:245–250.

200. Stavric S, Buchanan B, Gleeson TM. Intestinal colonization of young chicks with *Escherichia coli* O157:H7 and other verotoxin-producing serotypes. J. Appl. Bacteriol. 1993;74:557–563.

201. Doyle MP, Schoeni JL. Isolation of *Escherichia coli* O157:H7 from retail fresh meats and poultry. Appl. Environ. Microbiol. 1987;53:2394–2396.

202. Radu S, Ling OW, Rusul G, Karim MI, Nishibuchi M. Detection of *Escherichia coli* O157:H7 by multiplex PCR and their characterization by plasmid profiling, antimicrobial resistance, RAPD and PWWFGE analyses. J. Microbiol. Methods. 2001;46:131–139.

203. Manges AR, Smith SP, Lau BJ, Nuval CJ, Eisenberg JN, Dietrich PS, Riley LW. Retail meat consumption and the acquisition of antimicrobial resistant *Escherichia coli* causing urinary tract infections: A case-control study. Foodborne Pathog. Dis. 2007;4:419–431.

204. Yan S, Pendrak M, Abela-Ridder B, Punderson J, Fedorko D, Foley S. An overview of *Salmonella*typing public health perspectives. Clin. Applied Immunol. Rev. 2003;4:189–204.

CHAPTER 5

FOWLPOX: IDENTIFICATION AND ADOPTION OF PROPHYLACTIC MEASURES IN BACKYARD CHICKENS IN BAHIA, BRAZIL

Silva PS da[1] Batinga T de B[2] Sales TS[3] Herval EFG[4] Ramos I[5] Maia PCC[6] Fernandes LMB[7]

[1] DVM, Poultry Health Laboratory of Bahia (LASAB)/UFBA

[2] DVM, Poultry Health Laboratory of Bahia (LASAB)/UFBA

[3] DVM, graduate student in Tropical Animal Science, School of Veterinary Medicine / UFBA

[4] DVM, graduate student in Tropical Animal Science, School of Veterinary Medicine / UFBA

[5] DVM, Poultry Health Laboratory of Bahia (LASAB)/UFBA

[6] DVM, M. Sc. in Animal Pathology, Professor of the Departament of Preventive Veterinary Medicine, School of Veterinary Medicine /UFBA

[7] DVM, Ph.D. in Immunology, Professor of the Departament of Preventive Veterinary Medicine, School of Veterinary Medicine/ UFBA, coordinator of the Poultry Health Laboratory of Bahia (LASAB)/UFBA

ABSTRACT

This paper describes the identification of an outbreak of fowlpox in backyard chickens in two villages the state of Bahia, the intervention strategy to control the disease by adopting health measures and vaccination, as well as the impact of the intervention. The diagnosis was based in clinical and laboratory data. After the diagnosis was confirmed, control measures and the vaccination of non-infected birds were recommended. Finally, the impact of the intervention on re-incidence of the disease was evaluated. A number of 700 chickens was vaccinated, after which only 9% of the farmers reported the occurrence of new cases, and 70% informed the acquisition of new birds after vaccination. The information reported in this paper can be useful to design strategic plans to control fowlpox in backyard chickens.

INTRODUCTION

Fowlpox is a viral disease characterized by proliferative and nodular lesions in the featherless parts of the skin or fibrino-necrotic and proliferative in the mouth, esophagus, and mucous membrane of the upper respiratory tract (Hsieh, 2005). Clinical signs may vary according to host susceptibility, virulence of the virus strain, and lesion distribution (Tripathy & Reed, 2003). The disease has been described in chickens, turkeys, pigeons, ostriches, quails, pheasants, and canaries (Back *et al*., 1995), and the emergence of outbreaks is associated to environmental conditions, vector populations, and the habits of the affected species (Hansen, 1999; Van Ripper III *et al*., 2002).

Fowlpox is globally distributed (Isa *et al*., 2002; Tripathy & Reed, 2003; Pledger, 2005), despite being considered recent in North America (Pledger, 2005). The incidence is higher in tropical and subtropical countries (Beytut & Haligur, 2007). This disease is economically important in commercial poultry production, as it may cause decline in egg production, mortality (Isa *et al*., 2002; Ariyshi *et al*., 2003), and lower growth rate (Isa *et al*., 2002).

However, in addition to commercial poultry production, small farmers are also affected. Despite the increase in the number of backyard chicken farms in the last few years, little attention has been given to the health care and diseases of these birds (Santos, 2005).

According to Caporal & Costabeber (2000), rural extension is the process of intervention that has an educational and transforming character. This process is based on participating investigation-action methodologies that promote the development of social-economic-cultural practices, allowing the participants of the process to build and to systematize knowledge in order to consciously change reality. In this context, the Poultry Health Education Group (GESAV), which

Citation: Silva PS da1 Batinga T de B2 Sales TS3 Herval EFG4 Ramos I5 Maia PCC6 Fernandes LMB, Fowlpox: Identification and Adoption of Prophylactic Measures in Backyard Chickens in Bahia, Brazil, http://dx.doi.org/10.1590/S1516-635X2009000200007.

includes undergraduate students of the School of Veterinary Medicine of the Federal University of Bahia (EMEV/UFBA), has carried out research and extension activities in rural communities aiming at developing management and production practices for backyard chickens. The identification of health problems and the recommendation of prevention and control alternatives are emphasized (Batinga *et al.*, 2007).

This study aimed at reporting fowlpox incidence in backyard chickens in two villages in the state of Bahia, describing the prophylactic measures adopted to control the infection, and evaluating the impact of the intervention measures on the reemergence of the disease.

MATERIAL AND METHODS

The study was carried out in the villages of Terra Branca and Tatu, located in the district of Algodões, Quijingue, Bahia, Brazil. The municipality of Quijingue is located in the northeastern region of the state of Bahia, in the micro-region of Euclides da Cunha, located 322 km from the state capital city, Salvador.

The villages were visited three times. Terra Branca and Tatu were visited for the first time on November 3 and 4, 2006, respectively. During this first visit, the students organized a field day with the local farmers, when the participants discussed the most frequent problems found, and assessed the activities being carried out. The farmers' notes and observation indicated that most backyard birds from those villages could be suffering from fowlpox.

In order to investigate this suspicion, the students visited the local farms and the disease was clinically diagnosed by the lesions in the featherless skin parts of the birds. In addition, samples were collected and placed in formaldehyde at 10% for subsequent laboratory diagnosis. Samples were submitted to the Pathology Lab of the Veterinary Hospital of UFBA, and analyzed according to the method described by TIMM (2005).

Between January 16 and 20, 2007, the villages were visited a second time to provide the farmers with general guidelines for fowlpox prevention, and to vaccinate the birds against the disease. A freeze-dried vaccine against fowlpox (Hertape Calier) was applied. The flask was opened at the time of use, and was kept in a styrofoam box to ensure the preservation of the optimal temperature, as this is a live vaccine. Bird vaccination was carried out by a wing puncture using a vaccine applicator. Approximately 700 birds were vaccinated.

On April 29 and 30, 2007, meetings were carried out with the farmers of the two villages, and questionnaires were applied to assess the impact of the adopted prophylactic measures.

RESULTS AND DISCUSSION

The clinical signs observed in the flocks of the visited villages were similar to those reported by Jacob *et al.* (1998) in an extensive chicken rearing system in the USA. Those authors observed lesions in the skin and/or mouth and upper respiratory tract membranes, low growth rate, poor feed efficiency, and reduction of egg production. Beytut & Haligur (2007) described a similar condition in naturally-infected chickens in Turkey, where the birds presented conjutivitis, depression, anorexia, and crusts or nodules in the skin, comb, wattle, and eyelids.

In order to further investigate the problems, some farms were visited to observe the birds and the general conditions of the farms, looking for environmental factors that could favor the disease. Extensive crusty lesions were found on the corner of eyes and ears, which are consistent with fowlpox (Figure 1).

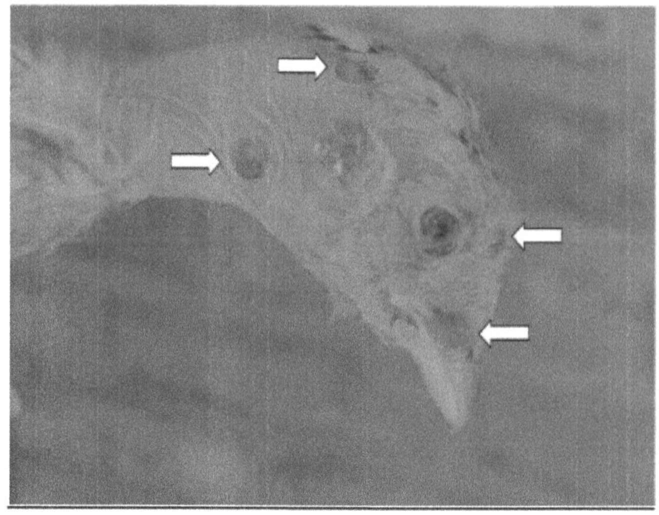

Figure 1: Fowlpox skin lesions in a backyard chicken of the village of Tatú.

Butcher & Rossi (1990) mention that fowlpox is a disease that can be readily diagnosed by veterinarians, based on the flock›s history and the presence of typical lesions. However, in some instances, the microscopic examination of the affected tissues may be required. During the visits to the flocks, material was collected for laboratory diagnosis. The material was stored according to the recommendations of Borja (2007), and subsequently processed at the Pathology Lab of the Veterinary School of UFBA. The histological examination confirmed the suspicion of fowlpox, revealing the presence of Bollinger bodies, which are characteristic of this viral infection (Figure 2). These inclusion bodies cause cytoplasmic distention, resulting in cell necrosis (Tanizaki*et al.*, 1986; Yoshikkawa & Alam, 2002; Beytut & Haligur, 2007).

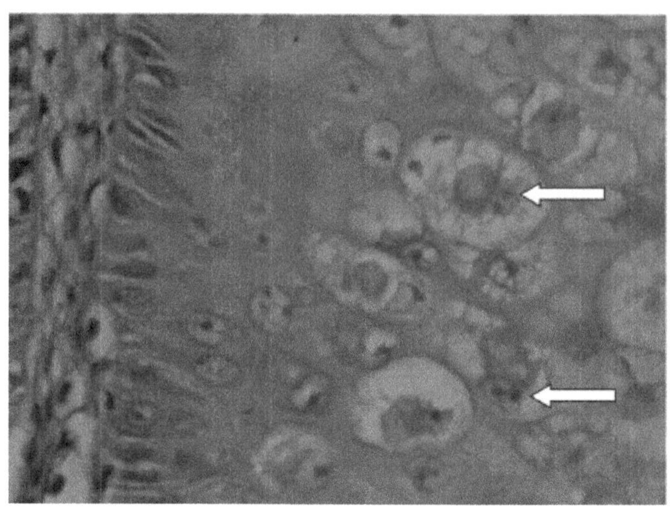

Figure 2: Presence of eosinopilic and circunscribed agglomerate (Bollinger bodies) in the cytoplams of some cells.

The main aim of the second visit - two months after the first visit - was to vaccinate birds and to check general management conditions. The representatives of the communities were previously contacted, and the vaccination day was scheduled. The farmers were asked to have the birds gathered the previous day, placing them in enclosures to make the vaccination process easier.

Butcher & Rossi (1990) suggest vaccination as a prevention measure against fowlpox, associated to insect control. Those authors emphasize, however, than only healthy birds should be vaccinated, as the vaccine induces mild infection.

There were no problems during vaccination. Most flocks were vaccinated, except for those which owners were not present or did not allow their birds to be vaccinated. Approximately 700 birds were immunized, and this number was considered satisfactory, as 93.9% of the flocks consisted of less than 30 birds.

Although vaccination is the main prevention strategy suggested in literature, many authors point out that the efficacy of the vaccination programs is very variable, and depend on epidemiological conditions (Butcher & Rossi, 1990; Figueiredo *et al.*, 2001; Permin & Pedersen, 2002).

The vaccine against fowlpox can be purchased in the capital city, Salvador, and other localities of the state of Bahia, where commercial poultry production is an important economic activity. Nevertheless, dwellers of distant villages have no knowledge of the existence of this vaccine, nor have veterinary technical services available.

Permin & Pedersen (2002), in studies carried out in Africa and Asia, observed that most small farmers did not vaccinate their birds against fowlpox.

When farmers do not have access to the vaccine to prevent the disease, farmers apply traditional home-made treatments when birds present skin lesions. The application of burnt oil, powder, or lemon is a common practice when warts emerge. Jugessur *et al.* (2006), in a study developed with small poultry farmers of the Republic of Mauritius, described a traditional treatment for fowlpox based on iodine, tomato, and cooking oil or shoe polisher.

However, to date, no single treatment for fowlpox has been successfully developed. Antibiotics can be used to control secondary bacterial infections, particularly in birds with respiratory and gastrointestinal lesions (Pledger, 2005).

The communities were visited again three months after vaccination. Between the second and the third visits, contact was made by telephone. During the third visits, meetings were held, and questionnaires were applied to assess the impact of the adoption of the prophylactic measures recommended. In both communities, the women are usually the family members responsible for bird care. This had already been observed in another study performed in the state of Bahia (Batinga, 2007) and it is consistent with information published by FAO (Food and Agriculture Organization) in 2006. The Coordinated Research Council (CRC) on Family Poultry Production of FAO concluded that, in 13 countries of Africa, women are also the main responsible people for the domestic rearing of chickens, and pointed out that better poultry performance may generate better life conditions to women and children (FAO/IAEA, 2006).

Table 1: Answers obtained in the questionnaires, in %

Items of the questionnaire	Yes	No
Women are responsible for bird care	81%	19%
Disease observation after vaccination	9%	91%
Introduction of new birds after vaccination	70%	30%

Butcher & Rossi (1990) stress that the fowlpox virus may remain stable for a long time in the environment, favoring the infection of new birds introduced in the affected farms.

Today, the disease is under control in both villages where the intervention was carried out, as farmers have not reported the incidence of new outbreak, as informed by local representatives. However, further work must be developed both in the studied villages and in other communities to develop prevention strategies and to implement health education programs, which should be coordinated by government authorities. These programs should enhance the capacity of disease identification, after which, in a partnership with the community, a control and prevention plan based on general and specific measures should be developed. The plan must consider environmental and management characteristics, such as rainfall period, and consequently the presence of vector insects, as well as the frequency of introduction of new birds in the flocks.

CONCLUSIONS

The present article describes the process of clinical and laboratory identification of fowlpox in backyard chickens reared in two villages in the state of Bahia, Brazil. Based on this identification, we report the recommended and applied prophylactic measures to control the disease, and discuss the impact of these measures on the reemergence of the disease. Although fowlpox is responsible for significant economic losses, particularly for small farmers, and can be controlled by vaccination and the implementation of hygiene measures, to date there are no established programs for the diagnosis and prevention of this disease in backyard chicken farming. Considering the importance of family poultry production to ensure food and income to small farmers, it is essential to develop strategies to reduce the losses caused by fowlpox.

REFERENCES

1. Ariyoshi R, Takase K, Matsuura Y, Deguchi K, Ginnaga A, Fujikawa H. Vaccination against fowlpox virus via drinking water. Journal of Veterinary Medical Science 2003; 65(10):1127-1130.
2. Back A, Soncini RA, Ruthes O, Madureira Júnior S, Flores R. An atypical fowl pox outbreak in broilers in southern Brazil. Avian Diseases 1995; 39:902-906.
3. Batinga TB. Análise sorológica e avaliação epidemiológica de salmoneloses e micoplasmoses em galinhas de quintal na Bahia [monografia]. Salvador (MG): Universidade Federal da Bahia; 2007.
4. Batinga TB, Silva PS, César AR, Ramos I, Fernandes L. Avaliação da ocorrência de Salmoneloses e Micoplasmoses, e de seu impacto, na criação de galinhas caipiras em pequenas propriedades rurais do Estado da Bahia. Anais do 1° Congresso Nordestino de Extensão Universitária; 2007; Salvador, Bahia. Brasil.

5. Beytut E, Haligur M. Pathological, immunochemical, and electron microscopic findings in the respiratory tract and skin of chickens naturally infected with avipoxvirus. Turkish Journal of Veterinary Animal Science 2007; 31(1):1-7.

6. Borja F. Métodos de estudos histológicos [citado em 12 set 2007]. Disponível em:http://www.cstr.ufcg.edu.br/histologia.

7. Butcher GD, Miles RD. Diseases prevention in commercial poultry [Fact Sheet CIR1079]. Gainsville: Florida Cooperative Extension Service, Institute of Food and Agricultural Sciences, University of Florida; 1993.

8. Butcher GD, Rossi F. Prevention and control of fowl pox in backyard chicken flocks [Fact Sheet VM65]. Gaisnville: Florida Cooperative Extension Service, Institute of Food and Agricultural Sciences, University of Florida; 1990.

9. Caporal FR, Costabeber JA. Agroecologia e desenvolvimento rural sustentável: perspectivas para uma nova Extensão Rural. Agroecologia e Desenvolvimento Rural Sustentável 2000; 1(1):16-37.

10. FAO - Food Agricultural Organization. Improving farmyard poultry production in Africa: interventions and their economic assessment. Vienna: IAEA; 2006.

11. Figueiredo EAP. Diferentes denominações e classificação brasileira de produção alternativa de frangos. Anais da Conferência de Ciência e Tecnologia Avícola; 2001; Campinas, São Paulo. Brasil. Campinas: Facta; 2001. p.209-222.

12. Hansen W. Avian pox. In: Friend M, Franson JC. Field manual of wildlife diseases: general field procedures and diseases of wild birds. Washington: US Department of the Interior, United States Geological Survey; 1999. p. 163-170.

13. Hsieh YC, Chen SH, Wang CW, Lee YF, Chung WC, Tsai MC, Chang TC, Lien YY, Tsai SS. Unsual pox lesions found in Chinese jungle mynahs (Acridotheres cristatellus). Avian Pathology 2005; 34(5): 415-417.

14. Isa G, Pfister K, Kaaden OR, Czerny CP. Development of a monoclonal blocking ELISA for the detection of antibodies against fowlpox virus. Journal of Veterinary Medicine 2002; 49:21-23.

15. Jacob JP, Wilson HR, Miles RD, Butcher GD, Mather FB. Factors affecting egg production in backyard chicken flocks [Fact Sheet PS 35]. Gainsville: Animal Science Department, Florida Cooperative Extension Service, Institute of Food and Agricultural Sciences, University of Florida; 1998.

16. Jugessur VS, Pillay MM, Ramnauth R, Allas MJ. The socio-economic importance of family poultry production in the republic of Mauritius. In:FAO/IAEA. Improving farmyard poultry production in Africa: Interventions and their economic assessment. Vienna: IAEA; 2006. p. 164-178.

17. Permin A, Pedersen G. The need for a holistic view on disease problems in free-range chickens. In: FAO/IAEA. Characteristics and parameters of family poultry production in Africa. Vienna: IAEA; 2002. p.1-8.

18. Pledger A. Avian pox virus infection in a mourning dove. Canadian Veterinay Journal 2006; 46:1143-1145.

19. Santos MSV. Biosseguridade em todos os níveis [cited 09 set 2005]. Available from:http://www.aviculturaindustrial.com.br

20. Tanizaki E, Kotani T, Odagiri Y. Pathological changes of tracheal mucosa in chickens infected with fowl pox virus. Avian Diseases 1986; 31(1):169-175.

21. Timm LL. Técnicas rotineiras de preparação e análise de lâminas histológicas. Caderno La Salle XI 2005; 2(1):231-239.

22. Tripathy DN, Reed WM. Pox. In: Saif YM. Diseases of poultry [CD-ROM]. 11th ed. Ames: Iowa State University Press; 2003. p. 253-269.

23. Van Riper III C, Van Riper SG, Hansen WR. Epizootiology and effect of avian pox on Hawaiian forest birds. The Auk 2002; 119(4):929-942.

24. Yoshikkawa MGT, Alam J. Histopathological studies of fowl pox in bantams. International Journal of Poultry Science 2002; 1(6):197-199.

CHAPTER 6

PATHOGENESIS AND DIAGNOSTIC APPROACHES OF AVIAN INFECTIOUS BRONCHITIS

Faruku Bande[1, 2] Siti Suri Arshad[1] Abdul Rahman Omar[1, 3] Mohd Hair Bejo[1, 3] Muhammad Salisu Abubakar[1] and Yusuf Abba[1]

[1]Department of Veterinary Pathology and Microbiology, Faculty of Veterinary Medicine, Universiti Putra Malaysia (UPM), 43400 Serdang, Selangor, Malaysia

[2]Department of Veterinary Services, Ministry of Animal Health and Fisheries Development, PMB 2109, Usman Faruk Secretariat, Sokoto 840221, Sokoto State, Nigeria

[3]Laboratory of Vaccine and Immunotherapeutics, Institute of Bioscience, Universiti Putra Malaysia (UPM), 43400 Serdang, Selangor, Malaysia

ABSTRACT

Infectious bronchitis (IB) is one of the major economically important poultry diseases distributed worldwide. It is caused by infectious bronchitis virus (IBV) and affects both galliform and nongalliform birds. Its economic impact includes decreased egg production and poor egg quality in layers, stunted growth, poor carcass weight, and mortality in broiler chickens. Although primarily affecting the respiratory tract, IBV demonstrates a wide range of tissues tropism, including the renal and reproductive systems. Thus, disease outcome may be influenced by the organ or tissue involved as well as pathotypes or strain of the infecting virus. Knowledge on the epidemiology of the prevalent IBV strains in a particular region is therefore important to guide control and preventions. Meanwhile previous diagnostic methods such as serology and virus isolations are less sensitive and time consuming, respectively; current methods, such as reverse transcription polymerase chain reaction (RT-PCR), Restriction Fragment Length Polymorphism (RFLP), and sequencing, offer highly sensitive, rapid, and accurate diagnostic results, thus enabling the genotyping of new viral strains within the shortest possible time. This review discusses aspects on pathogenesis and diagnostic methods for IBV infection.

INTRODUCTION

Infectious bronchitis (IB) causes significant economic losses to the poultry industry worldwide [1, 2]. The disease was first identified in North Dakota, USA, when Schalk and Hawn reported a new respiratory disease in young chickens [3]. Since then, IBV has been recognized widely, especially in countries with large commercial poultry populations. Apart from respiratory infections, IB affects the kidney and reproductive tract, causing renal dysfunction and decreased egg production, respectively. Although the disease first was believed to occur primarily in young chickens, however, chickens of all age are also susceptible [1].

Citation: Faruku Bande, Siti Suri Arshad, Abdul Rahman Omar, Mohd Hair Bejo, Muhammad Salisu Abubakar, and Yusuf Abba, "Pathogenesis and Diagnostic Approaches of Avian Infectious Bronchitis," Advances in Virology, vol. 2016, Article ID 4621659, 11 pages, 2016. doi:10.1155/2016/4621659.

AETIOLOGY AND MOLECULAR BIOLOGY

Infectious bronchitis is caused by infectious bronchitis virus (IBV), a single stranded positive sense, enveloped RNA virus of 27–32 kb length [4]. The virus has been classified under the Gammacoronavirus genus in the family Coronaviridae, order Nidovirales. Like other members of coronavirus family, the IBV genome is composed of structural and nonstructural proteins. Structural proteins include the spike [S] glycoprotein, envelope [E], matrix [M], and nucleocapsid [N]. These proteins together play different roles in viral attachment, replication, and inducing clinical disease. Of major structural proteins, the M protein is the most abundant transmembrane protein, which play vital role in coronavirus assembly through interaction with viral ribonucleocapsid and spike glycoprotein [5, 6]. IBV E protein is, however, scant and contains highly hydrophobic transmembrane N-terminal and cytoplasmic C-terminal domains. Studies have shown that the E protein is localized to the Golgi complex in IBV infected cells and is integrally associated with viral envelope formation, assembly, budding, ion channel activity, and apoptosis [7, 8]. Similar to other coronaviruses, the phosphorylated 409 amino acid of IBV-N protein is highly conserved between amino acid residues 238 and 293 [9]. IBV-N protein binds with the genomic RNA to form a helical ribonucleoprotein complex (RNP), thus aiding transcription, replication, translation, and packaging of the viral genome during replication [10]. The S1 portion of the spike glycoprotein plays important role in the attachment and entry of the virus into the cell via sialic acid receptors and has been considered as the determinant for viral diversity and immune protection [11]. This protein has been targeted for genotypic characterization as well as recombinant IBV serotypes vaccines [6,12, 13].

PATHOGENESIS

Infectious bronchitis virus infects primarily the respiratory system. However, some variants and several field isolates affect the reproductive, renal, and digestive systems of chickens. Disease pathogenesis differs according to the system involved, as well as the strain of the virus [1].

Host Susceptibility

Although domestic fowl (Gallus gallus) and pheasant (Phasianus spp.) are considered to be natural hosts for IBV [14], other IBV-like coronaviruses have been identified in nondomestic avian species including pheasant, peafowl, turkey, teal, geese, pigeon, penguins quail, duck, and Amazon parrot [15–18]. Antigenic similarities between turkey coronavirus (TCoV) and avian infectious bronchitis virus (AIBV) have also been demonstrated [19]. Antibodies to IBV have been demonstrated in humans with close contact to poultry, but the virus has not been reported to cause human clinical disease [20].

Age and Breed Predisposition

Chickens of all ages and breed types are susceptible to IBV infection, but the extent and severity of the disease is pronounced in young chicks, compared to adults. Similarly, resistance to infection was suggested to increase with increasing age [21]. Experimental evidence suggests that line C white leghorn chickens are more resistant to M41 IBV challenge, compared to line 151, although both lines had similar virus shedding rate [22, 23], perhaps influenced by genetic polymorphism in the chicken major histocompatibility complex (MHC), as observed between , , or chicken haplotypes [24].

Receptor and Entry

The IBV receptor-binding domain (RBD) in the S1-spike plays a major role in attachment of the virus to host cells [25, 26]. Thus, variation in the S1 glycoprotein partly determines tissue tropism and virulence [27, 28]. IBV affects trachea, kidney, and reproductive tract through interaction of S1 glycoproteins RBD (AAs 19–69 in M41) with α-2,3-sialic acid receptors on the surface of the cells [29, 30]. In addition to the sialic acid receptor, attenuated Baudette-IBV strain has been shown to interact with a putative heparan sulfate- (HS-) binding site that might contribute to its wide host range [31]. Following viral attachment, conformational changes occurring in the S1 glycoprotein mediate the membrane fusion activity of the S2 carboxylic acid terminal of the spike glycoprotein [1]. Subsequently, IBV enters the cell and releases its nucleocapsid into the cell's cytoplasm, thus triggering replication, virus budding, and release [32].

Infection and Transmission

The virus is transmitted via the respiratory secretions, as well as faecal droplets from infected poultry. Contaminated objects and utensils may aid transmission and spread of the virus from one flock to another. Evidence of virus was shown in trachea, kidney, and Bursa of Fabricius 24 hrs following aerosol transmission [33]. The nature of IBV persistence remains to be elucidated; however, detection of the virus in the caecal tonsils (up to 14 weeks) and from faeces (20 weeks) after infection might suggest a role of faecal shedding in viral transmission and persistence [34].

Incubation Period

Generally the short incubation period for IBV varies with infective dose and route of infection. For example, while infection via the tracheal route may take a course as short as 18 hours, ocular inoculation leads to an incubation period of 36 hours [33].

Clinical Course and Manifestations

In the host, initial infection occurs at epithelia of Harderian gland, trachea, lungs, and air sacs. The virus then moves to the kidney and urogenital tract, to establish systemic infection [33, 35]. In this regard, the severity and clinical features of IB depend on the organ or system involved. Infection of the respiratory system may result in clinical signs such as gasping, sneezing, tracheal rales, listlessness, and nasal discharges. Affected birds appeared listless and dull with ruffled feathers (Figure 1). Other signs may include weight loss and huddling of birds together under a common heat source [33].

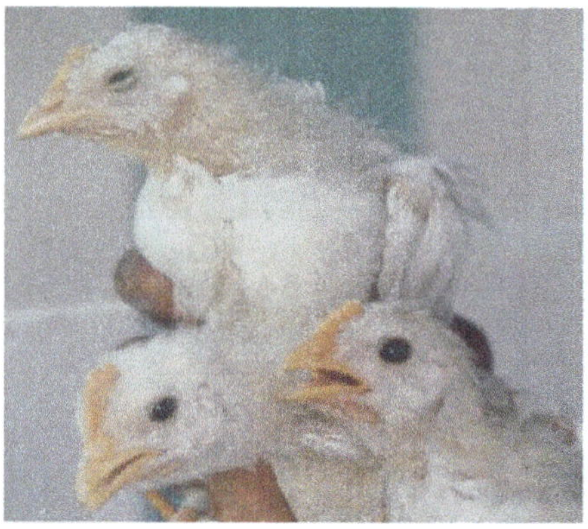

Figure 1: Dullness exhibited in chickens infected following experimental infection with IBV (courtesy: Siti Suri Arshad).

Other clinical outcomes associated with IB infection include frothy conjunctivitis, profuse lacrimation, oedema, and cellulitis of periorbital tissues. Infected birds may also appear lethargic, with evidence of dyspnoea and reluctance to move [36]. Nephropathogenic IBV strains are most described in broiler-type chickens. Clinical signs include depression, wet droppings, and excessive water intake. Infection of reproductive tract is associated with lesions of the oviduct, leading to decreased egg production and quality. Eggs may appear misshapen, rough-shelled, or soft with watery egg yolk (Figure 2). Unless effective measures are instituted, decline in egg production does not return to normal laying, thus contributing to high economic loss [1, 37].

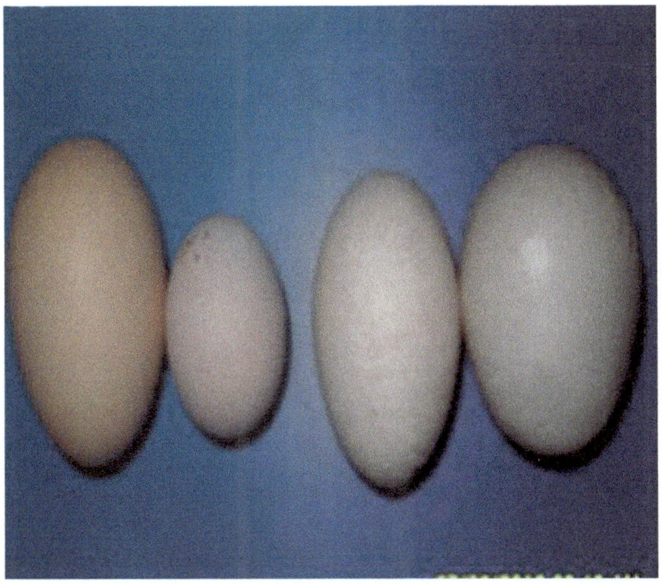

(a)

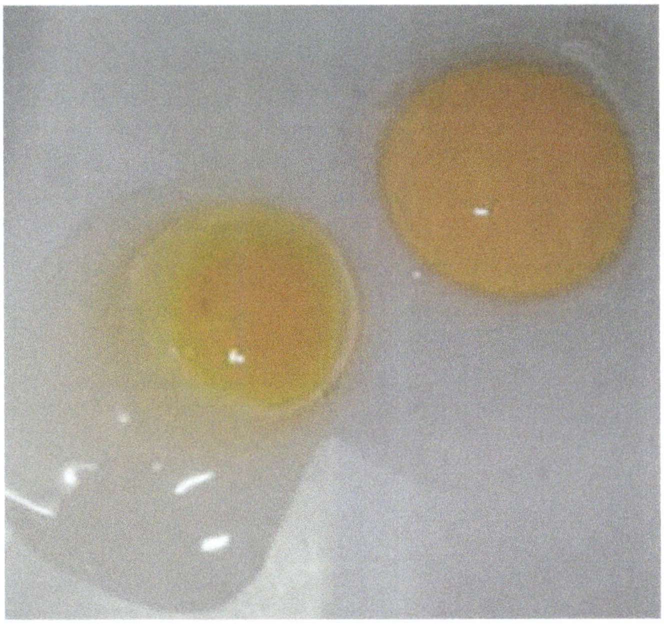

(b)

Figure 2: Irregularity in the shape and sizes of eggs from natural IBV infected breeder chickens (a). Watery albumen from IBV infected chicken ((b) left) compared to normal egg ((b) right).

Gross and Histopathology

Pathological changes observed grossly at necropsy include congestion and oedema of tracheal mucosa and extrapulmonary bronchi (Figure 3) [38, 39].

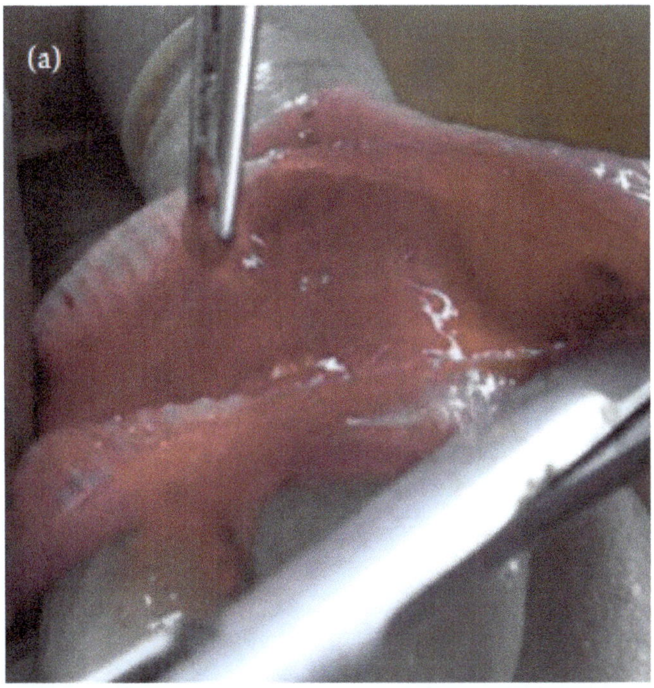

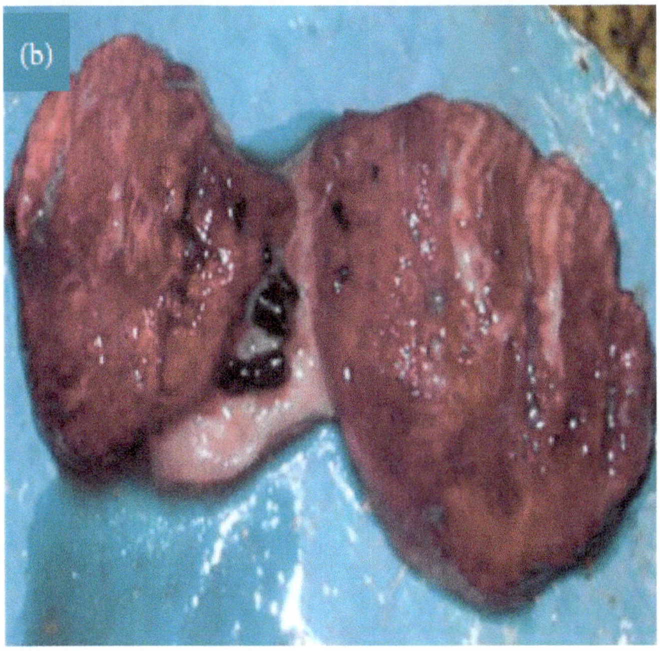

Figure 3: Gross lesions observed on respiratory organs of chicken naturally infected with IBV. Presence of mucoid secretion, congestion, and hyperaemia in the trachea (a); mild focal areas of lung consolidation (b).

Histopathological changes include loss of cilia, oedema, rounding and sloughing of epithelial cells, and infiltration by lymphocytes (Figure 4). Presence of Russell bodies in Harderian cells has been observed following infection with H120 IBV serotype [40].

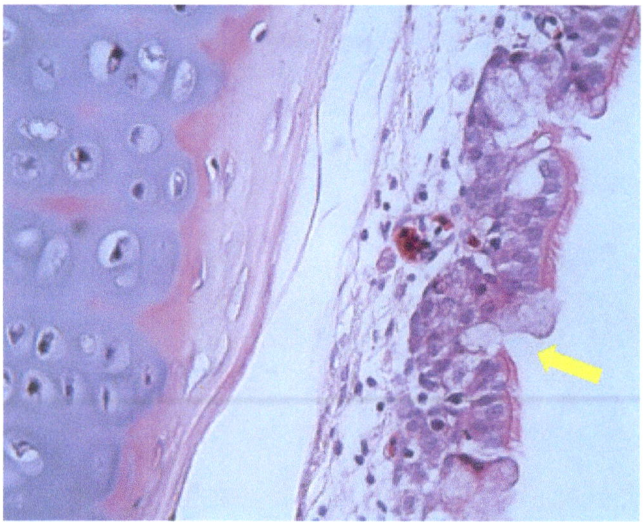

(a)

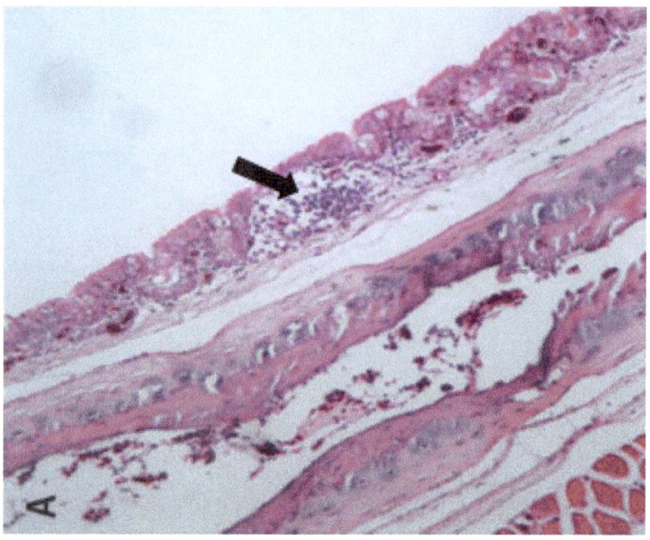

(b)

Figure 4: Histopathological changes in the trachea of naturally IBV infected chicken. Note: the marked infiltration of lymphocytes within the epithelia (black arrow (b)) and evidence of mucosal secretions of goblet cells (yellow arrow (a)).

Nephropathogenic IBV strains cause nephritis characterized by swelling and congestion of the kidney (Figure5), sometimes with pallor of ureters that contain urate deposits. Coinfection with bacterial pathogens such as E. coli may lead to a more complex outcome, usually associated with high morbidity and mortality. Similarly, infection with nephropathogenic IBV strains may result in pale, swollen, and mottled kidneys [39, 41]. Histological findings include interstitial nephritis, tubular degeneration, and infiltration by heterophils. In some cases, necrotic and dilated tubules are filled with urates and casts [33]. Experimental studies have shown that IBV-T-strain causes necrosis of the proximal convoluted tubule and distension of distal convoluted tubule. In addition, necrotic foci, heterophils, and lymphocytes are observed in the interstitial spaces. Oedema of Bowman's capsule and granulocytic infiltration has been reported in the collecting ducts and spheroids [42, 43].

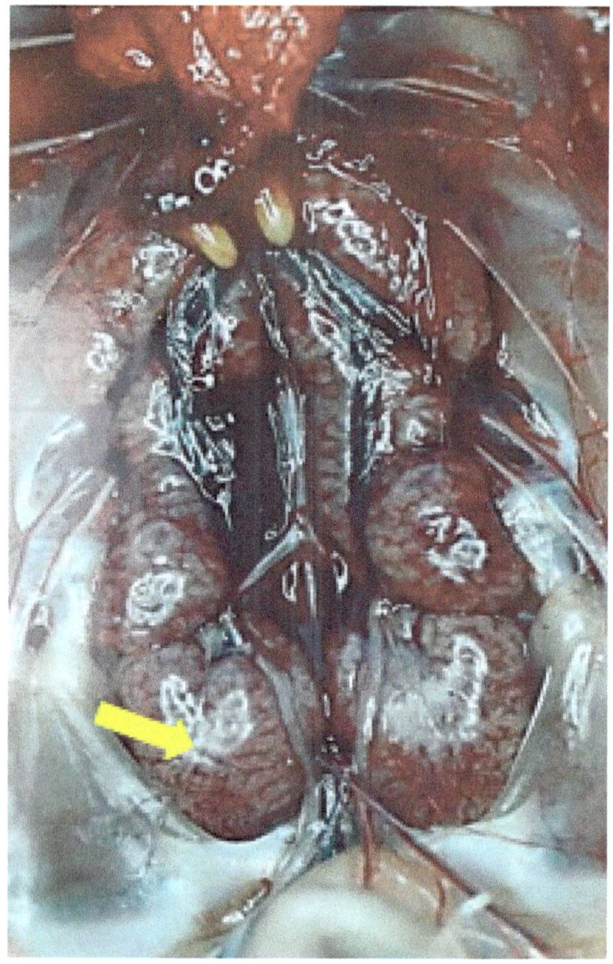

Figure 5: Gross lesions in kidney of chicken following experimental infection with a nephropathogenic infectious bronchitis virus. Note: swelling and congestion of the kidney (arrow) (courtesy: Siti Suri Arshad).

When the reproductive system is affected, there may be nonpatent and hypoglandular oviduct, especially in severely affected chickens [43, 44]. Large accumulation of yolk fluid may be seen in the abdominal cavity (Figure 6), often associated with bacterial infection in laying hens [45, 46]. Cystic oviduct has also been observed in young layers following infection with certain IBV strains (Figure 7).

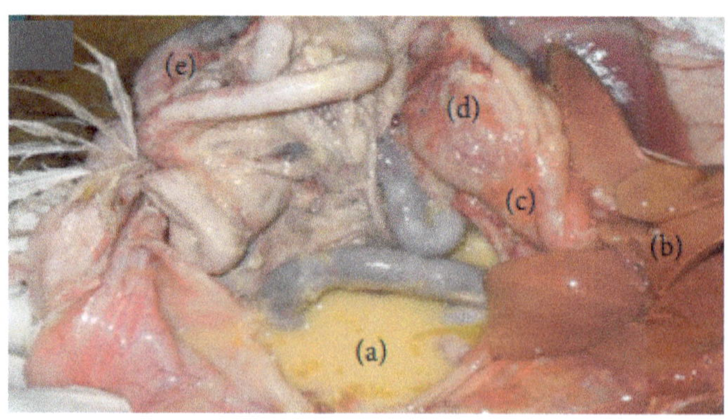

Figure 6: Chicken showing natural IBV infection. Accumulation of egg yolk in abdominal cavity (a); slightly enlarged, pale, friable liver (b) and multiple petechial haemorrhages on the serosal surfaces of proventriculus (c), gizzard (d), and small intestine (e).

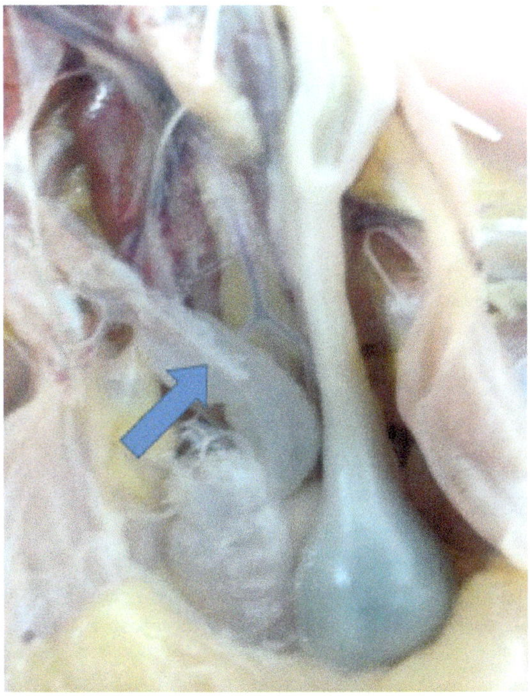

Figure 7: Cystic oviduct in 11-week-old chicken experimentally infected with a CR88 infectious bronchitis virus strain. Note the distention of the entire oviduct and fluid accumulation (arrow).

Morbidity and Mortality

Morbidity due to IBV infection can reach up to 100%. Mortality rate may range from 25 to 30% in young chicks but may increase to 80% as a result of factors that are host-associated (age, immune status), virus-associated (strain, pathogenicity, virulence, and tissue tropism), or environmental (cold and heat stresses, dust, and presence of ammonia). Secondary bacterial infections (E. coli) or coinfection with immunosuppressive viruses such as Marek's disease virus, infectious bursal disease virus (IBDV) [33, 47, 48], may worsen the outcomes of IBV infection. Generally, nephropathogenic IBV strain causes high mortality, compared with strains infecting only the respiratory or reproductive systems [49].

DIAGNOSIS

Conventional and more advanced methods have been used for the diagnosis of IBV infection. The choice of one test over another is guided by type of sample, availability of test materials and facilities, test reporting time, purpose of the test, and whether the test is carried out in the field or at the laboratory. Selected testing procedures are discussed below.

Serology

In the past, serological assays such as virus neutralization (VN) and haemagglutination inhibition (HI) were used widely for detecting and serotyping IBV strains. These tests also have been used to measure flock protection following vaccination [50, 51]. Serotype-specific antibodies usually are detected using HI, even though the HI test is less reliable [51]. On the other hand, ELISA assays are more sensitive and easily applied for field use and in monitoring antibody response following vaccination or exposure. However, emergence of different IBV serotypes that do not cross-react with commonly available antisera generally made serological tests less applicable and nonconclusive in classifying new or emerging IBV isolates [52, 53].

Virus Isolation and Identification

Virus isolation has been the gold standard for the diagnosis of IBV [54, 55]. Taking samples during early onset of the disease and ensuring the right sampling techniques are important keys for successful isolation of IBV. To support successful virus isolation from swabs, recommended to place swab sample in buffered solutions of media or PBS before transporting them to the laboratory. If tissue samples are to be collected, recommended tissues are trachea, kidney, proventriculus, tonsil, and oviduct. Tissue samples must be collected aseptically from scarified chickens or immediately upon death, placed in sterile, tightly sealed plastic specimen bags, and transported to the laboratory on ice for further processing [56]. The stringent technique requirements and factors, such as the time required for several passages of virus in egg or cell culture, limit the use of virus isolation as a diagnostic method of choice for IBV infection. Notwithstanding, different laboratories use various isolation methods, as described below.

Embryonated Chicken Egg

Most IBV strains grow well when inoculated into the allantoic cavity of a 9–11-day-old chicken embryo. Clinical samples from tracheal swab, broth, or tissue homogenate (10% w/v) are inoculated into the allantoic cavity of specific pathogen-free eggs and incubated at 34–37°C, after inoculation. Eggs are candled daily to monitor embryo viability; death within 24 hrs is considered nonspecific. After 48–72 hrs, allantoic fluid (AF) is harvested from representative eggs that were chilled overnight and tested for the presence of IBV using serological tests or RT-PCR assay. Sometimes the allantoic fluid needs to be subjected to several passages to allow the virus to adapt and replicate to high titre, thus increasing the period that is needed to obtain results. The latter may vary among viral strains [54]. After 5–7 days, inoculated eggs are opened and observed for characteristic IB lesions such as curling and dwarfism of the infected embryo (Figure 8). It is important to note that such findings are suggestive, but not pathognomonic [57].

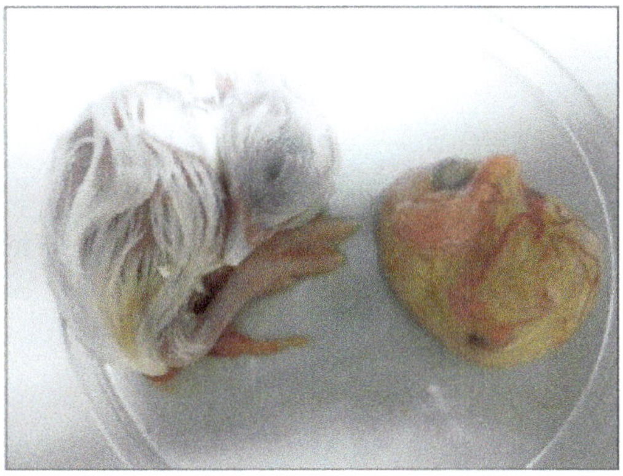

Figure 8: Embryo development at 17 days old following inoculations with IBV-CR88 strain. Note evidence of dwarfism and curling of the toes in IBV infected embryo (right) compared to a noninfected control embryo (left).

Cell Cultures

Isolation of IBV has been attempted in various primary and secondary cells, such as chicken embryo kidney fibroblast and Vero cells, respectively [58, 59]. Infected cultures are characterized by rounding, development of syncytia, and subsequent detachment from the surface of the plate [59]. A major limitation of cell culture methods for IBV isolation is that not all strains of IBV are easily adapted in cell culture. Even for some cell culture adaptable IBV (M41, Iowa 97, and NZ) strains, growth of the virus often requires primary isolation in embryonated eggs and several passages, prior to adaptation. In some cases, attempts to grow IBV in various cell lines either failed or resulted in very low viral titre [58].

Organ Cultures

Tracheal organ culture (TOC) can be used to propagate both embryo-adapted and non-embryo-adapted IBV strains. TOC is prepared from tracheal rings of 20-day-old chicken embryo. The tracheal rings are maintained in a roller bottle and infected with IBV-suspected samples. The culture is observed microscopically for evidence of ciliostasis under light microscope. Complete impairment of ciliary activity usually is considered as a positive culture [60]. Successful growth of IBV has been demonstrated in organ cultures derived from kidney, intestine, proventriculus, and oviduct. However, susceptibility of these organs to IBV can be influenced by the strain of the virus and the amount of virus presence in the sample (infective dose). While a study suggested the universality of using kidney, bursa, and proventriculus in growing IBV, a poor result was obtained when IBV was propagated in cultures derived from different intestinal segments [61]. An advantage of this method includes easy titration and serotyping of IBV, since no virus adaptation is required [62]. Possible constraints include lack of affinity of some IBV strain for some organ cells and difficulty in differentiating ciliostasis arising from other viruses, such as Newcastle disease virus and avian adenovirus [33].

Electron Microscopy

Electron microscopy provides a direct means of detecting and identifying IBV in biological samples based on morphological characteristics of coronavirus. Positive cultures are confirmed based on the presence of coronavirus-like pleomorphic structures with spike projections, following negative staining with phosphotungstic acid (Figure 9). Importantly, the shape and diameter (120 nm) of the virus are taken into consideration when making diagnostic judgements. Apart from the negative staining method, transmission electron microscopy (TEM) is also a useful tool which enables the visualization of virus-like particles in infected cells [59, 63]. However, this method is often applied to understand viral attachment and entry into the cell but is not a specific diagnostic test [35].

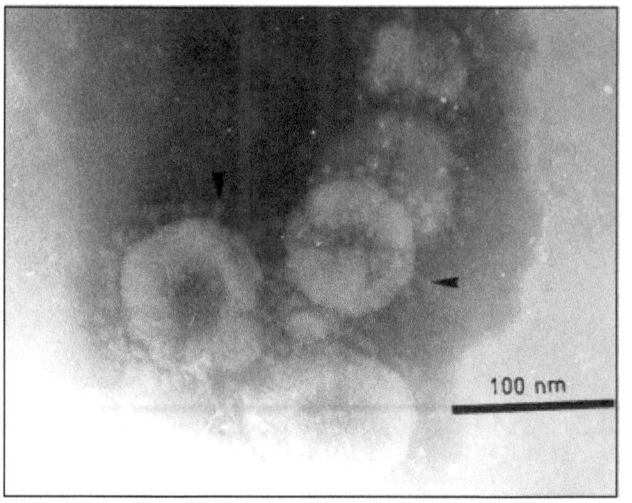

Figure 9: Negative staining electron microscope showing spherical shape of virus with typical spike projections (arrow) surrounding the virion of avian infectious bronchitis virus (courtesy: Siti Suri Arshad).

Immunohistochemistry

Immunoperoxidase and immunofluorescence are two important histochemistry methods for detection and confirmation of IBV antigen from infected tissue and/or cells. These methods work based on antigen-antibody reactions [64, 65]. Immunoperoxidase methods such as the avidin-biotin complex (ABC) have been used successfully to localize IBV antigen in tissue samples [66]. Likewise, indirect immunofluorescent assay is the most frequently used fluorescent technique [66, 67].

Molecular Diagnostic Assays

In view of their increased sensitivity and reduced reporting time, molecular methods, such as Reverse Transcriptase Polymerase Chain Reaction (RT-PCR), real-time PCR, Restriction Fragment Length Polymorphism (RFLP), and genome sequencing, have nearly replaced conventional serology and virus cultivation methods of IBV diagnosis [68, 69].

RT-PCR Methods

This approach uses viral RNA, amplified either directly (one-step RT-PCR) or following cDNA synthesis (two-step RT-PCR). An RT-PCR assay was designed and introduced in 1991 for detecting the IBV-S2 gene [70]. Subsequently, general and serotype-specific RT-PCR assays were designed to target different regions and/or fragments (Figure 10) in the IBV viral genome [71–73]. The UTR and N-gene-based RT-PCR are used for universal detection, because of the conserved nature of the target region in many IBV serotypes [68, 71]. A pan-coronavirus primer, targeting a conserved region of different coronavirus isolates, could also be used in one-step RT-PCR amplification of IBV strains [55]. However, amplification and sequencing of the S1 gene provide a reliable means for genotypic classification of new IBV strains [74]. A serotype-specific PCR assay has been designed to enable differentiation of Massachusetts, Connecticut, Arkansas, and Delaware field isolates [73].

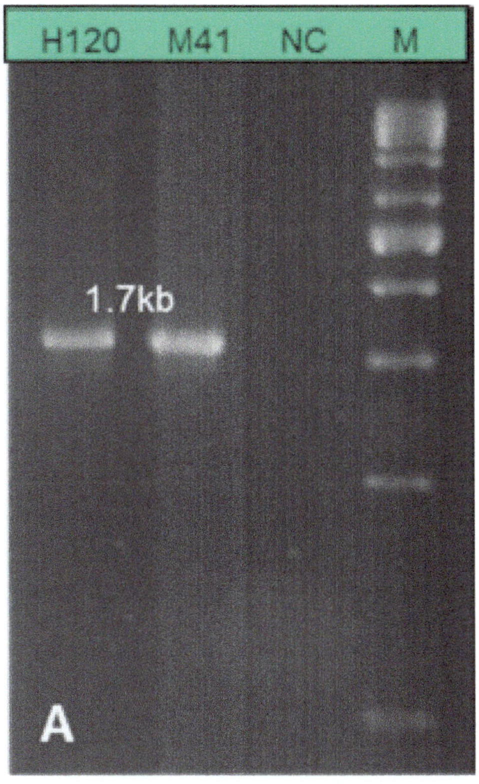

(a)

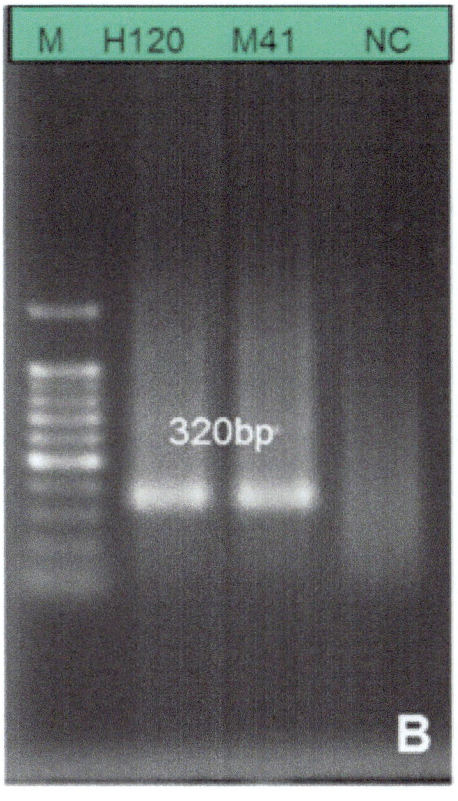

(b)

Figure 10: Electropherogram showing 1.7 kb RT-PCR amplified S1 genes from vaccine (H120) and virulent (M41) IBV strains (a) compared to a 320 bp RT-PCR amplified N-gene (b) of H120 and M41 IBV serotypes. Lane kb molecular ladder (a) and 100 bp ladder (b); lane NC: negative control (no template control).

Restriction Fragment Length Polymorphism (RFLP)

This is an IBV genotyping method carried out to differentiate different known strains of IBV and to identify new variants following RT-PCR amplification [75]. Full-length sequence of IBV S1 glycoprotein could be targeted for amplification and enzymes analysis [72, 76]. RFLP allows differentiation of various known IBV strains, based on their unique electrophoresis banding patterns defined by restriction enzyme digestion [72,77]. The assay was found to be comparable with traditional virus neutralization assay, although some strains such as the Gray and JMK strains were reportedly difficult to differentiate using arrays of restriction enzymes, thus limiting the universal application of this method [72].

Real-Time RT-PCR and Other Forms of PCR Assays

For increased test sensitivity and specificity, real-time RT-PCR assays [78, 79] have been introduced for detecting IBV. Apart from detection, it is possible to quantify IBV viral load from tissue and/or clinical samples by real-time RT-PCR assays based on viral copy number or fold changes [80, 81]. Likewise, differentiation of Massachusetts from non-Massachusetts is possible by real-time RT-PCR assay targeting S1 glycoprotein gene [79, 82]. Recently, a high resolution melt curve analysis (HRM) was also developed to allow differentiation of field from vaccine IBV strains as well as for rapid and sensitive detection of recombinant variants [83, 84]. Meir et al. [85] reported that real-time RT-PCR was comparable to virus isolation and one or two times more sensitive in detecting M41 IBV than ordinary N-gene and S1 gene specific RT-PCR assays. On the other hand, real-time RT-PCR was tenfold more sensitive compared to virus isolation and 30- or 40-fold compared to N-gene or S1 gene-based RT-PCR, respectively. The authors, however, reported variations in sensitivity when either N-gene or S1 genes were targeted as well as when different samples are used for viral amplification. Other forms of PCR methods used in detecting IBV include nested PCR [68]; multiplex PCR [86]; and reverse transcription loop-mediated isothermal amplification (RT-LAMP) [87]. While these methods are more sensitive than standard RT-PCR, they are more expensive as well and might be beyond the financial capacity of many producers.

Sequence and Phylogenetic Analyses

For genotyping, S1 gene usually is amplified using RT-PCR, sequenced, and subjected to bioinformatics analyses [88, 89]. Following S1 gene sequencing, isolates are characterized through bioinformatics analyses based on their phylogenetic relatedness with reference sequences available in sequence databases such as the NCBI, EMBL, and DDBJ (Figure 11). Lack of method standardization among laboratories, particularly with respect to the S1 gene segment length that is used in phylogenetic analysis, limits genotyping to some extent. Currently, molecular methods such as next generation sequencing (NGS) have been introduced to sequence whole genomes within limited periods of time, though this approach has been used only in the laboratory.

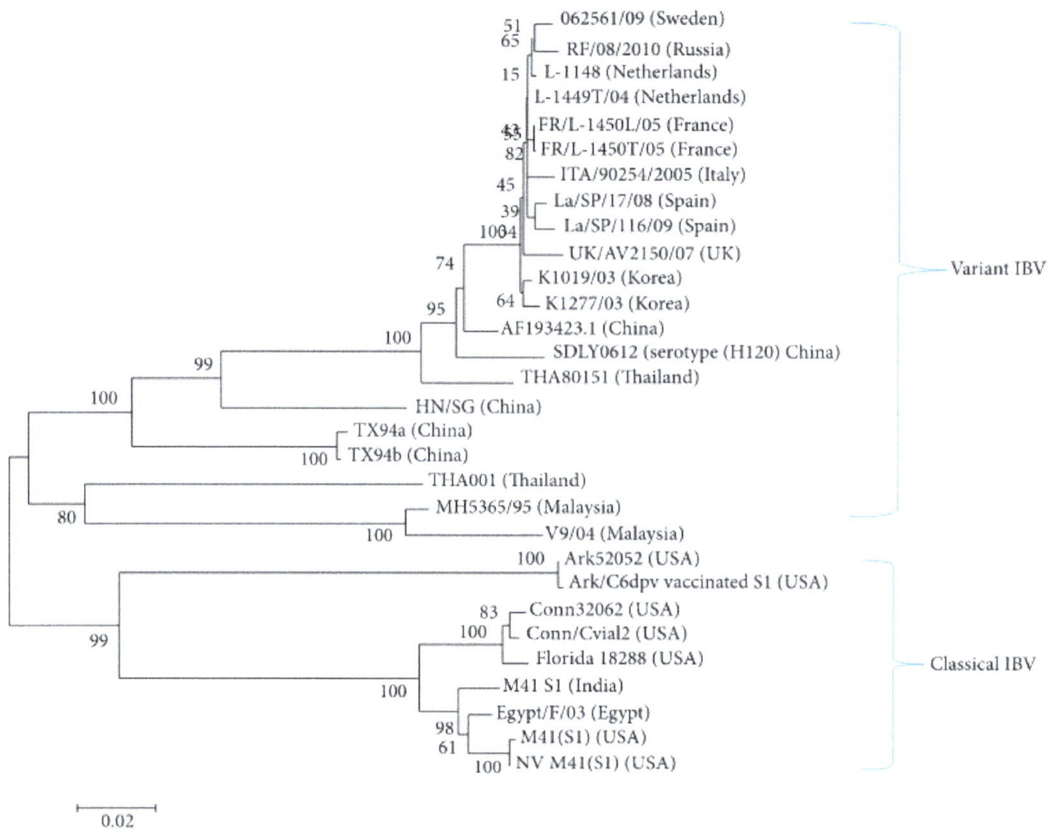

Figure 11: Neighbour joining phylogenetic analysis based on nucleotide acid sequence of S1-spike gene of classical and variant IBV strains identified in different countries. The tree was drawn with MEGA5 software using 1000 bootstrap replicates.

DIFFERENTIAL DIAGNOSIS

Several respiratory diseases, such as Newcastle disease (ND), infectious laryngotracheitis, infectious coryza, avian metapneumovirus (aMPV), and avian influenza (AI), may produce clinical signs similar to avian infectious bronchitis. However, certain clinical features, including neurological signs and diarrhoea in ND, high mortality in AI, and pronounced head swelling in coryza, are uncommon in IBV infection and thus may be used in ruling out or arriving at narrowed tentative differential list [33, 90].

CONCLUSION

Ever since the first identification of IBV in 1930s, the poultry industry has suffered a growing number of emerging IBV serotypes. Importantly, the newly evolved strains have been favoured by selection pressure, mutation, and/or recombinations, thus allowing them to avoid detection, evade host immune response, and cause diverse pathological outcomes. Lack of effective diagnostic methods and vaccines that could easily tackle the menace caused by multiple IBV serotypes is partly blamed for the serious economic losses as results of infectious bronchitis disease. Conventional detection assays such as virus neutralization and virus isolation have been used extensively, but, due to lack of sensitivity and specificity of serological assays and laborious nature of virus isolation methods, these assays have gradually been replaced by the new sensitive and specific assays such as RT-PCR, RFLP, and qRT-PCR that enable rapid genotyping and identification of new IBV strains. However, there is a need for standardization across laboratories with respect to the type and length of target gene to be considered for genotyping so as to ensure common understanding of genotype distributions in order to guide vaccine selection for prevention and control.

AUTHORS' CONTRIBUTION

Faruku Bande conceived the idea, collected and studied published papers, drafted the review paper, and made all uncited photos from cases handled in his Ph.D. work available. Siti Suri Arshad, Abdul Rahman Omar, Mohd Hair Bejo, Yusuf Abba, and Muhammad Salisu Abubakar all participated in conceptualization of the idea, study design, review, and editing of paper. Siti Suri Arshad provided photos used in Figures 1, 5, and 9. All authors have read and agreed with submission of final paper to the journal.

ACKNOWLEDGMENTS

The authors would like to thank the Universiti Putra Malaysia and Ministry of Science, Technology and Innovation (MOSTI), Project no. 02-01-04-SF1070 for funding supports. Dennis F. Lawler also provided paper-editing assistance.

REFERENCES

1. D. Cavanagh, "Coronavirus avian infectious bronchitis virus," Veterinary Research, vol. 38, no. 2, pp. 281–297, 2007. · ·
2. S. S. Arshad, "Infectious bronchitis," in Diseases of Poultry in South East Asia, M. Zamri-Saad, Ed., pp. 199–206, Universiti Putra Malaysia Press, Serdang, Malaysia, 2006.

3. A. Schalk and M. Hawn, "An apparently new respiratory disease of baby chicks," Journal of the American Veterinary Medical Association, vol. 78, pp. 413–422, 1931.

4. M. M. Lai and D. Cavanagh, "The molecular biology of coronaviruses," Advances in Virus Research, vol. 48, pp. 1–100, 1997. ·

5. C. A. M. de Haan, H. Vennema, and P. J. M. Rottier, "Assembly of the coronavirus envelope: homotypic interactions between the M proteins," Journal of Virology, vol. 74, no. 11, pp. 4967–4978, 2000. · ·

6. F. Bande, S. S. Arshad, M. Hair Bejo, H. Moeini, and A. R. Omar, "Progress and challenges toward the development of vaccines against avian infectious bronchitis," Journal of Immunology Research, vol. 2015, Article ID 424860, 12 pages, 2015, 10.1155/2015/424860.

7. E. Corse and C. E. Machamer, "The cytoplasmic tails of infectious bronchitis virus E and M proteins mediate their interaction," Virology, vol. 312, no. 1, pp. 25–34, 2003. · ·

8. L. Wilson, P. Gage, and G. Ewart, "Hexamethylene amiloride blocks E protein ion channels and inhibits coronavirus replication," Virology, vol. 353, no. 2, pp. 294–306, 2006. · ·

9. A. K. Williams, W. Li, L. W. Sneed, and E. W. Collisson, "Comparative analyses of the nucleocapsid genes of several strains of infectious bronchitis virus and other coronaviruses," Virus Research, vol. 25, no. 3, pp. 213–222, 1992. · ·

10. J. Jayaram, S. Youn, and E. W. Collisson, "The virion N protein of infectious bronchitis virus is more phosphorylated than the N protein from infected cell lysates," Virology, vol. 339, no. 1, pp. 127–135, 2005. · ·

11. M. W. Jackwood, D. Hall, and A. Handel, "Molecular evolution and emergence of avian gammacoronaviruses," Infection, Genetics and Evolution, vol. 12, no. 6, pp. 1305–1311, 2012. · ·

12. Z. J. Wei, P. Wei, M. L. Mo, M. Li, T. C. Wei, and K. R. Li, "Genetic variation of S1 gene hypervariable region I of infectious bronchitis viruses isolated in different periods in Guangxi," Chinese Journal of Virology, vol. 24, no. 2, pp. 126–132, 2008.

13. X.-M. Shi, Y. Zhao, H.-B. Gao et al., "Evaluation of recombinant fowlpox virus expressing infectious bronchitis virus S1 gene and chicken interferon-7 gene for immune protection against heterologous strains," Vaccine, vol. 29, no. 8, pp. 1576–1582, 2011. · ·

14. D. Cavanagh, K. Mawditt, D. D. B. Welchman, P. Britton, and R. E. Gough, "Coronaviruses from pheasants (Phasianus colchicus) are genetically closely related to coronaviruses of domestic fowl (infectious bronchitis virus) and turkeys," Avian Pathology, vol. 31, no. 1, pp. 81–93, 2002. · ·

15. S. Dea and P. Tijssen, "Detection of turkey enteric coronavirus by enzyme-linked immunosorbent assay and differentiation from other coronaviruses," American Journal of Veterinary Research, vol. 50, no. 2, pp. 226–231, 1989. ·

16. C. M. Jonassen, T. Kofstad, I.-L. Larsen et al., "Molecular identification and characterization of novel coronaviruses infecting graylag geese (Anser anser), feral pigeons (Columbia livia) and mallards (Anas platyrhynchos)," Journal of General Virology, vol. 86, no. 6, pp. 1597–1607, 2005. · ·

17. D. Cavanagh, "Coronaviridae: a review of coronaviruses and toroviruses," in Coronaviruses with Special Emphasis on First Insights Concerning SARS, pp. 1–54, Birkhäuser, Basel, Switzerland, 2005. ·

18. E. Circella, A. Camarda, V. Martella, G. Bruni, A. Lavazza, and C. Buonavoglia, "Coronavirus associated with an enteric syndrome on a quail farm," Avian Pathology, vol. 36, no. 3, pp. 251–258, 2007. · ·

19. J. S. Guy, "Turkey coronavirus is more closely related to avian infectious bronchitis virus than to mammalian coronaviruses: a review," Avian Pathology, vol. 29, no. 3, pp. 207–212, 2000. · ·

20. L. T. Miller and V. J. Yates, "Neutralization of infectious bronchitis virus human sera," American Journal of Epidemiology, vol. 88, no. 3, pp. 406–409, 1968. ·

21. R. A. Crinion and M. S. Hofstad, "Pathogenicity of four serotypes of avian infectious bronchitis virus for the oviduct of young chickens of various ages," Avian Diseases, vol. 16, no. 2, pp. 351–363, 1972. · ·

22. K. Otsuki, M. Huggins, and J. K. Cook, "Comparison of the susceptibility to avian infectious bronchitis virus infection of two inbred lines of white leghorn chickens," Avian Pathology, vol. 19, no. 3, pp. 467–475, 1990. ·

23. N. Bumstead, "Genetic resistance to avian viruses," OIE Revue Scientifique et Technique, vol. 17, no. 1, pp. 249–255, 1998. ·

24. L. D. Bacon, D. B. Hunter, H. M. Zhang, K. Brand, and R. Etches, "Retrospective evidence that the MHC (B haplotype) of chickens influences genetic resistance to attenuated infectious bronchitis vaccine strains in chickens," Avian Pathology, vol. 33, no. 6, pp. 605–609, 2004. · ·

25. G. J. Babcock, D. J. Esshaki, W. D. Thomas Jr., and D. M. Ambrosino, "Amino acids 270 to 510 of the severe acute respiratory syndrome coronavirus spike protein are required for interaction with receptor,"Journal of Virology, vol. 78, no. 9, pp. 4552–4560, 2004. · ·

26. N. Promkuntod, R. E. W. van Eijndhoven, G. de Vrieze, A. Gröne, and M. H. Verheije, "Mapping of the receptor-binding domain and amino acids critical for attachment in the spike protein of avian coronavirus infectious bronchitis virus," Virology, vol. 448, pp. 26–32, 2014. · ·

27. R. Casais, B. Dove, D. Cavanagh, and P. Britton, "Recombinant avian infectious bronchitis virus expressing a heterologous spike gene demonstrates that the spike protein is a determinant of cell tropism," Journal of Virology, vol. 77, no. 16, pp. 9084–9089, 2003. · ·

28. D. E. Wentworth and K. V. Holmes, Coronavirus Binding and Entry. Coronaviruses: Molecular and Cellular Biology, Caister Academic Press, Norfolk, UK, 2007.

29. C. Winter, C. Schwegmann-Weßels, D. Cavanagh, U. Neumann, and G. Herrler, "Sialic acid is a receptor determinant for infection of cells by avian infectious bronchitis virus," Journal of General Virology, vol. 87, no. 5, pp. 1209–1216, 2006. · ·

30. K. Shahwan, M. Hesse, A.-K. Mork, G. Herrler, and C. Winter, "Sialic acid binding properties of soluble coronavirus spike (S1) proteins: differences between infectious bronchitis virus and transmissible gastroenteritis virus," Viruses, vol. 5, no. 8, pp. 1924–1933, 2013. · ·

31. I. G. Madu, V. C. Chu, H. Lee, A. D. Regan, B. E. Bauman, and G. R. Whittaker, "Heparan sulfate is a selective attachment factor for the avian coronavirus infectious bronchitis virus Beaudette," Avian Diseases, vol. 51, no. 1, pp. 45–51, 2007. · ·

32. V. C. Chu, L. J. McElroy, V. Chu, B. E. Bauman, and G. R. Whittaker, "The avian coronavirus infectious bronchitis virus undergoes direct low-pH-dependent fusion activation during entry into host cells,"Journal of Virology, vol. 80, no. 7, pp. 3180–3188, 2006. · ·

33. D. Cavanagh and J. Gelb, "Infectious bronchitis," in Diseases of Poultry, pp. 117–135, Wiley-Blackwell, 12th edition, 2008.

34. D. J. Alexander and R. E. Gough, "Isolation of avian infectious bronchitis virus from experimentally infected chickens," Research in Veterinary Science, vol. 23, no. 3, pp. 344–347, 1977. ·

35. S. Arshad, K. Al-Salihi, and M. Noordin, "Ultrastructural pathology of trachea in chicken experimentally infected with infectious bronchitis Virus-MH-5365/95," Annals of Microscopy, vol. 3, pp. 43–47, 2002.

36. C. Terregino, A. Toffan, M. Serena Beato et al., "Pathogenicity of a QX strain of infectious bronchitis virus in specific pathogen free and commercial broiler chickens, and evaluation of protection induced by a vaccination programme based on the Ma5 and 4/91 serotypes," Avian Pathology, vol. 37, no. 5, pp. 487–493, 2008. · ·

37. R. W. Winterfield, H. L. Thacker, and S. F. Badylak, "Effects of subtype variations in the Holland strain of infectious bronchitis virus when applied as a vaccine," Poultry Science, vol. 63, no. 2, pp. 246–250, 1984.· ·

38. D. A. Purcell and J. B. McFerran, "The histopathology of infectious bronchitis in the domestic fowl,"Research in Veterinary Science, vol. 13, no. 2, pp. 116–122, 1972. ·

39. Z. Boroomand, K. Asasi, and A. Mohammadi, "Pathogenesis and tissue distribution of avian infectious bronchitis virus isolate IRFIBV32 (793/B serotype) in experimentally infected broiler chickens," The Scientific World Journal, vol. 2012, Article ID 402537, 6 pages, 2012. · ·

40. H. Toro, V. Godoy, J. Larenas, E. Reyes, and E. F. Kaleta, "Avian infectious bronchitis: viral persistence in the harderian gland and histological changes after eyedrop vaccination," Avian Diseases, vol. 40, no. 1, pp. 114–120, 1996. · ·

41. F. Cong, X. Liu, Z. Han, Y. Shao, X. Kong, and S. Liu, "Transcriptome analysis of chicken kidney tissues following coronavirus avian infectious bronchitis virus infection," BMC Genomics, vol. 14, no. 1, article 743, 2013. · ·

42. K. K. Chousalkar, J. R. Roberts, and R. Reece, "Histopathology of two serotypes of infectious bronchitis virus in laying hens vaccinated in the rearing phase," Poultry Science, vol. 86, no. 1, pp. 59–62, 2007. · ·

43. K. K. Chousalkar and J. R. Roberts, "Ultrastructural study of infectious bronchitis virus infection in infundibulum and magnum of commercial laying hens," Veterinary Microbiology, vol. 122, no. 3-4, pp. 223–236, 2007. · ·

44. K. K. Chousalkar, J. R. Roberts, and R. Reece, "Comparative histopathology of two serotypes of infectious bronchitis virus (T and N1/88) in laying hens and cockerels," Poultry Science, vol. 86, no. 1, pp. 50–58, 2007. · ·

45. R. W. Winterfield and S. B. Hitchner, "Etiology of an infectious nephritis-nephrosis syndrome of chickens," American Journal of Veterinary Research, vol. 23, pp. 1273–1279, 1962. ·

46. J. J. de Wit, J. Nieuwenhuisen-van Wilgen, A. Hoogkamer, H. vande Sande, G. J. Zuidam, and T. H. F. Fabri, "Induction of cystic oviducts and protection against early challenge with infectious bronchitis virus serotype D388 (genotype QX) by maternally derived antibodies and by early vaccination," Avian Pathology, vol. 40, no. 5, pp. 463–471, 2011. · ·

47. M. P. Ariaans, M. G. R. Matthijs, D. van Haarlem et al., "The role of phagocytic cells in enhanced susceptibility of broilers to colibacillosis after infectious bronchitis virus infection," Veterinary Immunology and Immunopathology, vol. 123, no. 3-4, pp. 240–250, 2008. · ·

48. R. A. Gallardo, V. L. van Santen, and H. Toro, "Effects of chicken anaemia virus and infectious bursal disease virus-induced immunodeficiency on infectious bronchitis virus replication and genotypic drift,"Avian Pathology, vol. 41, no. 5, pp. 451–458, 2012. · ·

49. J. Ignjatovic, D. F. Ashton, R. Reece, P. Scott, and P. Hooper, "Pathogenicity of Australian strains of avian infectious bronchitis virus," Journal of Comparative Pathology, vol. 126, no. 2-3, pp. 115–123, 2002. · ·

50. D. King and D. Cavanagh, "Infectious bronchitis," Diseases of Poultry, vol. 9, pp. 471–484, 1991.

51. OIE, Avian Infectious Bronchitis, chapter 2. 3. 2., 2008.

52. D. Cavanagh, P. J. Davis, and J. K. Cook, "Infectious bronchitis virus: evidence for recombination within the Massachusetts serotype," Avian Pathology, vol. 21, no. 3, pp. 401–408, 1992. ·

53. A. Kant, G. Koch, D. J. Van Roozelaar, J. G. Kusters, F. A. J. Poelwijk, and B. A. M. Van der Zeijst, "Location of antigenic sites defined by neutralizing monoclonal antibodies on the S1 avian infectious bronchitis virus glycopolypeptide," Journal of General Virology, vol. 73, no. 3, pp. 591–596, 1992. · ·

54. F. Beaudette and C. Hudson, "Cultivation of the virus of infectious bronchitis," Journal of the American Veterinary Medical Association, vol. 90, pp. 51–60, 1937.

55. C. B. Stephensen, D. B. Casebolt, and N. N. Gangopadhyay, "Phylogenetic analysis of a highly conserved region of the polymerase gene from 11 coronaviruses and development of a consensus polymerase chain reaction assay," Virus Research, vol. 60, no. 2, pp. 181–189, 1999. · ·

56. J. Gelb Jr., W. A. Nix, and S. D. Gellman, "Infectious bronchitis virus antibodies in tears and their relationship to immunity," Avian Diseases, vol. 42, no. 2, pp. 364–374, 1998. · ·

57. L. N. Loomis, C. H. Cunningham, M. L. Gray, and F. Thorp Jr., "Pathology of the chicken embryo infected with infectious bronchitis virus," American Journal of Veterinary Research, vol. 11, no. 40, pp. 245–251, 1950. ·

58. K. Otsuki, H. Yamamoto, and M. Tsubokura, "Studies on avian infectious bronchitis virus (IBV)—I. Resistance of IBV to chemical and physical treatments," Archives of Virology, vol. 60, no. 1, pp. 25–32, 1979. · ·

59. S. S. Arshad, A study on two malaysian isolates of infectious bronchitis virus [Ph.D. thesis], Universiti Pertanian Malaysia, 1993.

60. B. V. Jones and R. M. Hennion, "The preparation of chicken tracheal organ cultures for virus isolation, propagation, and titration," Methods in Molecular Biology, vol. 454, pp. 103–107, 2008. · ·

61. P. S. Bhattacharjee and R. C. Jones, "Susceptibility of organ cultures from chicken tissues for strains of infectious bronchitis virus isolated from the intestine," Avian Pathology, vol. 26, no. 3, pp. 553–563, 1997. · ·

62. M. Armesto, S. Evans, D. Cavanagh, A.-B. Abu-Median, S. Keep, and P. Britton, "A recombinant Avian infectious bronchitis virus expressing a heterologous spike gene belonging to the 4/91 serotype," PLoS ONE, vol. 6, no. 8, Article ID e24352, 2011. · ·

63. S. Patterson and R. W. Bingham, "Electron microscope observations on the entry of avian infectious bronchitis virus into susceptible cells," Archives of Virology, vol. 52, no. 3, pp. 191–200, 1976. · ·

64. A. Bezuidenhout, S. P. Mondal, and E. L. Buckles, "Histopathological and immunohistochemical study of air sac lesions induced by two strains of infectious bronchitis virus," Journal of Comparative Pathology, vol. 145, no. 4, pp. 319–326, 2011. · ·

65. S. S. Arshad and K. A. Al-Salihi, "Immunohistochemical detection of infectious bronchitis virus antigen in chicken respiratory and kidney tissues," in Proceedings of the 12th Federation of Asian Veterinary Associations Congress/14th Veterinary Association Malaysia Scientific Congress, p. 51, August 2002.

66. A. S. Abdel-Moneim, P. Zlotowski, J. Veits, G. M. Keil, and J. P. Teifke, "Immunohistochemistry for detection of avian infectious bronchitis virus strain M41 in the proventriculus and nervous system of experimentally infected chicken embryos," Virology Journal, vol. 6, article 15, 2009. ·

67. K. Yagyu and S. Ohta, "Detection of infectious bronchitis virus antigen from experimentally infected chickens by indirect immunofluorescent assay with monoclonal antibody," Avian Diseases, vol. 34, no. 2, pp. 246–252, 1990. · ·

68. A. Adzhar, K. Shaw, P. Britton, and D. Cavanagh, "Universal oligonucleotides for the detection of infectious bronchitis virus by the polymerase chain reaction," Avian Pathology, vol. 25, no. 4, pp. 817–836, 1996. · ·

69. A. Adzhar, R. E. Gough, D. Haydon, K. Shaw, P. Britton, and D. Cavanagh, "Molecular analysis of the 793/B serotype of infectious bronchitis virus in Great Britain," Avian Pathology, vol. 26, no. 3, pp. 625–640, 1997. · ·

70. Z. Lin, A. Kato, Y. Kudou, K. Umeda, and S. Ueda, "Typing of recent infectious bronchitis virus isolates causing nephritis in chicken," Archives of Virology, vol. 120, no. 1-2, pp. 145–149, 1991. · ·

71. K. A. Zwaagstra, B. A. M. van der Zeijst, and J. G. Kusters, "Rapid detection and identification of avian infectious bronchitis virus," Journal of Clinical Microbiology, vol. 30, no. 1, pp. 79–84, 1992. ·

72. H. M. Kwon, M. W. Jackwood, and J. Gelb Jr., "Differentiation of infectious bronchitis virus serotypes using polymerase chain reaction and restriction fragment length polymorphism analysis," Avian Diseases, vol. 37, no. 1, pp. 194–202, 1993. · ·

73. C. L. Keeler Jr., K. L. Reed, W. A. Nix, and J. Gelb Jr., "Serotype identification of avian infectious bronchitis virus by RT-PCR of the peplomer (S-1) gene," Avian Diseases, vol. 42, no. 2, pp. 275–284, 1998. · ·

74. J. G. Zhu, H. D. Qian, Y. L. Zhang, X. G. Hua, and Z. L. Wu, "Analysis of similarity of the S1 gene in infectious bronchitis virus (IBV) isolates in Shanghai, China," Archivos de Medicina Veterinaria, vol. 39, no. 3, pp. 223–228, 2007. ·

75. Z. Lin, A. Kato, Y. Kudou, and S. Ueda, "A new typing method for the avian infectious bronchitis virus using polymerase chain reaction and restriction enzyme fragment length polymorphism," Archives of Virology, vol. 116, no. 1–4, pp. 19–31, 1991. · ·

76. K. Mardani, A. H. Noormohammadi, J. Ignatovic, and G. F. Browning, "Typing infectious bronchitis virus strains using reverse transcription-polymerase chain reaction and restriction fragment length polymorphism analysis to compare the 3′ 7.5 kb of their genomes," Avian Pathology, vol. 35, no. 1, pp. 63–69, 2006. · ·

77. M. D. F. S. Montassier, L. Brentano, H. J. Montassier, and L. J. Richtzenhain, "Genetic grouping of avian infectious bronchitis virus isolated in Brazil based on RT-PCR/RFLP analysis of the S1 gene," Pesquisa Veterinaria Brasileira, vol. 28, no. 3, pp. 190–194, 2008. ·

78. K. K. Chousalkar, B. F. Cheetham, and J. R. Roberts, "LNA probe-based real-time RT-PCR for the detection of infectious bronchitis virus from the oviduct of unvaccinated and vaccinated laying hens,"Journal

of Virological Methods, vol. 155, no. 1, pp. 67–71, 2009. · ·

79. A. M. Acevedo, C. L. Perera, A. Vega et al., "A duplex SYBR Green I-based real-time RT-PCR assay for the simultaneous detection and differentiation of Massachusetts and non-Massachusetts serotypes of infectious bronchitis virus," Molecular and Cellular Probes, vol. 27, no. 5-6, pp. 184–192, 2013. · ·

80. M. W. Jackwood, D. A. Hilt, and S. A. Callison, "Detection of infectious bronchitis virus by real-time reverse transcriptase-polymerase chain reaction and identification of a quasispecies in the Beaudette strain," Avian Diseases, vol. 47, no. 3, pp. 718–724, 2003. · ·

81. S. A. Callison, D. A. Hilt, T. O. Boynton et al., "Development and evaluation of a real-time Taqman RT-PCR assay for the detection of infectious bronchitis virus from infected chickens," Journal of Virological Methods, vol. 138, no. 1-2, pp. 60–65, 2006. · ·

82. R. M. Jones, R. J. Ellis, W. J. Cox et al., "Development and validation of RT-PCR tests for the detection and S1 genotyping of infectious bronchitis virus and other closely related gammacoronaviruses within clinical samples," Transboundary and Emerging Diseases, vol. 58, no. 5, pp. 411–420, 2011. · ·

83. K. Hewson, A. H. Noormohammadi, J. M. Devlin, K. Mardani, and J. Ignjatovic, "Rapid detection and non-subjective characterisation of infectious bronchitis virus isolates using high-resolution melt curve analysis and a mathematical model," Archives of Virology, vol. 154, no. 4, pp. 649–660, 2009. · ·

84. K. A. Hewson, G. F. Browning, J. M. Devlin, J. Ignjatovic, and A. H. Noormohammadi, "Application of high-resolution melt curve analysis for classification of infectious bronchitis viruses in field specimens,"Australian Veterinary Journal, vol. 88, no. 10, pp. 408–413, 2010. · ·

85. R. Meir, O. Maharat, Y. Farnushi, and L. Simanov, "Development of a real-time TaqMan® RT-PCR assay for the detection of infectious bronchitis virus in chickens, and comparison of RT-PCR and virus isolation," Journal of Virological Methods, vol. 163, no. 2, pp. 190–194, 2010. · ·

86. H.-W. Chen and C.-H. Wang, "A multiplex reverse transcriptase-PCR assay for the genotyping of avian infectious bronchitis viruses," Avian Diseases, vol. 54, no. 1, pp. 104–108, 2010. · ·

87. H.-T. Chen, J. Zhang, Y.-P. Ma et al., "Reverse transcription loop-mediated isothermal amplification for the rapid detection of infectious bronchitis virus in infected chicken tissues," Molecular and Cellular Probes, vol. 24, no. 2, pp. 104–106, 2010. · ·

88. Z. M. Zulperi, A. R. Omar, and S. S. Arshad, "Sequence and phylogenetic analysis of S1, S2, M, and N genes of infectious bronchitis virus isolates from Malaysia," Virus Genes, vol. 38, no. 3, pp. 383–391, 2009. · ·

89. S. H. Abro, L. H. M. Renström, K. Ullman et al., "Emergence of novel strains of avian infectious bronchitis virus in Sweden," Veterinary Microbiology, vol. 155, no. 2–4, pp. 237–246, 2012. · ·

90. R. Droual and P. Woolcock, "Swollen head syndrome associated with E. coli and infectious bronchitis virus in the Central Valley of California," Avian Pathology, vol. 23, no. 4, pp. 733–742, 1994. ·

CHAPTER 7

MODELLING MAREK'S DISEASE VIRUS (MDV) INFECTION: PARAMETER ESTIMATES FOR MORTALITY RATE AND INFECTIOUSNESS

Katherine E Atkins[1,4], Andrew F Read[2], Nicholas J Savill[1], Katrin G Renz[3], Stephen W Walkden-Brown[3] and Mark EJ Woolhouse[1]

[1] Centre for Infectious Diseases, University Of Edinburgh, West Mains Road, EH9 3JT, UK

[2] Center for Infectious Disease Dynamics, Departments of Biology and Entomology, 208 Mueller Laboratory, The Pennsylvania State University, University Park, PA 16802, USA

[3] Centre for Animal Health and Welfare, School of Environmental and Rural Science, The University of New England, Armidale NSW 2351, Australia

[4] Department of Epidemiology and Public Health, Yale School of Medicine, New Haven

ABSTRACT

Background

Marek's disease virus (MDV) is an economically important oncogenic herpesvirus of poultry. Since the 1960s, increasingly virulent strains have caused continued poultry industry production losses worldwide. To understand the mechanisms of this virulence evolution and to evaluate the epidemiological consequences of putative control strategies, it is imperative to understand how virulence is defined and how this correlates with host mortality and infectiousness during MDV infection. We present a mathematical approach to quantify key epidemiological parameters. Host lifespan, virus latent periods and host viral shedding rates were estimated for unvaccinated and vaccinated birds, infected with one of three MDV strains. The strains had previously been pathotyped to assign virulence scores according to pathogenicity of strains in hosts.

Results

Our analyses show that strains of higher virulence have a higher viral shedding rate, and more rapidly kill hosts. Vaccination enhances host life expectancy but does not significantly reduce the shedding rate of the virus. While the primary latent period of the virus does not vary with challenge strain nor vaccine treatment of host, the time until the maximum viral shedding rate is increased with vaccination.

Conclusions

Our approach provides the tools necessary for a formal analysis of the evolution of virulence in MDV, and potentially simpler and cheaper approaches to comparing the virulence of MDV strains.

Citation: Katherine E Atkins, Andrew F Read, Nicholas J Savill1, Katrin G Renz, Stephen W Walkden-Brown and Mark EJ Woolhouse, Modelling Marek's Disease Virus (MDV) infection: parameter estimates for mortality rate and infectiousness, DOI: 10.1186/1746-6148-7-70.

BACKGROUND

Marek's Disease Virus (MDV) is an oncogenic poultry herpesvirus of considerable economic importance to the poultry industry. Virus strains have become increasingly virulent since the 1960s [1, 2]. The causes of this viral evolution are unclear [3]. Quantification of patterns of viral shedding and virus-induced host mortality are necessary for a rigorous understanding of the epidemiology of a disease, not least to identify increases in virulence. Here we develop methods to do this.

MDV is an airborne pathogen with infection occurring via inhalation [4]. Virus shedding occurs by infected feather follicle epithelium [5]. The resulting dust and dander from dead stratified cells and moulted feathers can then remain in the environment and act as a reservoir for chicken infection. Clinical signs are varied and result in significant morbidity and mortality depending on host genetic susceptibility and virulence of the MDV strain [6]. Symptoms include polyneuritis (an enlargement of multiple peripheral nerves), visceral lymphoma (tumours affecting organs such as the heart, liver, spleen etc.), acute transient paralysis, immunosuppression, brain oedema and acute rash. There has been a change in the types of clinical signs since the disease was first noted [7, 8], when chronic polyneuritis was the only sign. Since then, the list of clinical signs described above expanded gradually over the decades [2].

Almost all industrialised countries have experienced MD losses in their poultry industry and a crude estimate of the cost of Marek's disease is said to be in the range of US $1-2 billion annually [7]. Control of Marek's disease is predominantly via vaccination of chickens. Crucially the MDV vaccine was the first vaccine to be developed against any cancer [9]. Three types of vaccine have been developed for use against MD. These are herpesvirus of turkeys (HVT), non-pathogenic serotype 2 MDV and non-pathogenic serotype 1 [10]. These vaccines have been used in different sequences in different countries and the vaccine types have also been commonly combined in bivalent or trivalent vaccines.

Definitions of virulence are numerous and varied [11]. Microbiologists equate virulence with the notions of both infectivity and severity of disease, whereas evolutionary biologists focus on evolutionary fitness of either the pathogen or the host [12]. Zoologists tend to focus on host fitness [13, 14] with most mathematical models describing this specifically as host mortality [14, 15].

There have been various attempts to define virulence in the context of MDV [16]. For example, Witter [1] relates the percentage of HVT or Bivalent (HVT + serotype 2) vaccinated chickens, that when infected with a particular strain develop gross lesions or die of Marek's disease within eight weeks to the figure in unvaccinated chickens challenged with the same strain. This percentage score uses the protective effect of vaccines as its metric for virulence. In addition, [17] use neurovirulence as a tool for pathotyping MDV strains, noting that many of the very virulent strains are synonymous with high levels of neuropathology. This method circumvents the need for both vaccine-based definitions and therefore high numbers of birds, and also may cut the experiment time. In the first pathotyping regime, there are four recognised MDV serotype 1 pathotypes, each occupying part of the 'continuum of virulence' [1] defined as: mild, m; virulent, v; very virulent, vv; very virulent plus, vv+. This grouping correlates very well with the second pathotyping regime [18].

Control strategies for MDV require an understanding of the epidemiology of the disease, in particular how virulence relates to key parameters such as viral shedding rates and duration of infectious period. There have been efforts to find correlates with virulence of MDV isolates, most notably with viral load (virus within a bird tissue). This has been achieved by cell culture techniques [19] and intra-cellular detection during the first 10 days of infection [20]. However, the relationship between viral load (or replication) and virulence has not been convincingly tested [16]. PCR testing methods have been developed in order to quantify viral loads [20, 21, 22,23, 24, 25, 26], which have enabled the viral loads in shed dust to be directly measured [27, 28]. The infectious period is defined as the total time in which an infected bird sheds virus [29]. This is determined by the clearance rate and the lifespan of the individual host. Since there is no recovery from MDV infection, the infectious period is defined by a total of four parameters: the disease-induced mortality, the latent period (the time between infection and infectiousness of a host) and two other non-disease associated parameters, namely non-disease induced mortality and the maximum lifespan of an individual (the farm slaughter time in the case of broilers).

Here we present methods for parameter estimation for MDV isolates, allowing a formal quantification of infected host lifespan, viral shedding rates and viral latent periods. The parameters determined from the analysis allow comparison between isolates of different virulence in both unvaccinated and vaccinated birds. It is anticipated that the parameter estimates will be used for a better understanding of the pathology and aetiology of the disease itself and as a platform for investigation into the causes of virulence evolution.

RESULTS

In the first section, we used survival analysis with a Weibull mortality function to build a statistical model for the lifespan of birds infected with MDV. In the second section, we developed a dynamic model to simulate the shedding of virus by a group of birds and used Bayesian techniques to estimate the four key infectiousness parameters: primary and secondary latent periods and viral shedding rates.

Mortality

An additive covariate Weibull regression model was fitted to the bird survival data, since the interaction terms were not significant. The model estimates are given in Table 1. The Weibull model captures the data significantly better with the covariates used than without ($p < 0.01$). The resulting graphs showing the data and Weibull model fit are displayed in Figure 1. The model showed that host lifespan decreased with virulence score and increased with vaccination (Figure 2 and Table 1), although there was no significant difference between the effect of the two vaccines on lifespan (Table 1). On most days there were either zero or one birds dying from MDV-related illness from the initial 52 or 53 individual birds in each group (Figure 1). These data and further information are published in separate experimental work [30].

Table 1: Survival analysis: Estimated coefficients of the covariates in the survival analysis

Symbol	**Coefficient**	**Value (95% CI via McMC)**	z	p
r	Shape Parameter	4.18 (3.38,4.99)	-11.60	< 0.001
β_0	Intercept	4.54 (4.23,4.87)	26.08	< 0.001
β_1	Virulence Score	-0.53 (-1.01,-0.06)	-2.04	0.040
β_2	HVT vaccine	0.44 (0.24,0.66)	3.95	< 0.001
β_3	Bivalent vaccine	0.35 (0.19,0.52)	4.28	< 0.001

The transformed virulence score is a continuous covariate and the vaccine treatment is a categorical covariate in an additive regression, giving the test statistic, z and the corresponding p value. The numbers in brackets are the 95% credible intervals.

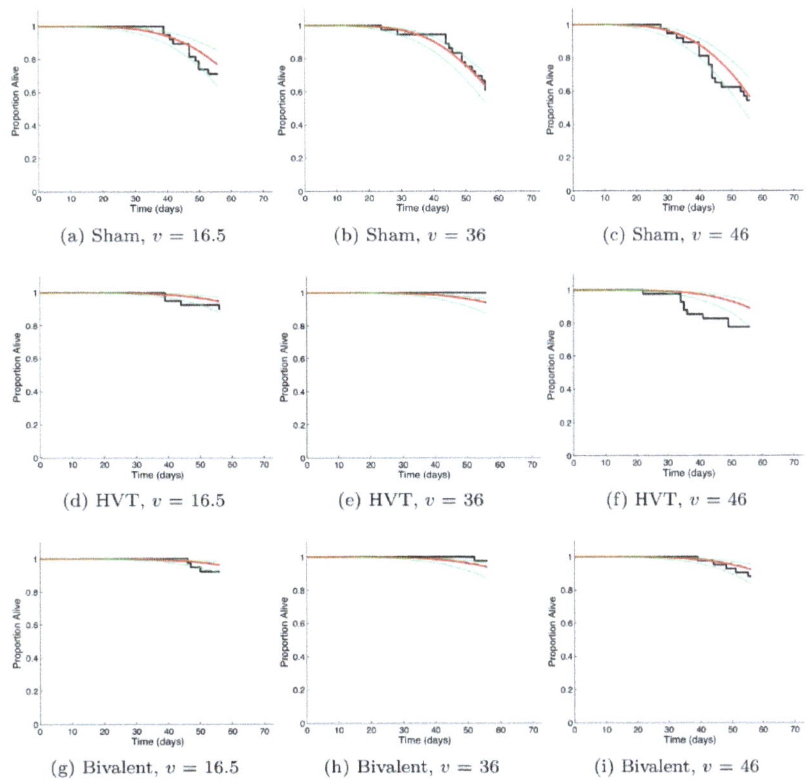

Figure 1: Mortality: Three different treatments crossed with three different virulence scores as stated. Graphs show data (black), maximum likelihood estimate of Weibull distribution (red) and 95% credible interval (green). Transformed virulence score (continuous) and vaccine treatment (categorical) are the (additive) covariates.

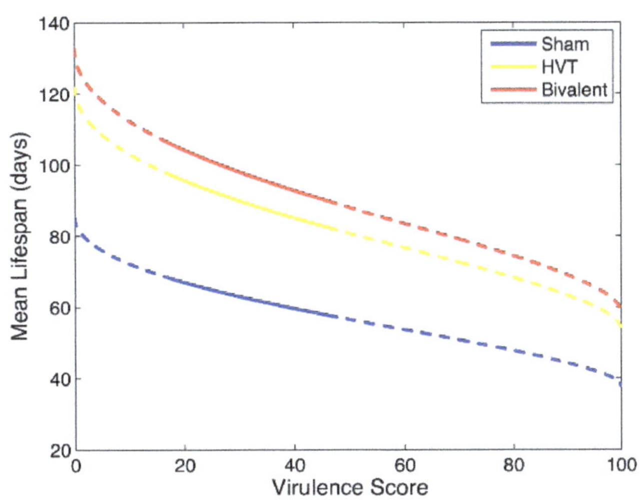

Figure 2: Mortality: Maximum likelihood estimates of and r give the mean lifespan ($\lambda\Gamma(1+1r)$, where $\Gamma(z)$ is the Gamma function as it varies with virulence score. The dashed lines represent extrapolation outside virulence scores given in data.

Shedding

The dynamic model output records the density of virus (measured in viral copy number (VCN)/mg dust), which fitted to the data from each isolator independently. The model fits can be compared directly in Figures 3, 4and 5, which give the day of sampling and the sample value. These data and further information are published in a separate experimental paper [30].

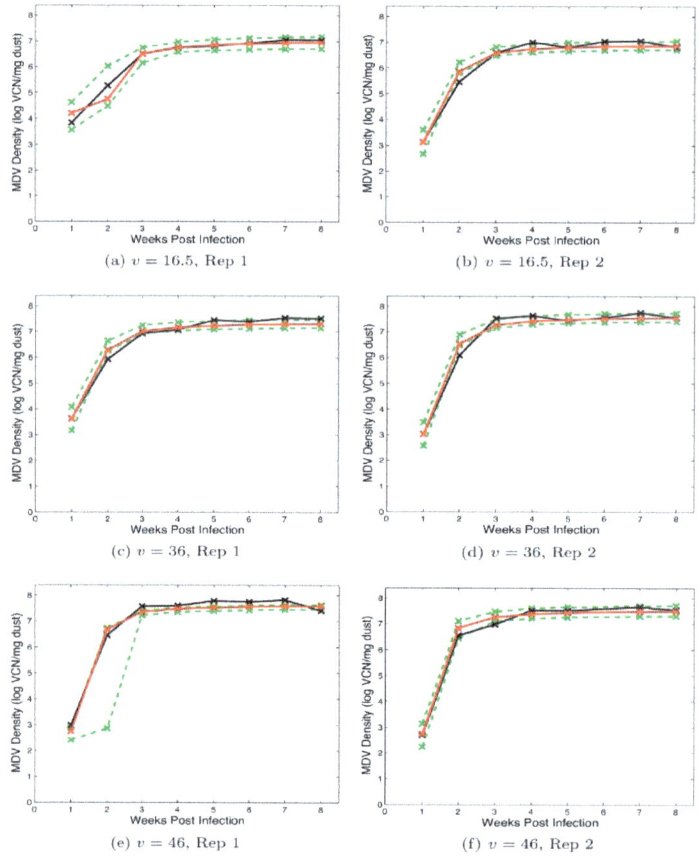

Figure 3: Viral Shedding: Sham vaccinated treatments. Graphs include the data (black), the maximum likelihood realisation (red) and the 95% credible interval (green). The panels show each replicate for the virus strains which have been given the virulence score, v as denoted in the caption.

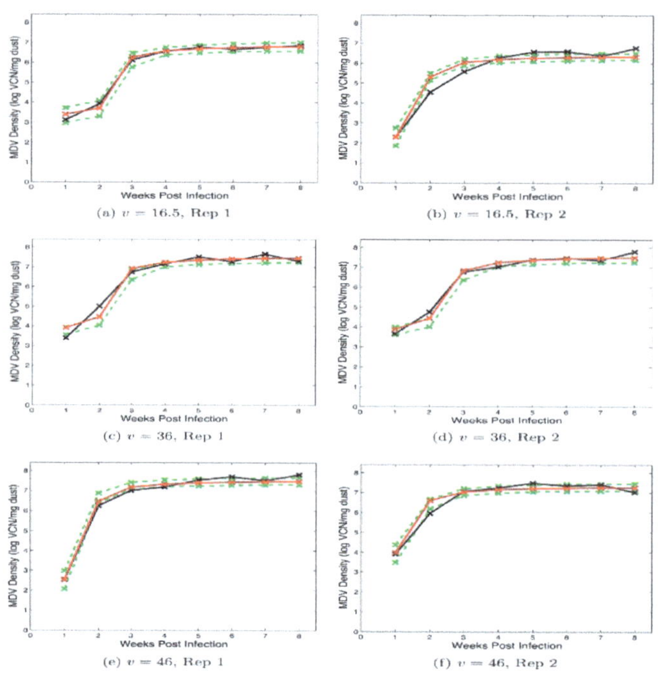

Figure 4: Viral Shedding: HVT vaccinated treatments. Graphs include the data (black), the maximum likelihood realisation (red) and the 95% credible interval (green). The panels show each replicate for the virus strains which have been given the virulence score, v as denoted in the caption.

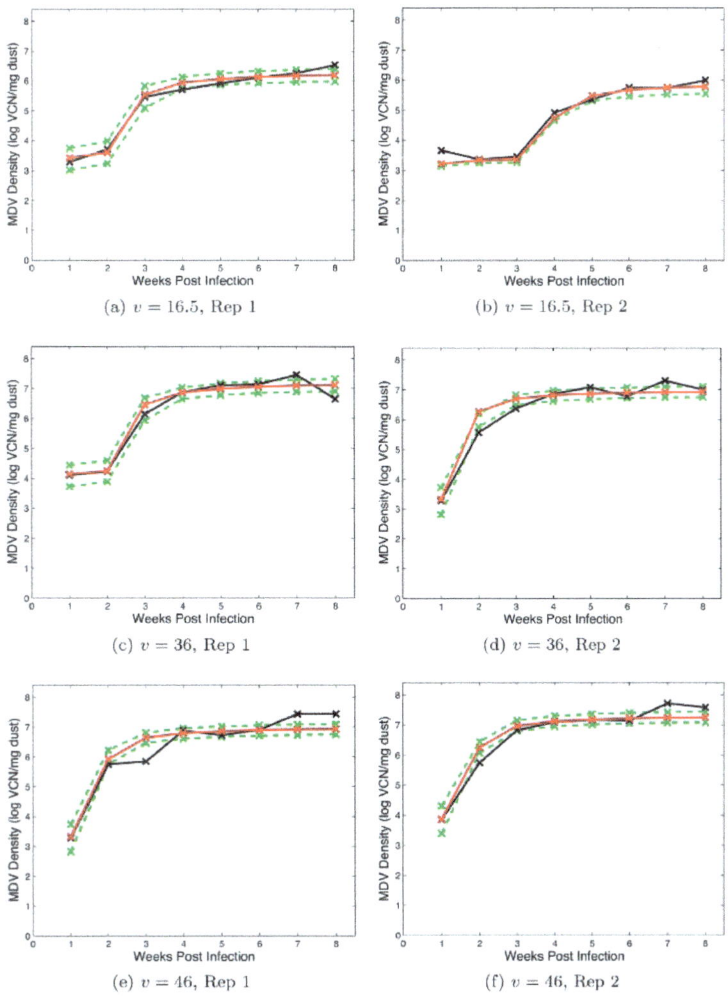

Figure 5: Viral Shedding: Bivalent vaccinated treatments. Graphs include the data (black), the maximum likelihood realisation (red) and the 95% credible interval (green). The panels show each replicate for the virus strains which have been given the virulence score, *v* as denoted in the caption.

For each isolator, the median of the posterior distribution for the four parameters in the model (two latent periods and two rates of viral shedding) are given in Tables 2, 3 and 4, where the number of air changes per hour, , is set to 15. Assuming ∈ [5, 25], the results obtained in the McMC method did not change, whatever value of is chosen.

Table 2: Viral shedding unvaccinated: median and 95% credible intervals for the posterior distribution of the four parameters for both replicates of the sham vaccinated factorial study for different virulence scores, *v*

			VIRULENCE SCORE			
PARAMETER	**16.5**		**36**		**46**	
	Rep 1	**Rep 2**	**Rep 1**	**Rep 2**	**Rep 1**	**Rep 2**
1 Latent Period (days)	6 (2,6)	4 (0,6)	4 (0,6)	4 (0,6)	3 (0,6)	3 (0,6)
2 Latent Period (days)	10 (7,14)	9 (6,13)	9 (6,13)	9 (6,13)	9 (6,13)	9 (5,13)
1 Shedding Rate (logVCN/mg dust)	4.87 (3.79,5.25)	3.37 (2.79,4.05)	3.86 (3.30,4.56)	3.28 (2.71,3.95)	3.20 (2.64,3.90)	2.89 (2.34,3.59)
2 Shedding Rate (logVCN/mg dust)	6.99 (6.72,7.21)	6.89 (6.72,7.07)	7.34 (7.17,7.51)	7.58 (7.41,7.76)	7.69 (7.51,7.85)	7.52 (7.32,7.72)

The numbers in brackets are the 95% credible intervals.

Table 3: Viral shedding HVT vaccination: median and 95% credible intervals for the posterior distribution of the four parameters for both replicates of the HVT vaccinated factorial study for different virulence scores, *v*

			VIRULENCE SCORE			
PARAMETER	**16.5**		**36**		**46**	
	Rep 1	**Rep 2**	**Rep 1**	**Rep 2**	**Rep 1**	**Rep 2**
1 Latent Period (days)	5 (0,6)	2 (0,6)	6 (4,6)	6 (2,6)	3 (0,6)	3 (0,6)
2 Latent Period (days)	12 (8,17)	10 (7,13)	11 (8,14)	12 (8,16)	10 (6,13)	9 (6,13)
1 Shedding Rate (logVCN/mg dust)	3.79 (3.34,4.20)	2.44 (1.93,3.02)	4.58 (4.19,4.92)	4.56 (4.13,4.91)	2.70 (2.16,3.42)	4.15 (3.58,4.82)
2 Shedding Rate (logVCN/mg dust)	6.83 (6.61,7.04)	6.35 (6.18,6.52)	7.49 (7.28,7.70)	7.53 (7.31,7.75)	7.50 (7.32,7.67)	7.29 (7.11,7.46)

The numbers in brackets are the 95% credible intervals.

Table 4: Viral shedding bivalent vaccination: median and 95% credible intervals for the posterior distribution of the four parameters for both replicates of the Bivalent vaccinated factorial study for different virulence scores, *v*

			VIRULENCE SCORE			
PARAMETER	**16.5**		**36**		**46**	
	Rep 1	**Rep 2**	**Rep 1**	**Rep 2**	**Rep 1**	**Rep 2**
1 Latent Period (days)	4 (0,6)	2 (0,5)	3 (0,6)	3 (0,6)	3 (0,6)	3 (0,6)
2 Latent Period (days)	14 (9,19)	23 (18,27)	15 (10,19)	9 (6,13)	10 (6,13)	10 (6,13)
1 Shedding Rate (logVCN/mg dust)	4.87 (3.27,5.19)	3.37 (3.27,3.83)	3.86 (2.92,4.70)	3.28 (2.93,4.14)	3.20 (2.94,4.18)	2.89 (2.49,4.69)
2 Shedding Rate (logVCN/mg dust)	6.23 (6.02,6.45)	5.85 (5.61,6.09)	7.16 (6.94,7.37)	6.95 (6.78,7.13)	6.96 (6.78,7.12)	7.28 (7.11,7.45)

The numbers in brackets are the 95% credible intervals.

A linear model was fitted to account for the variation in the primary and secondary latent periods, with the latent period as the response variable and arcsine square-root transformed virulence score and vaccine treatment as multiplicative covariates. For the primary latent period, none of the results were significant ($p = 0.41$), showing that the primary latent period did not differ among virus strains and nor was it altered by vaccine treatment. For the secondary latent period, neither virulence score nor HVT vaccine affected the duration of the latent period, however, Bivalent vaccine increased the duration of the second latent period significantly and to a greater extent for smaller virulence scores (see Table 5).

Table 5: Secondary latent period: linear regression results for effect of transformed virulence score and vaccine treatment on the secondary latent period (days)

	Estimate	**Std. Error**	**t value**	**Pr(> |*t*|)**
Intercept	10.16	4.30	2.36	0.04
Virulence Score	-1.64	6.98	-0.24	0:82
VaccHVT	2.60	6.10	0.43	0:68
VaccBiv	19.29	6.10	3.16	< 0.01
Virulence Score:VaccBiv	-24.82	9.88	-2.51	0.03
Virulence Score:VaccHVT	-1.82	9.88	-0.18	0.86

Adjusted $R^2 = 0.54$, $p = 0.01$.

An association between the virulence score and the estimated viral shedding rates was found. A linear regression was used to estimate the viral shedding rate as a function of arcsine square-root transformed virulence score and vaccine treatment. There was no significant association between the primary viral shedding rate and HVT or Bivalent vaccine treatment (p = 0.085, 0.10 respectively) nor virulence score (p = 0.055). There was, however, a strong positive association between the virulence score of a strain and the secondary viral shedding rate (p = 0.00076). There was no association between the secondary viral shedding rate and either HVT or Bivalent vaccine treatment (p = 0.66, 0.39 respectively, see Table 6). Figure 6 shows the estimated secondary viral shedding rate as a function of virulence score for different vaccine treatments.

Table 6: Secondary viral shedding: linear regression results for effect of transformed virulence score and vaccine treatment on the second viral shedding rate (VCN/mg dust)

	Estimate	Std. Error	t value	Pr(> |*t*|)
Intercept	-3.24×10^7	1.35×10^7	-0.24	0.03
Virulence Score	9.79×10^7	2.19×10^7	4.47	< 0.01
VaccHVT	8.51×10^6	1.91×10^7	0.45	0.66
VaccBiv	1.70×10^7	1.91×10^7	0.89	0.39
Virulence Score:VaccBiv	-5.73×10^7	3.19×10^7	-0.19	0.09
Virulence Score:VaccHVT	-2.37×10^7	3.10×10^7	-0.77	0.46

Adjusted $R^2 = 0.74$, $p < 0.01$.

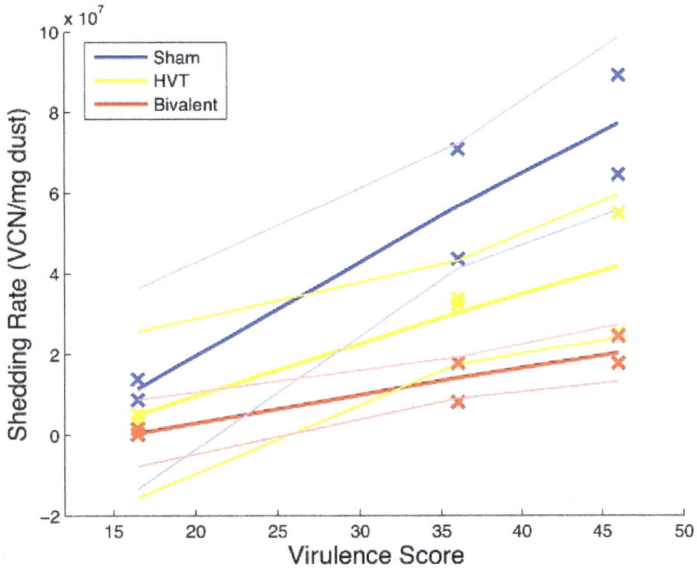

Figure 6: Viral Shedding: Linear regression analysis of the virulence score and the corresponding estimated secondary viral shedding rate for all treatments. The 95% confidence intervals for the mean response are given in fainter lines. The linear regression results are shown in Table 6.

DISCUSSION

The survival model fits the nine survival curves well on the whole, with both replicates combined into one fit. The delay which characterises the mortality profile for Marek's disease is captured well by the Weibull model. In most cases, the viral shedding model captures the data well.

The viral shedding model assumes that all birds become initially infected with MDV. While it is difficult to model individual birds based on the resolution of the data available, we do point out that the assumption that all birds become infected precipitates the estimated per bird viral shedding rates being perhaps an over-estimate of the actual rates. On the other hand, the qPCR methods used estimate total viral copies which is not necessarily equivalent to total infectious material and therefore serves as an upper limit of viable infectious DNA.

Our estimate of the primary latent period of between 2 and 6 days is much shorter than earlier estimates of around 13 days [31] but only slightly shorter than more recent estimates based on new PCR techniques which have detected significant quantities of virus in feather tips [32] and feather dander [27, 28] at 7 days post infection. This discrepancy may be due to a number of factors: detectability of virus at low quantities, the sampling time of the experiments and heterogeneities between the experiments. The estimates here also have confidence intervals between 0-6 days which suggest the data are not able to give a great deal of certainty on the exact time of onset of viral shedding. Further analysis might take into account biological knowledge through prior distributions to get a more exact value, and past experimental studies would suggest shedding begins towards the end of the estimated interval [27, 28].

The pathotyping of MDV isolates, similar to that pioneered by Witter and colleagues [1, 16], is a useful tool for comparing the pathogenicity of strains with respect to others in vaccinated birds. However several of the more recent isolated, highly virulent strains have ranks above 80, in some cases 90 on Witter's ranking system. Should more virulent strains emerge, it will be difficult to categorise them via this method, as the scale is truncated at 100. The method of fitting a Weibull distribution proposed in this paper allows for a greater flexibility of pathotyping, in that an isolate may be categorised according to its mean time to kill the host. The subsequent effect of vaccination of the host on this metric can then be established.

Biologically, it may seem more sustainable to pathotype according to the lifespan of an unvaccinated bird, but experimentally it may also be a solution to the costly procedure of having two or three groups of birds, each vaccinated with a different treatment. Even a simple 'time to death' metric can be performed in relatively few birds, as was the case for the myxoma virus in rabbits in Australia. Myxoma strains were pathotyped effectively when the case fatality rate proved experimentally intensive and ineffective in discriminating between similarly virulent strains [33, 17] noted this restriction of current pathotyping regimes, instead favouring a system based on neuropathology to circumvent these methodological and experimental limitations. The analysis presented here differs from both of these past approaches due to its epidemiological focus on virulence. However, we point out that the methodology adopted here only analyses three distinct strains. Therefore, a wider range of strain virulences and places of origin will be required to sufficiently extrapolate the current results to the whole virulence spectrum.

CONCLUSIONS

This paper uses a mathematical approach to estimate key epidemiological parameters for Marek's Disease Virus (MDV). We used survival analysis with a Weibull mortality function to build a statistical model for the lifespan of birds infected with MDV. We were able to compare the relative impact of virulence score and vaccine covariates by calculating credible intervals via Bayesian methods. We developed a dynamic model to simulate the shedding of virus by a group of birds and used Bayesian techniques to estimate the four key infectiousness parameters: primary and secondary latent periods and viral shedding rates.

We applied these methods to the data for three MDV strains varying moderately in virulence. From the survival analysis, we found that increasing the virulence score of a virus strain decreases the lifespan of the host (Figure 2). Vaccinating the host with either the first or second generation vaccine increases its lifespan, but neither one to any greater degree (Table 1). From the viral shedding analysis, we concluded primary latent period is not affected by vaccination or virulence score, however, secondary latent period increases with Bivalent vaccine treatment (Table 5). Secondary (long term) viral shedding rate (measured in VCN per mg dust) is higher for strains of higher virulence (Table 5 and Figure 6). Vaccination does not reduce long term viral shedding rate significantly. Together, these results imply that more virulent viruses shed more infectious material into the environment and Bivalent vaccines reduce the infectious period, especially for less virulent strain infections.

The results described here are qualitatively in line with current thinking on MDV pathogenesis, but the new methods presented allow a formal comparison of strains in an epidemiological meaningful way. It is anticipated that this analysis will allow a more quantitative understanding of the aetiology of MDV and the mechanisms governing a functional rise in virulence for a strain. With this analysis it is hoped that a more epidemiologically significant classification of MDV strains will emerge which will eventually provide not only insight into the reasons for evolution to highly virulent strains but also a metric to evaluate future risks and the efficacy of possible control strategies.

METHODS

Experimental Data

We look at a single experiment [30] with two response variables measured. Groups of maternal antibody positive IsaBrown layer chicks were inoculated with one of three vaccine treatments: sham (diluent only), HVT (first generation industry vaccine) or Bivalent (second generation industry vaccine) at one day old. At 5 days post vaccination, the birds were challenged with 500 pfu (plaque forming units) of one of three MDV strains: 04CRE, MPF57 and 02LAR. These independently sampled isolates were Australian in origin and have been pathotyped with virulence scores (the percentage of HVT or Bivalent vaccinated chickens infected with a particular strain which develop gross lesions or die of MDV within eight weeks [34]) of 16.5, 36 and 46 respectively. The viruses were all isolated from field outbreaks and used at passage level 4 to 7 in chick kidney cells. The experiment was therefore a 3×3 factorial design study, with vaccine type fully cross-factored against virus strain. Each treatment combination was replicated in two separate isolators resulting in 26 or 27 birds per combination for the pathotyping component of the study. The air in each isolator was changed 8-20 times per hour. Further details can be found in [30]. The experiment was approved by the University of New England Animal Ethics Committee with approval number AEC05/076. Due to Animal Ethics regulations, birds thought to be nearing death were euthanised and classified as mortality in the experimental results. The experiment lasted 56 days post infection (dpi) and all birds were humanely killed and examined for MD lesions on the last day. Therefore for the purposes of this analysis, the data were censored after day 55. All birds were given a large dose of MDV (500 pfu) via intra-abdominal injection and it was therefore assumed that all the birds were infected and would shed the virus. Differences between unvaccinated and vaccinated birds in detection of MD have been reported [35], but these have been in studies where infection has been by injection with 50 pfu. Increasing the MDV dose fourfold (from 50 to 200 pfu) significantly increased the detected incidence of MD in unvaccinated birds from 64% to 81% [27].

The two variables recorded were the time to death of a bird (measured in days) and the density of virus within each isolator every week (measured in logVCN per mg of dust in the environment). The virus titres in the dust were determined via quantitative real-time PCR of dust collected from the isolator exhaust ducts, the methods of which have been discussed in separate studies [25]. The data are shown in Figures 1 (mortality), 3, 4 and 5 (shedding).

Parameter Estimates

We assumed that each infected bird starts shedding virus after an initial delay, then after a further delay, the rate at which it sheds virus rises to a long-term stable value. We estimated five key epidemiological parameters: host lifespan, primary latent period (the time until an infected bird becomes infectious), secondary latent period (the delay between an infectious bird first shedding virus and when it sheds virus at its secondary long term rate) and viral shedding rates (both primary and secondary, measured in VCN/mg dust). A survival analysis was undertaken for the mortality data because multiple covariates were needed to find the host lifespan. These covariates were vaccine treatment and virus virulence score. Latent period and rate of viral shedding could not be estimated directly from the data since the response variable (measured weekly in VCN per mg dust) could vary with the number of birds housed together, which changed as birds died. Therefore a dynamic model capturing this variability was used to estimate the two infectiousness parameters.

For ease of notation, log is written to represent $\log_{10}$ throughout the paper.

Mortality

The biology of Marek's disease suggests that the probability of death by MDV infection changes through time, since the virus undergoes lytic, latent stage (this is a description of an MDV pathogenesis stage and not equivalent to the 'latent periods' in the epidemiological context which this study estimated), late lytic (where infection is extended to other organs of the host), and transformative (tumour-induction) stages. These stages are pathologically distinct and may lead to a different mortality rate. Therefore, a Weibull distribution was chosen as a candidate distribution for modelling survivorship curves, which is often used for time to death data since it is flexible and can mimic other distributions but only has two parameters in its non-location form. We therefore assumed that time to death can be modelled as a random variable, T, such that $T \sim W(r, \lambda)$ where$r, \lambda > 0$ are the shape and scale parameters respectively. The associated probability density function is

$$f(t) = \begin{cases} \frac{r}{\lambda}\left(\frac{t}{\lambda}\right)^{r-1} e^{-\left(\frac{t}{\lambda}\right)^r} & \text{if } t \geq 0 \\ 0 & \text{if } t < 0 \end{cases}$$

A Weibull model was fitted to the survival data in the study. In the case when $r = 1$, the distribution collapses to an exponential distribution. When $r > 1$ or $r < 1$ there is an increasing or decreasing chance of death over time respectively. Coefficients, $\boldsymbol{\beta}$, are such that $\lambda = \exp(\boldsymbol{\beta} \cdot \mathbf{x})$, where $\boldsymbol{\beta} = [\beta_0, \beta_1, \beta_2, \beta_3]$ are the covariate coefficients and $\mathbf{x} = [1, x_1, x_2, x_3]^T$ are the covariates. In this analysis, there were three covariates (one continuous: the transformation of the virulence score of an isolate (x_1) and two binary: the presence or absence of HVT (x_2) and Bivalent (x_3) vaccine). Therefore there were 9 combinations on the set of possible covariates, thus $\lambda_j = \boldsymbol{\beta} \cdot \mathbf{x}_j$ where $j \in [1, 9]$ The likelihood function can therefore be written

$$\mathcal{L}(\boldsymbol{\lambda}, r) = \prod_{j=1}^{9} \prod_{i=i}^{n} \left\{ \frac{r}{\lambda_j} \left(\frac{t_i}{\lambda_j} \right)^{r-1} \right\}^{\delta_i} \exp\left(-\frac{t_i}{\lambda_j} \right)^r$$

where δ_i is zero when the ith observation is censored and unity elsewhere. This function was maximized via the Newton-Raphson algorithm such that $\mathcal{L}(\tilde{\boldsymbol{\lambda}}, \tilde{r}) = \max \mathcal{L}(\boldsymbol{\lambda}, r)$ where $\tilde{\boldsymbol{\lambda}}$ and $\tilde{r}$ are the maximum likelihood estimates. Note that the virulence score, v, of an isolate is a percentage measure and to be used as an explanatory variable in a regression analysis, it should be transformed such that $v_T = \arcsin \sqrt{0.01v}$. The regression fitted the maximum likelihood estimates for $\boldsymbol{\beta}$, however further Bayesian analysis was required to estimate the associated credible intervals when the covariate covariance matrix does not approximate the identity matrix. An McMC framework was set up in WinBUGS [36] to calculate the posterior distributions and the credible intervals of the Weibull survival function.

The prior distributions of each parameter were assumed to be uninformative and were thus taken as uniform, to ensure equivalence to maximum likelihood estimation. The burn-in was set to 22,000 iterations with every 10th sample taken from the subsequent 100,000 iterations [37, 38].

Viral Shedding

The dynamic model tracked the density of MDV over time in each isolator. In this model it is assumed:

1. After MDV infection, there is a delay before virus is first shed [31]. This is termed the primary latent period.
2. After this primary latent period, virus is shed at a constant rate (the primary viral shedding rate, measured in VCN per mg dust) for a set period of time, termed the secondary latent period.
3. Once this secondary latent period is over, virus is shed at a constant rate (the secondary viral shedding rate) until the termination of the experiment.

Additionally, the density of virus (VCN per mg dust) was calculated at the end of each day and any removal of birds was assumed to occur at the start of the day. While all parameters are assumed to be constant across all the birds in a single isolator, they can vary between isolators.

There are therefore four parameters estimated per isolator: the primary/secondary latent periods (in days) and the primary/secondary rates of viral shedding (VCN/mg dust). The primary and secondary latent periods are denoted by T^1 and T^2 respectively. Birds shed virus at a rate, a^1 (VCN per mg dust) from T^1+1 to T^1+T^2 days post infection; and at a rate a^2 (VCN per mg dust) from T^2+1 until the end of the experiment (at 8 weeks post infection). The density of MDV in the dynamic model could be compared to the amount of virus recorded in the data (sampled every 7 days). We therefore estimated $a_j^1(v), a_j^2(v), T_j^1(v)$ and $T_j^2(v)$ for each virulence score $v \in \{16.5, 36, 46\}$ and each vaccine status $j \in \{Sham, HVT, Bivalent\}$.

The model accounts for the removal of birds given in the mortality data and the number of complete hourly air changes (varied as a parameter α). The daily quantity of dust shed per bird was calculated by fit ting a cubic spline to dust MDV data provided from the same experiment [30].

To calculate the measurement error of a quantity of virus in a sample of dust we noted that a final MDV density was reached some time before the end of the sampling period. Such data can therefore be assumed to be identically and independently distributed. If Y_1 and Y_2 are samples from the experiment when the virus density and the data are lognormally distributed then:

$$logY_1, logY_2 \sim N(\mu, \sigma^2)$$
$$\Rightarrow logY_1 - logY_2 \sim N(0, 2\sigma^2)$$

To find the time point after which the data is assumed to have plateaued, four sets of points were examined: weeks 5, 6, 7 and 8. The differences between the logged data of weeks 7-8 provided the highest probability of both being drawn from a normal distribution (p = 0.8, Anderson-Darling n = 18) and that the distribution has a mean of zero (p = 0.40). The resulting standard deviation of the difference between log-transformed data was estimated to be 0.33 logVCN/mg dust.

Posterior distributions were found by means of McMC realisations by calculating the likelihood of the data given the parameter values, with lognormal errors of $^{2} = 0.33^{2}/2$. The burn-in time was set to 30,000 iterations and the posterior distribution was taken as every 10th sample from the following 90,000 iterations [37, 38].

DECLARATIONS

Acknowledgements

We thank BBSRC, Pfizer, the Australian Poultry CRC, R. Howey for supplying Bayesian sampling code and M. Chase-Topping for statistical advice.

Authors' contributions

KEA performed the statistical analysis and drafted the manuscript. AFR was involved in the drafting and revision of the manuscript for intellectual content. NJS was involved in the Bayesian statistical analysis. SWB and KGR were involved in supplying data and associated technical advice. SWB was involved in the revision of the manuscript for intellectual content. MEJW was involved in design of the statistical analysis and the drafting and revision of the manuscript for intellectual content. All authors approved the final manuscript.

REFERENCES

4. Witter RL: Increased virulence of Marek's disease virus field isolates. Avian Diseases. 1997, 41: 149-163. 10.2307/1592455.

5. Osterrieder N, Kamil JP, Schumacher D, Tischer BK, Trapp S: Marek's disease virus: from miasma to model. Nature Res Microbiology. 2006, 4: 753-761.

6. Witter RL: The changing landscape of Marek's disease. Avian Pathology. 1998, 27: S46-S53. 10.1080/03079459808419292.

7. Calnek BW, Adldinger HK, Kahn DE: Feather Follicle Epithelium: a Source of Enveloped and Infectious Cell-Free Herpesvirus from Marek's Disease. Avian Diseases. 1970, 14 (2): 219-233. 10.2307/1588466.

8. Carrozza JH, Fredrickson TN, Prince RP, Luginbuhl RE: Role of desquamated epithelial cells in transmission of Marek's disease. Avian Diseases. 1973, 17: 767-781. 10.2307/1589045.

9. Baigent SJ, Smith LP, Nair VK, Currie RJW: Vaccinal control of Marek's disease: current challenges, and future strategies to maximize protection. Veterinary Immunology and Immunopathology. 2006, 112: 78-86. 10.1016/j.vetimm.2006.03.014.

10. Morrow C, Fehler F: Marek's disease: a worldwide problem. Marek's disease: an Evolving Problem. Elsevier Academic Press 2004.

11. Nair V, Kung HJ: Marek's disease virus oncogenicity: molecular mechanisms. Marek's Disease: an Evolving Problem. Elsevier Academic Press 2004.

12. Churchill A, Payne L, Chubb R: Immunization against Marek's Disease using a live attenuated virus. Nature. 1969, 221 (5182): 744-747. 10.1038/221744a0.

13. Bublot M, Sharma J: Vaccination against Marek's disease. Marek's Disease: an Evolving Problem. Edited by: Nair V, Davison F. Elsevier Academic Press 2004.

14. Dieckmann U: Adaptive dynamics of pathogen-host interactions. Adaptive Dynamics Of Infectious Diseases: In Pursuit of Virulence Management. Cambridge University Press 2002.

15. Read AF: The Evolution of Virulence. Trends in Microbiology. 1994, 2: 73-76. 10.1016/0966-842X(94)90537-1.

16. Levin S, Pimentel D: Selection of Intermediate Rates of Increase in Parasite-Host Systems. American Naturalist. 1981, 117: 308-315. 10.1086/283708.

17. Anderson RM, May RM: Directly transmitted diseases: Control by vaccination. Science. 1982, 215 (4536): 1053-1060. 10.1126/science.7063839.

18. Tompkins DM, Dobson AP, Arneberg P, Begon ME, Cattadori IM, Greenman JV, Heesterbeeck JAP, Hudson PJ, Newborn D, Pugliese A, Rizzoli AP, Rosa R, Rosso F, Wilson K: Parasites and Host Population Dynamics. The Ecology of Wildlife Diseases. Oxford University Press 2002.

19. Witter RL, Calnek BW, Buscaglia C, Gimeno IM, Schat KA: Classification of Marek's disease viruses according to pathotype: philosophy and methodology. Avian Pathology. 2005, 34 (2): 75-90. 10.1080/03079450500059255.

20. Gimeno IM, Witter RL, Neumann U: Neuropathotyping: A New System to Classify Marek's Disease Virus. Avian Diseases. 2002, 46 (4): 909-918. 10.1637/0005-2086(2002)046[0909:NANSTC]2.0.CO;2. [http://www.jstor.org/stable/1593315]

21. Gimeno IM, Witter RL, Hunt HD, Reddy SM, Lee LF, Silva RF: The pp38 gene of Marek's disease virus (MDV) is necessary for cytolytic infection of B cells and maintenance of the transformed state but not for cytolytic infection of the feather follicle epithelium and horizontal spread of MDV. Journal of Virology. 2005, 79 (7): 4545-4549. 10.1128/JVI.79.7.4545-4549.2005.

22. Calnek BW, Witter RL: Marek's disease - a model for herpesvirus oncology. CRC Critical Res of Microbiology. 1986, 12: 293-319.

23. Yunis R, Jarosinski KW, Schat KA: Association between rate of viral genome replication and virulence of Marek's

disease herpesvirus strains. Virology. 2004, 328: 142-150. 10.1016/j.virol.2004.07.017.

24. Baigent SJ, Petherbridge LJ, Howes K, Smith LP, Currie RJW, Nair VK: Absolute quantification of Marek's disease virus genome copy number in chicken feather and lymphocyte samples using real-time PCR. Journal of Virological Methods. 2005, 123: 53-64. 10.1016/j.jviromet.2004.08.019.

25. Bumstead N, Sillibourne J, Rennie M, Ross N, Davison F: Quantification of Marek's disease virus in chicken lymphocytes using the polymerase chain reaction with fluorescence detection. Journal of Virological Methods. 1997, 65: 75-81. 10.1016/S0166-0934(96)02172-6.

26. Burgess SC, Davison TF: A quantitative duplex PCR technique for measuring amounts of cell-associated Marek's disease virus: difference s in two populations of lymphomas cells. Journal of Virological Methods. 1999, 82: 27-37. 10.1016/S0166-0934(99)00075-0.

27. Islam A, Harrison B, Cheetham BF, Mahony TJ, Young PL, Walkden-Brown SW: Differential amplification and quantification of Marek's disease viruses using real-time polymerase chain reaction. Journal of Virological Methods. 2004, 119: 103-113. 10.1016/j.jviromet.2004.03.006.

28. Islam A, Cheetham BF, Mahony TJ, Young PL, Walkden-Brown SW: Absolute quantification of Marek's disease virus and herpesvirus of turkeys in chicken lymohocyte, feather tip and dust samples using real-time PCR. Journal of Virological Methods. 2006, 132: 127-134. 10.1016/j.jviromet.2005.10.009.

29. Reddy SM, Witter RL, Gimeno I: Development of quantitative-competitive polymerase chain reaction assay for serotype 1 Marek's disease virus. Avian Diseases. 2000, 44: 770-775. 10.2307/1593048.

30. Islam AFMF, Walkden-Brown SW, Groves PJ, Underwood GJ: Effects of vaccine dose, virus challenge dose and interval from vaccination to challenge on protection of broiler chickens against Marek's disease virus challenge. Australian Veterinary Journal. 2007, 85 (9): 348-355. 10.1111/j.1751-0813.2007.00195.x.

31. Islam AFMF, Walkden-Brown SW, Groves PJ, Underwood GJ: Kinetics of Marek's disease virus (MDV) infection in broiler chickens 1: effect of varying vaccination to challenge interval on vaccinal protection and load of MDV and herpesvirus of turkey in the spleen and feather dander over time. Avian Pathology. 2008, 37 (3): 225-235. 10.1080/03079450701802230.

32. Witter R, Solomon JJ, Nazerian Champion: Long-term studies of Marek's disease infection in individual chickens. Avian Diseases. 1971, 15 (2): 346-65. 10.2307/1588707.

33. Renz KG: In vitro and in vivo characterisation of selected Australian isolates of Marek's disease virus. 2008, Ph.D Thesis, University of New England, Australia, [https://e-publications.une.edu.au/vital/access/services/Download/une:1909/SOURCE04?=true]

34. Baigent SJ, Davison F: Marek's disease virus: Biology and life cycle. Marek's Disease: an Evolving Problem. Elsevier Academic Press 2004.

35. Baigent SJ, Smith LP, Currie RJW, Nair VK: Replication kinetics of Marek's disease vaccine virus in feathers and lymphoid tissus using PCR and virus isolation. Journal of General Virology. 2005, 86: 2989-2998. 10.1099/vir.0.81299-0.

36. Fenner F, Fantini B: Biological Control of Vertebrate Pests: The History of Myxomatosis - an Experiment in Evolution. CABI Publishing 1999.

37. Walkden-Brown S, Cooke J, Islam A, Renz K, Hussain Z, Islam A, Tannock G, Groves P: Pathotyping of Australian isolates of MDV. Proceedings of the 8th International Marekís Disease Symposium: 6-10th July, Townsville, Australia. 2008

38. Islam AFMF, Walkden-Brown SW, Wong CW, Groves PJ, Burgess SC, Arzey KE, Young PL: Influence of vaccine deposition site on post-vaccinal viraemia and vaccine efficacy in broiler chickens following *in ovo* vaccination against Marek's disease. Avian Pathology. 2001, 30: 525-533. 10.1080/03079450120078725.

39. Lunn D, Thomas A, Best N, Spiegelhalter D: WinBUGS Bayesian modelling framework: concepts, structure, and extensibility. Statistics and Computing. 2000, 10: 325-337. 10.1023/A:1008929526011.

40. Raftery A, Lewis S: How many iterations in the Gibbs sampler?. Bayesian Statistics. Oxford University Press, 4: 1992.

41. Carlin B, Lewis T: Bayesian Methods for Data Analysis. Chapman & Hall/CRC 2008.

CHAPTER 8

OUTBREAK OF MAREK'S DISEASE IN A VACCINATED BROILER BREEDING FLOCK DURING ITS PEAK EGG-LAYING PERIOD IN CHINA

Xinyu Zhuang[1], Haitao Zou[1], Huoying Shi[1,2,3], Hongxia Shao[1,2,3], Jianqiang Ye[1,2,3], Ji Miao[2], Genghua Wu[2] and Aijian Qin[1,2,3]

[1] Ministry of Education Key Laboratory for Avian Preventive Medicine, Yangzhou University, No. 12 East Wenhui Road, Yangzhou, Jiangsu 225009, P.R. China

[2] Key Laboratory of Jiangsu Preventive Veterinary Medicine, Yangzhou University, Yangzhou 225009, P.R. China

[3] Jiangsu Co-innovation Center for the Prevention and Control of Important Animal Infectious Diseases and Zoonoses, Yangzhou 225009, P.R. China.

ABSTRACT

Background

Outbreaks of Marek's disease (MD), caused by Marek's disease virus (MDV), primarily occur in 10–12-week-old hens.

Case presentation

We report a case of MD in a breeding flock of 24–30-week-old vaccinated broilers in China. The clinical signs in the affected chickens appeared at 24 weeks, and the incidence of tumours peaked at 30 weeks. The morbidity and mortality of the hens were 5 % and 80 %, respectively. Hematoxylin–eosin staining of the tissues showed the typical characteristics of MD. MDV infection was confirmed in the hens with an agar gel diffusion precipitation assay for the MD antigen in the feather follicle epithelium. An MDV strain, designated AH1410, was isolated from the blood lymphocytes. Sequence analyses of the pp38, meq, and gB genes revealed that strain AH1410 had molecular features consistent with a virulent, previously identified MDV.

Conclusion

Our data provide evidence that not only is MDV becoming more virulent, but that the period of its onset in chickens is expanding. These findings provide the basis the molecular surveillance and further study of virulent MDV mutants and control strategies for MD in China.

BACKGROUND

Marek's disease (MD) is caused by Marek's disease virus (MDV), of the family *Herpesviridae*. MD was first reported in 1907 by Josef Marek and is characterised by T-cell lymphomas in the peripheral nerves or organs of 10–12-week-old hens [1]. MDV is currently distributed worldwide. Although vaccination plays a vital role in the prevention and control of MD globally, MDVs of increased virulence have been frequently isolated in some countries, even among vaccinated chickens, calling into question the current vaccination program against MDVs. The virulent MDVs (vMDVs) usually carry mutations in genes such

Citation: Xinyu Zhuang, Haitao Zou, Huoying Shi, Hongxia Shao, Jianqiang Ye, Ji Miao, Genghua Wu and Aijian Qin, Outbreak of Marek's disease in a vaccinated broiler breeding flock during its peak egg-laying period in China, DOI 10.1186/s12917-015-0493-7.

as *pp38*, *meq*, or *gB*, that are associated with the oncogenicity and and their immune evasion [2, 3].

In China, a vaccine has been widely used to prevent MD in the poultry industry. However, the MD vaccine program has frequently failed, and vMDVs are occasionally isolated in vaccinated chickens [4]. In this study, we report a recent outbreak of MD in a vaccinated breeding broiler flock in China during its peak egg-laying period.

CASE PRESENTATION

Clinical symptoms and pathological lesions

The sick chickens were obtained from a large farm in Anhui Province, China. The owner of the chickens gave permission for their animals to be included in this study. The chickens were 24–30 weeks old. Tumours were found in their organs and skin. The occurrence of tumours increased progressively and reached its highest level (5 %) during the peak egg-laying period (30 weeks old), after which it began to decline. In the majority of sick chickens, the cysts first appeared between the toes (Fig. 1a) and then in the tarsometatarsus. All the chickens were hens. Tumours were observed in almost all tissues, particularly the liver (Fig. 1b). Immature infiltrated lymphocytes were observed in the liver and spleen during the histopathological diagnosis, ultimately destroying the tissue structure. Most of the darkly stained cells were lymphocytes, among which red eosinophilic granules were spotted. Many multinucleate cells with infiltrated lymphoid cells were present in the compartment of the liver (Fig. 1c), corresponding to the classical lesions of MDV.

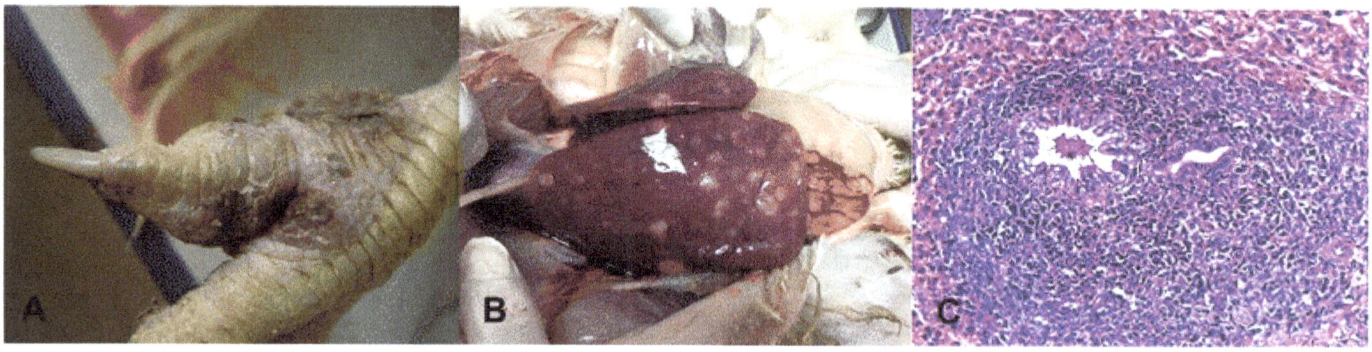

Figure 1: Clinical symptoms and pathological lesions. **a**: Cysts appeared in the toes; **b**: tumors appeared in the liver; **c**: histopathological tissue (HE, 400×).

MDV antigen found in feathers

A band of MDV antigen was precipitated from the feather epithelia of the sick chickens. However, no band representing MDV antigen was found in the sera of the sick chickens. This suggests that the feather tips of the chickens excrete MDV particles. The anti-MDV antibody titres in the sera of the chickens were too low to detect with the agar gel diffusion precipitation (AGP) assay.

Isolation and identification of MDV in the flock

After two blind passages of chicken embryo fibroblast (CEF) cells, the presence of MDV (designated strain AH1410) in the CEF was confirmed when the typical cytopathic effect (CPE) appeared on the third day after infection (Fig. 2a). The infected cells became round and were highly refractive. When the cells were analysed with an anti-gB monoclonal antibody (Mab) BA4, specific uniform fluorescence was observed in both the nuclei and cytoplasm of the infected cells, but not in the CEF, suggesting that the cells showing the CPE reacted with the MDV-1 gB-specific Mab BA4 (Fig. 2b).

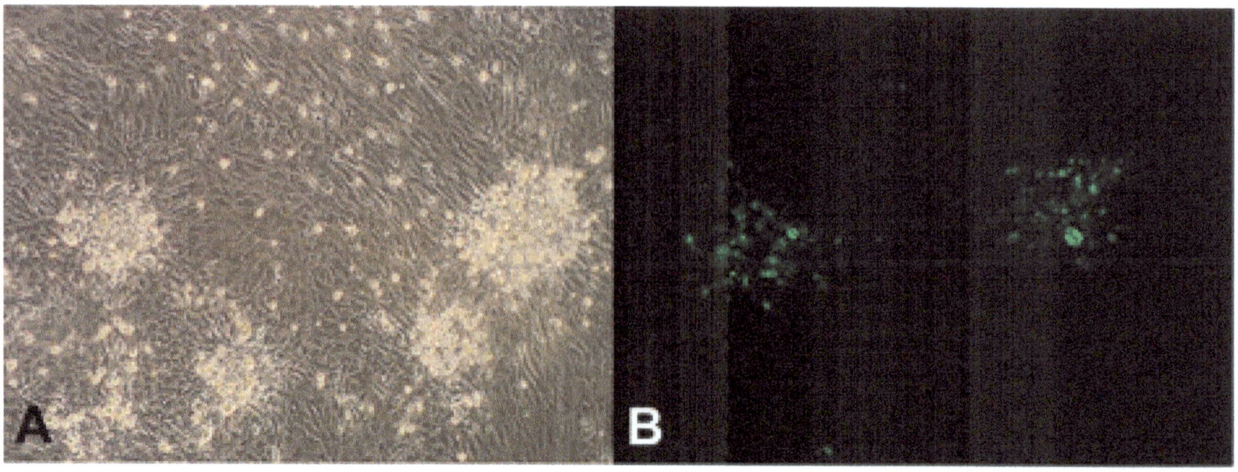

Figure 2: Viruses in CEF cells and indirect immunofluorescence assay with an MAb directed against MDV. **a**: MDV CPE in the CEF; **b**: immunofluorescence-positive cells tested with MAb BA4 against MDV-1.

MDV isolate has molecular features of vMDVs

The genomic DNA was extracted from CEF infected with the isolated virus. The complete sequences of the*meq*, *gB*, and *pp38* genes were successfully amplified with PCR (Fig. 3a). A sequence analysis revealed that the*pp38* gene of AH1410 shared 99.3 %–100.0 % identity with those of reference strains, with only a single amino acid mutation at position 109 (E→G) in the deduced amino acid sequence (Fig. 3b). When we compared the*meq* sequences of reference strains published in the National Center for Biotechnology Information database with that of isolate AH1410, we found an insertion of 59 amino acids at position 194 of MEQ in the vaccine strain CVI988, so that its ORF encodes 398 amino acids. However, isolate AH1410 and other vMDVs all have ORFs encoding 339 amino acids in their *meq* genes, with 99.7 %–100.0 % homology. Only four amino acid mutations, at residues 80 (D→Y), 115 (V→A), 139 (T→A), and 176 (P→R), were found in isolate AH1410, which are identical to those in strain GX0101 (Fig. 3c). Analysis of the *gB* gene indicated that it was 100.0 % homologous between isolate AH1410 and other MDVs, with no mutations.

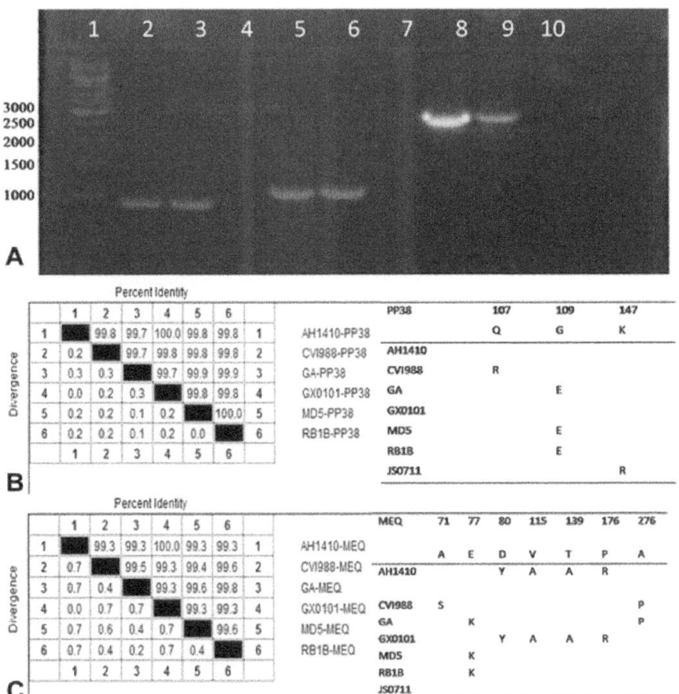

Figure 3: MDV genes amplified with PCR and the corresponding homology analyses. **a**: PCR results for the *meq*, *pp38*, and *gB*genes. Lane 1: 1-kb marker; lanes 4, 7, 10: negative controls; lanes 2 and 3: amplified *meq* gene; lanes 5 and 6: amplified *pp38* gene; lanes 8 and 9: amplified *gB* gene. **b**: Homology analysis and mutations of*pp38*. **c**: Homology analysis and mutations of *meq*.

DISCUSSION

Marek's disease is one of the most significant infectious diseases in poultry. In birds, it can result in tumours or immunosuppression, making the birds more sensitive to other pathogens. Although MD vaccines have been widely used in China for a long time, failures of MD vaccination occur frequently on some poultry farms. The improper selection of a vaccine could be the cause of vaccine failure [5]. Birds are also more susceptible to MDV mutants that have emerged in regions with more-virulent strains than to previous MDV isolates.

The *pp38* gene encodes a phosphoprotein of approximately 38 kDa that is necessary for both cell transformation and viral reactivation in the latent period [6, 7]. The *pp38* gene is conserved in all strains of MDV so far isolated. Previously, it was believed that *pp38* was not present in MDV strain CVI988 [8], but in recent years, the gene was shown to be expressed by CVI988, and a mutation at residue 107 (Q→R) is identified with Mab H19 [9, 10]. In this study, we found no mutation at residue 107 of the PP38 protein of the isolated strain AH1410. The *pp38* gene sequence was identical to that of the vMDVs. However, at residue 109 of pp38 in the vMDVs and the very virulent MDVs (vvMDVs), such as strains GA, MD5, and RB1B, glutamate is replaced by glycine, which differs from the sequence of strain AH1410, which is similar to that of other virulent viruses isolated in China, such as GX0101 and JS0711. Therefore, the isolated virus AH1410 is not the vaccine strain.

The MEQ protein, which is considered to be the major factor responsible for the occurrence of tumours, contains 339 amino acids [4]. However, the *meq* gene of CVI988 has an insertion of 177 bp compared with the genes of the vMDVs, which results in a 59-amino-acid insertion relative to the MEQ proteins of the vMDVs [11,12, 13], that inhibits the expression of the *meq* gene [14]. Research has also indicated that mutations at positions 71 and 77 of the MEQ protein could be distinct in the vvMDVs [15]. Compared with CVI988, position 71 of strain AH1410 is mutated (S→A), as in the vMDVs, whereas position 77 is conserved. No deletion or insertion was found at position 194 and the ORF of AH1410 *meq* encodes 339 amino acids. We also found mutations at positions 80, 115, 139, and 176 of MEQ in our isolate AH1410, similar to those in GX0101 [16], suggesting that this type of strain has been circulating in China for many years.

With sequence alignments of the *meq*, *pp38*, and *gB* genes of strain AH1410 and other MDV isolates, we found that GX0101 and AH1410 are completely identical in these three genes. A previous study demonstrated that the virulence of GX0101 was at a level between those of GA and Md5 [16]. Collectively, these data indicate that the pathogenicity of isolate AH1410 may be similar to that of isolate GX0101.

The mutations and increasing virulence of MDV are thought to be responsible for the occurrence of MD on vaccinated farms. The failure of MD vaccination may be one reason for the outbreak reported here. Notably, the onset of MD in broilers generally starts at 4–6 weeks of age. In hens, MD usually occurs at 10–12 weeks of age [17]. However, in this case, the rate of tumours reached its highest level during the peak egg-laying period (30 weeks old).

Outbreaks among egg-laying chickens have also been reported in the mining area of Karnataka, India [18], and excessive losses from MD have recently been reported in adult laying flocks over the age of 40 weeks in Japan [19]. The data indicate that these birds may have contracted these infections later in life, with subsequent clinical signs. We also found that the feathers of the chickens were positive for the virus, whereas their sera were negative for MDV antigen, indicating that the chickens' immune responses may have been suppressed in other ways, an unusual phenomenon and a disquieting trend. Another interesting observation is that all the diseased chickens were hens, which is consistent with an observation by Heier et al., who noted that males tended to be more resistant to MD than females [20].

It is necessary to strengthen the surveillance of circulating MDVs because new variants of virulent MDVs may appear at any time, and better vaccines against MD must be developed.

CONCLUSION

Our data provide evidence that not only is MDV becoming more virulent, but that the period of its onset in chickens is also expanding. These findings provide the basis for the molecular surveillance of MDV, and further study of its virulence mutants and the control strategies required for MDV in China.

METHODS

CHICKENS AND SAMPLES

All the chickens were obtained from a breeding broiler chicken farm in Anhui, China. The chickens were immunized with the CVI988 vaccine at 1 day old. This vaccine had been used on the chicken farm for many years by skilled workers who vaccinate the chickens according to standard procedures. The clinical symptoms presented between 24 and 30 weeks. The morbidity and mortality of the hens were 5 % and approximately 80 %, respectively. Samples were obtained from the sick chickens. *Avian leukosis virus* and*Reticuloendotheliosis virus* infections were detected with PCR and virus isolation in our initial pathogen screening. The chickens reported here were negative for both viruses. All the experiments complied with institutional animal care guidelines and were approved by the University of Yangzhou Animal Care Committee.

Histochemical assay

A histopathological assay and hematoxylin–eosin (HE) staining of the tissues were performed as previously described [21]. In brief, the livers and spleens of the sick chickens were fixed in 10 % neutral formalin, dehydrated in alcohol, and embedded in paraffin. They were then stained with HE and screened with light microscopy.

AGP assay

An AGP test was performed on 1 % agar plates containing 8 % NaCl. In the AGP test, CEF cells infected with MDV strain RB1B were used as the positive control antigen, and preserved sera from the MDV-infected chickens were used as the positive control sera. The positive antigen (20 µl) was placed in the central well, and the same volumes of positive sera and samples were placed in the surrounding wells. The feather follicle epithelium was tested for the presence of MDV antigen. The plates were then placed in a humidified cabinet at 37 °C, and the precipitation lines were examined after 72 h.

Virus isolation

Lymphocytes were separated with Lymphocyte Separation Medium (Tianjin Haoyang Biological Manufacture Co., Ltd) from the anticoagulant blood samples collected from the chickens. Primary CEF cultures were prepared from 10-day specific-pathogen-free embryos and inoculated in six-well plates with Dulbecco's modified Eagle's medium (DMEM) containing 5 % foetal bovine serum (FBS) in a total volume of 2 ml and incubated for 24 h. Then 60 µl of lymphocytes was added to the six-well plates that had been spread with the CEF. The plates were incubated at 37 °C in 5 % CO_2. After 24 h, the DMEM was replaced with DMEM maintenance medium containing 1 % FBS. The plates were then incubated in a culture chamber for 6 days with 2–3 blind passages.

Indirect immunofluorescence assay

The CEF with CPE were fixed with acetone: ethanol solution (3:2) for 10 min and washed once with PBS. After the fixed cells were blocked with 1 % BSA in PBS, they were incubated with the MDV-specific Mab BA4 [22] for 30 min at 37 °C. After three washes with PBS, the cells were incubated with fluorescein isothiocyanate (FITC)-conjugated goat anti-mouse antibody (Sigma-Aldrich, USA) for another 30 min. After three washes with PBS, the cells were examined under a fluorescence microscope.

PCR and sequence analysis

The *meq*, *pp38*, and *gB* genes of the isolates were amplified with the primers listed in Table 1. The DNA extracted from CEF infected with the isolate was used as the template. In the PCR system, 50 µl of reaction volume was used, consisting of 5 µl of 10×*LA Taq* PCR buffer, 2 µl each of the two primers, 0.5 µl of *LA Taq*DNA polymerase, 38.5 µl of ddH_2O, and 2 µl of the DNA template. The PCR parameters for the *pp38* and *meq*genes were: 95 °C for 5 min, 30 cycles of 94 °C for 60 s, 55 °C for 60 s, and 72 °C for 60 s, and then 72 °C for 10 min. The PCR parameters for the *gB* gene were: 95 °C for 5 min, 30 cycles of 94 °C for 60 s, 55 °C for 60 s, and 72 °C for 2 min, and then 72 °C for 10 min. The PCR products were separated on a 1 % DNA gel and then sequenced by Genscript (Nanjing, China). All the sequences were aligned and analysed with DNAStar.

Table 1: Primers used to amplify MDV genes

Target	Name	Sequence	Length
pp38	pp38-F	5-AATGGATCCATGGAATTCGAAGCAGAAC-3	903 bp
	pp38-R	5-ATTGTCGACAACATCGGGTACGGCTAC-3	
meq	meq-F	5-CGCGAATTCTACAGGTGTAAAGAGATG-3	1058 bp
	meq-R	5-TAACTCGAGTGCTGAGAGTCACAATGC-3	
gB	gB-F	5-CAGTCGACTATGCACTATTTTAG-3	2.8 kb
	gB-R	5-CAGGAATTCACAAGGAAAGCATCG-3	

DECLARATIONS

Acknowledgements

This research was supported by the National Natural Science Foundation of China (31472192), the Major Basic Research Department of the Natural Science Foundation of Jiangsu Higher Education Institutions of China (grant no. 12KJA23001), and the Priority Academic Program Development of Jiangsu Higher Education Institutions.

Authors' contributions

XYZ carried out the molecular genetic studies, the immunoassays, AGP test and Virus isolation, participated in the sequence alignment and drafted the manuscript. HYS carried out the histochemistry assay. HTZ participated in the sequence alignment. AJQ designed the study, analyzed the results and drafted the manuscript. JQY, HXS discussed and revised the manuscript. JM and GHW conceived of the study, and participated in its design and coordination. All authors read and approved the final manuscript.

REFERENCES

1. Calnek BW. Pathogenesis of Marek's disease virus infection. Curr Top Microbiol Immunol. 2001;255:25–55.
2. Afonso CL, Tulman ER, Lu Z, Zsak L, Rock DL, Kutish GF. The genome of turkey herpesvirus. J Virol. 2001;75(2):971–8.
3. Lupiani B, Lee LF, Reddy SM. Protein-coding content of the sequence of Marek's disease virus serotype 1. Curr Top Microbiol Immunol. 2001;255:159–90.
4. Zhang YP, Liu CJ, Zhang F, Shi W, Li J. Sequence analysis of the Meq gene in the predominant Marek's disease virus strains isolated in China during 2006–2008. Virus Genes. 2011;43(3):353–7.
5. Gong Z, Zhang L, Wang J, Chen L, Shan H, Wang Z, et al. Isolation and analysis of a very virulent Marek's disease virus strain in China. Virol J. 2013;10:155.
6. Gimeno IM, Witter RL, Hunt HD, Reddy SM, Lee LF, Silva RF. The pp 38 gene of Marek's disease virus (MDV) is necessary for cytolytic infection of B cells and maintenance of the transformed state but not for cytolytic infection of the feather follicle epithelium and horizontal spread of MDV. J Virol. 2005;79(7):4545–9.
7. Ross NL. T-cell transformation by Marek's disease virus. Trends Microbiol. 1999;7(1):22–9.
8. Witter RL, Silva RF, Lee LF. New serotype 2 and attenuated serotype 1 Marek's disease vaccine viruses: selected biological and molecular characteristics. Avian Diseases. 1987;31(4):829–40.
9. Davidson I, Borovskaya A, Perl S, Malkinson M. Use of the polymerase chain reaction for the diagnosis of natural infection of chickens and turkeys with Marek's disease virus and reticuloendotheliosis virus. Avian Pathol. 1995;24(1):69–94.
10. Cui Z, Qin A, Lee LF, Wu P, Kung HJ. Construction and characterization of a H19 epitope point mutant of MDV CVI988/Rispens strain. Acta Virol. 1999;43(2–3):169–73.
11. Chang KS, Ohashi K, Onuma M. Diversity (polymorphism) of the meq gene in the attenuated Marek's disease virus (MDV) serotype 1 and MDV-transformed cell lines. J Vet Med Sci. 2002;64(12):1097–101.
12. Lee LF, Wu P, Sui D, Ren D, Kamil J, Kung HJ, et al. The complete unique long sequence and the overall genomic organization of the GA strain of Marek's disease virus. Proc Natl Acad Sci U S A. 2000;97(11):6091–6.
13. Spatz SJ, Petherbridge L, Zhao Y, Nair V. Comparative full-length sequence analysis of oncogenic and vaccine (Rispens) strains of Marek's disease virus. J Gen Virol. 2007;88(Pt 4):1080–96.
14. Chang KS, Ohashi K, Onuma M. Suppression of transcription activity of the MEQ protein of oncogenic Marek's disease virus serotype 1 (MDV1) by L-MEQ of non-oncogenic MDV1. J Vet Med Sci. 2002;64(12):1091–5.
15. Shamblin CE, Greene N, Arumugaswami V, Dienglewicz RL, Parcells MS. Comparative analysis of Marek's disease virus (MDV) glycoprotein-, lytic antigen pp 38- and transformation antigen Meq-encoding genes: association of meq mutations with MDVs of high virulence. Vet Microbiol. 2004;102(3–4):147–67.
16. Zhang Z, Cui Z. Isolation of recombinant field strains of Marek's disease virus integrated with reticuloendotheliosis virus genome fragments. Sci China C Life Sci. 2005;48(1):81–8.
17. Okwor EC, Eze DC. Outbreak and Persistence of Marek's Disease in Batches of Birds Reared in a Poultry Farm Located in Nsukka, South East Nigeria. Int J Poult Sci. 2011;10(8):617–20.
18. Muniyellappa HK, Satyanarayana ML, Isloor S, Shivakumar Gowda NK. Marek's disease outbreak among vaccinated commercial layer flocks in the mining area of Karnataka, India. Vet Rec. 2013;172(17):452.
19. Ikezawa M, Goryo M, Sasaki J, Haridy M, Okada K. Late Marek's disease in adult chickens inoculated with virulent Marek's disease virus. J Vet Med Sci. 2010;72(12):1539–45.
20. Heier BT, Jarp J, Kaldhusdal MI, Schaller G, Forus IB. A longitudinal field study of mortality and Marek's disease in Norwegian and imported white Leghorns. Prev Vet Med. 1999;40(3–4):207–19.
21. Zhang W, Li Y, Lin J, Wan S, Gao H, Zhang L, et al. Comparison of hematoxylin-eosin staining and methyl violet staining for displaying ghost cells. Eye Sci. 2013;28(3):140–3.
22. Liu L, Qu Y, Wang T, Wang G, Wang F, Liu S. Skin involvement in lymphomas caused by Marek's disease virus infection in Silkie chickens. J Vet Diagn Invest. 2014;26(2):302–7.

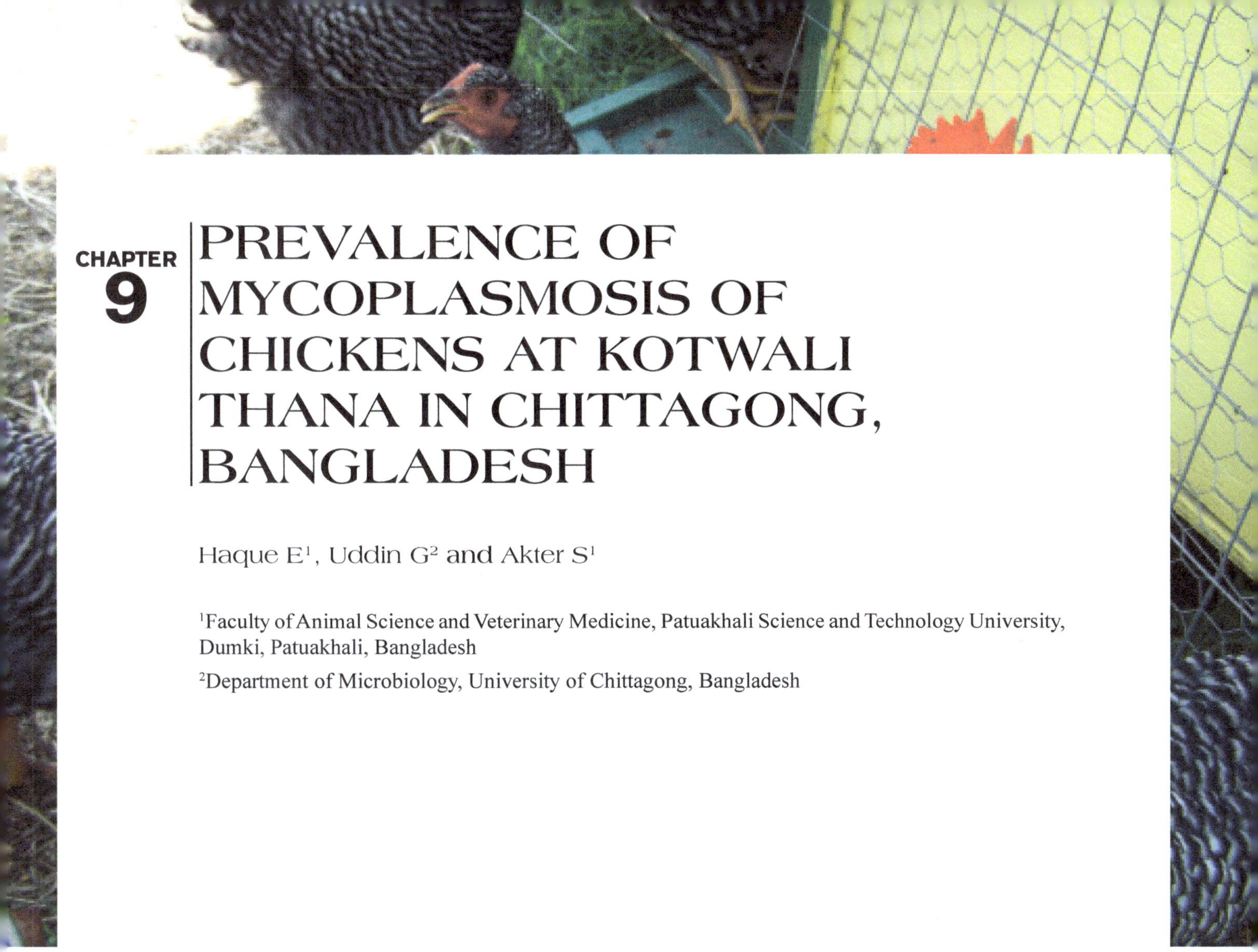

CHAPTER 9

PREVALENCE OF MYCOPLASMOSIS OF CHICKENS AT KOTWALI THANA IN CHITTAGONG, BANGLADESH

Haque E[1], Uddin G[2] and Akter S[1]

[1]Faculty of Animal Science and Veterinary Medicine, Patuakhali Science and Technology University, Dumki, Patuakhali, Bangladesh

[2]Department of Microbiology, University of Chittagong, Bangladesh

ABSTRACT

A study of prevalence of mycoplasmosis of chicken at kotwali thana in Chittagong was conducted from 23rd November, 2010 to 22nd March, 2011. A total of 455 either dead or sick birds were examined during the period. Diagnosis was based on history, clinical signs, serum plate agglutination (SPA) test and postmortem lesions. The overall prevalence of mycoplasmosis was 15.38%. The prevalence was 73% in broiler and 27% in layer. The result further revealed that highest number of cases were recorded in the age group of 8-21 days (49%) followed by 22-35 days age group (21%), 0-7 days age group (21%), 36-60 days age group (6%) and over 60 days age group (3%). It was also demonstrated that during the study period the highest prevalence of mycoplasmosis was recorded in January (33%) followed by February (30%), March (23%), and December (13%) and lowest in November (1%).

INTRODUCTION

Poultry industry is one of the rapidly developing areas in the livestock sector of Bangladesh. This industry is playing an important role in the economy of Bangladesh. At present, one of the most important sources of protein in Bangladesh is poultry meat and eggs. Over the years commercial poultry farming has been developed introduce some high yielding strains of chicken are reared in intensive system. The total number of domestic chicken in Bangladesh is about 195 million [1]. Moreover poultry sub-sector has provided job opportunity to the unemployed young people. But at present this profitable sub-sector is seriously interrupted by a number of infectious and contagious diseases such as Newcastle disease, Infectious bursal disease, mycoplasmosis, Salmonellosis, Fowl cholera, Avian leucosis complex, Marek´s disease, Infectious laryngotracheitis, Infectious coryza, Aspergillosis, Coccidiosis, Necrotic enteritis and mycotoxicosis. Among these infectious diseases, mycoplasmosis is of great importance. In Bangladesh, the sero-prevalence of Mycoplasma gallisepticum was reported in exotic hybrid chickens by Amin [2]. Mycoplasmosis is a chronic and slow spreading contagious disease in birds characterized by obstinate hacking cough, sneezing and tracheal rales [3]. The economic loss often incurred results from poor feed conversion ratio of broiler, declining of egg production in layer, reduction of hatchability in breeder flock, down-grading of broiler meat and condemnations of carcasses. The disease can be transmitted both horizontally and vertically and remain in the flock constantly as subclinical form [4]. The present study was undertaken to determine the prevalence of mycoplasmosis in chickens at Kotwali Thana in Chittagong.

Citation: Haque E, Uddin G, Akter S (2015) Prevalence of Mycoplasmosis of Chickens at Kotwali Thana in Chittagong, Bangladesh. J Fisheries Livest Prod 3:151. doi:10.4172/2332-2608.1000151.

MATERIALS AND METHODS

A pathological investigation on the prevalence of mycoplasmosis was conducted at the Thana Livestock Hospital at Kotwali in Chittagong region from 23rd November, 2010 to 22nd March, 2011. Serological test was conducted in the laboratory of Thana Livestock Office at Kotwali in Chittagong. A total of 455 dead or sick birds of different poultry farms of Kotwali Thana at Chittagong region, were used for this study. These birds were brought to the Thana Livestock Office at Kotwali in Chittagong. Diagnosis of disease was made on the basis of history, clinical signs, serological test and postmortem lesions.

Diagnosis of mycoplasmosis

Diagnosis of mycoplasmosis was made on the basis of clinical signs of infected chickens and postmortem changes in dead chickens. The birds were examined systematically and the postmortem changes were recorded during necropsy.

Clinical signs

The disease was diagnosed based on clinical signs including nasal discharge, coughing, and rales. Depression, conjunctivitis, swollen eye, eyelid edema and other more general signs were included such as in appetence, depression, weight loss and a drop in egg production. The highest morbidity and mortality occurred in the presence of concurrent infections and environmental stress.

Serological analysis

In live birds, blood samples (2 mL) were collected from wing vein by using fresh disposable plastic syringe (5 mL) and collected blood was kept at room temperature for about 1 to 2 hours.

A clean straw color serum was seen around the clotted clump and after centrifugation (252 g for 10 minutes) the serum was stored at -20°C until used.

Serum plate agglutination (SPA) test

The SPA test was conducted with crystal violet stained M. gallisepticum commercial antigen (Nobilis® MG) obtained from Intervet Company Ltd. (The Netherlands). Following the manufacturer›s instruction, antigen (0.03 mL) and crude or diluted serum (0.03 mL) was placed side by side with pipette in a glass plate and mixed well by stirring with glass rod, followed by rocking. Results were read within 2 minutes [5,6]. In positive cases granules were formed slowly which could be seen during rocking. In the negative case, no such granules were formed. All SPA results were recorded.

Postmortem changes

Diagnosis was confirmed by post-mortem examination of dead chickens. Lesions comprising catarrhal exudates in the nasal passages, infraorbital sinuses, trachea, and bronchi, Caseous exudates in the air sacs, fibrinous or fibrinopurulent pericarditis, perihepatitis and congestion in lungs were observed.

Data analysis

Clinical and postmortem data were categorized according to age, month of study period and types of chicken (layer and broiler). Data were analyzed by normal tabular method with Microsoft office excel 2007.

RESULTS

A total number of 455 chickens were examined and mycoplasmosis was diagnosed in 70 chickens. Among them 51 broiler birds (73%) followed by 19 layer birds (27%) were positive to mycoplasma. The overall prevalence of mycoplasma was 15.38% (Figure 1).

The result revealed that highest number of cases were recorded in the age group (Table 1) of 8-21 days 34 (49%) followed by 22-35 days age group 15 (21%), 0-7 days age group 15 (21%), 36-60 days age group 4 (6%) and over 60 days age group 2 (3%) of chicken.

The prevalence of mycoplasmosis on different months (Table 2) of study period during which prevalence was recorded highest in January 23 (33%) followed by February 21 (30%), March 16 (23%) and December 9 (13%) and lowest in November 1 (1%).

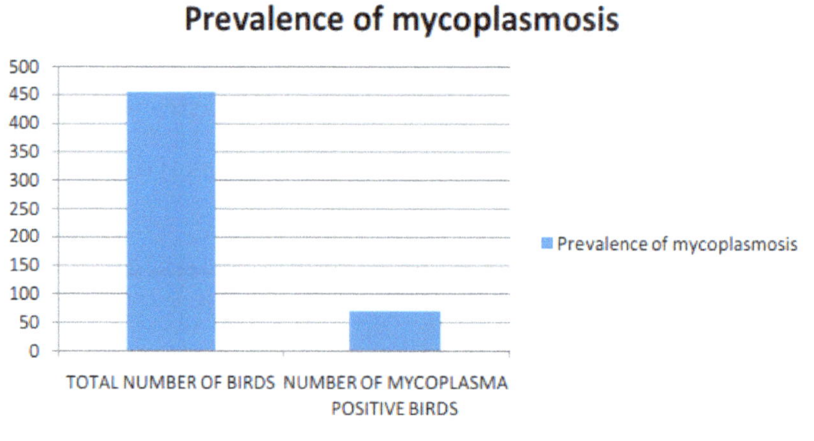

Figure 1 represents prevalence of mycoplasmosis. Total numbers of birds were 455 and mycoplasma positive birds were 70. It was observed that the overall prevalence of mycoplasmosis in chickens was (15.38%).

Figure 1: Prevalence of mycoplasmosis.

Table 1: Prevalence of mycoplasmosis on different age groups

Age of birds	0-7 Days	8-21 Days	22-35 Days	35-60 Days	Over 60 days
Positive case	15	34	15	4	2
Percentage	21%	49%	21%	6%	3%

Table 2: Prevalence of mycoplasmosis on different month of the study period

Different month of the study period	Number of positive case	Percentage
November	1	1%
December	9	13%
January	23	33%
February	21	30%
March	16	23%

DISCUSSION

Prevalence of mycoplasmosis was estimated on the Thana Livestock Office at Kotwali in Chittagong. The present study revealed 15.38% of mycoplasmosis in Chittagong region which did not vary significantly with earlier investigations. 11.55% of cases of mycoplasmosis at Chittagong and Mymensingh region, but prevalence of the present study is higher than previous study, reported 5.32% on Sylhet. This variation may be due to cold environmental condition.

The overall prevalence of mycoplasmosis was lower than that of earlier report of 55.83% [7], 52% [8] and 13-22% [2]. The present findings were also differed with the previous results reported by Kelly et al. [9] in Zimbabwe, Chrysostome et al. [10] in Benin, Shah-Majid [11] in Malaysia, Pandey and Hasegawa [12] in Zambia. Bencina et al. [13] and Godoy et al. [14] reported 56.54, 57.15 and 59.10% seroprevalence of MG infection in chickens, respectively. This might be due increase awareness about vaccination against mycoplasma among the farmers around the Thana Livestock Office at Kotwali in Chittagong. Only postmortem and serological based diagnosis of mycoplasmosis was might be another reason.

In the present study, seasonal variation in MG seroprevalence was observed. Variation of prevalence of mycoplasmosis on different month of the study period was observed at the present study. The prevalence was higher 33% in January followed by 30% in February, 23% in March 13% in December and 1% in November which was in agreement with the result of Pradhan et al. [15]. The prevalence was highest in winter and lowest in summer which was in agreement with the results. It was probable that the cold weather depress the natural resistance of birds, leading to an increased susceptibility to infections.

In the present investigation the prevalence was also found to have decreased with the increase of age. Similar report was demonstrated highest MG infection (71.42%) at 18 weeks of age and lowest (55.17%) at 63 weeks of age. This finding also supports the report of Sarkar et al. [16] who recorded 73.80% MG infection at 20 weeks of age in comparison to 45.16% at 55 weeks of age. Similar report was demonstrated the prevalence of MG infection significantly decreased with the increase of age. It might be due to the seasonal influence as during the winter birds were younger than in summer season [17]. Highest infection in the young chickens is probably due to the vertical transmission of this organism.

CONCLUSION

In this Study, it was well mentioning that the prevalence of MG was higher in broiler then layer birds. Age and seasonal variation plays an important role in occurrence of this disease. So more attention should be given at the age and season as mycoplasmosis is the most economically significant disease in poultry industry of Bangladesh which causes serious economic losses in poultry farm, reduce feed efficiency, decrease growth and reduce egg production. The present study is a preliminary work on the mycoplasmosis which was identified only on the basis of history, clinical signs, Serum plate agglutination (SPA) test and postmortem lesions. However, the result of this study will certainly help the future researchers to provide guidance in carrying out further detail study on mycoplasmosis of poultry in Bangladesh.

REFERENCES

1. Dolberg F (2008)Poultry Sector Country Review: Bangladesh.
2. Amin MM, Sidique M, Rahman MM (1992)Investigation on chronic respiratory disease in chickens: part-II. BUA Research Progress6: 519-526.
3. Chakraborty D, Sadhukahan T, Guha D, Chatarjee A (2001)Seroprevalence of Mycoplasmagallisepticumin West Bengal. Indian Veterinary Journal 78: 855-856.
4. Bencina D, Tadina T, Dorrer D (1988) Natural infection of geese with Mycoplasma gallisepticumand Mycoplasma synoviae and egg transmission of the mycoplasmas. AvianPathology 17: 925-928.
5. Pakpinyo S, Pitayachamrat P, Saccavadit S, Santaswang T, Tawatsin Tet al. (2006) Laboratory diagnosis of Mycoplasma gallisepticum(MG) infection in experimental layer chicken receiving MG vaccines and MG organisms. Thai J vet Med 36: 29-37.
6. Ley DH, Yoder HWJr (1997)Mycoplasma gallisepticuminfection. In: Calnek BW, Barnes H,Beard

CW, McDougald LR, Saif YM (eds) Diseases of poultry. Iowa StateUniversity Press.

7. Islam M, Hassan J, Khan MSR (2014)Seroprevalence of Mycoplasma gallisepticuminfection in backyard and commercial layer chickens in Bhola district, Bangladesh. J Adv Vet Anim Res 1: 11-15.
8. Dulali RS (2003)Seroprevalence and Pathology of Mycoplasmosis in Sonali chickens.
9. Kelly PJ, Chitauro D, Rhode C, Rukwava J, Majok A, et al. (1994) Diseases and management of backyard chicken flocks in chiturgwiza. Avian Dis 38: 626-629.
10. Chrysostome CAAM, Bell JG, Demey F, Verhulst A (1995)Seroprevalence to three diseases in village chickens in Benin. Prevent Vet Med 22: 257-261.
11. Shah-Majid M (1996) Detection of Mycoplasma gallisepticumantibodies in sera of village chickensby the enzyme linked immunosorbent assay. TropAnim Heal Prod 28: 181-182.
12. Pandey GS, Hasegawa M (1998) Serological survey of Mycoplasma gallisepticumandMycoplasma synoviaeinfection in chickens Zambia.Bull Anim Heal ProdAfr46:113-117.
13. Bencina D, Mrzel I, Tadina T, Dorrer D (1987) Mycoplasma species in chicken flocks with different management systems. AvPathol16: 599-608.
14. Godoy A, Andrade LF, Colmenares O, Bermudez V, Herrera A, et al. (2001) Prevalence of Mycoplasma gallisepticum in egg-laying hens. Vet Trop26: 25-33.
15. PradhanMAM, Amin MM, Taimur MJF (2000)Asero-prevalence study of avian mycoplasmosis in Bangladesh.
16. Sarkar SK, Rahman MB, Rahman M, Amin KMR, Khan MFR, et al. (2005)Seroprevalence of Mycoplasmagallisepticuminfection in chickens in model breeder poultry farms of Bangladesh. Inter J PoultSci4: 32-35.
17. Nunoya T, Yagihashi T, Tajima M, Nagasawa Y (1995) Occurrence ofkerato-conjunctivitis apparently caused by Mycoplasma gallisepticumin layer chickens. Veterinary Pathology 32: 11-18.

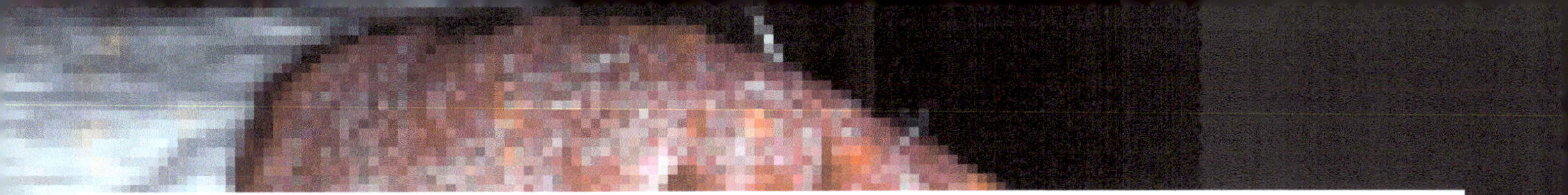

CHAPTER 10

THE SUCCESSFUL EXPERIMENTAL INDUCTION OF NECROTIC ENTERITIS IN CHICKENS BY CLOSTRIDIUM PERFRINGENS: A CRITICAL REVIEW

Bahram Shojadoost[1], Andrew R Vince[2] and John F Prescott[2]

[1] Department of Clinical Sciences, Faculty of Veterinary Medicine, University of Tehran, Tehran, Iran

[2] Department of Pathobiology, University of Guelph, Guelph, Ontario N1G 2W1, Canada

ABSTRACT

Necrotic enteritis (NE) is one of the most important enteric diseases in poultry and is a high cost to the industry worldwide. It is caused by avian-specific, Necrotic Enteritis Beta toxin (NetB)-producing, strains ofClostridium perfringens that also possess in common other virulence-associated genes. In Europe the disease incidence has increased since the ban on in-feed "growth promoting" antibiotics. Because of this, many recent studies of NE have focused on finding different ways to control the disease, and on understanding its pathogenesis. Frustratingly, reproduction of the disease has proven impossible for some researchers. This review describes and discusses factors known to be important in reproducing the disease experimentally, as well as other considerations in reproducing the disease. The critical bacterial factor is the use of virulent,netB-positive, strains; virulence can be enhanced by using tpeL- positive strains and by the use of young rather than old broth cultures to increase toxin expression. Intestinal damaging factors, notably the use of concurrent or preceding coccidial infection, or administration of coccidial vaccines, combined with netB-positive C. perfringens administration, can also be used to induce NE. Nutritional factors, particularly feeding high percentage of cereals containing non-starch polysaccharides (NSP) (wheat, rye, and barley) enhance disease by increasing digesta viscosity, mucus production and bacterial growth. Animal proteins, especially fish meal, enhance C. perfringens proliferation and toxin production. Other factors are discussed that may affect outcome but for which evidence of their importance is lacking. The review compares the different challenge approaches; depending on the aim of particular studies, the different critical factors can be adjusted to affect the severity of the lesions induced. A standardized scoring system is proposed for international adoption based on gross rather than histopathological lesions; if universally adopted this will allow better comparison between studies done by different researchers. Also a scoring system is provided to assist decisions on humane euthanasia of sick birds.

INTRODUCTION

Necrotic enteritis (NE) in chickens, first reported by Parish [1], is an enteric disease caused by *C. perfringens*, a Gram-positive anaerobic spore-forming, rod-shaped bacterium [2]. According to the current classification, *C. perfringens* has five toxinogenic types (A, B, C, D, E), which are differentiated according to the production of four different major toxins (Alpha, Beta, Epsilon, Iota) [3]. The discovery in recent years of new toxins (Beta2, NetB, TpeL) in *C. perfringens* shows the need for an enhanced classification scheme. NE is caused by type A isolates [3] and rarely by type C isolates [4,5]. The recently discovered new toxin, NetB, is crucial for development of the disease [6,7].

Citation: Bahram Shojadoost, Andrew R Vince and John F Prescott, The successful experimental induction of necrotic enteritis in chickens by Clostridium perfringens: a critical review, doi: 10.1186/1297-9716-43-74.

Keyburn et al.'s [6] seminal discovery of the crucial role of the pore-forming toxin NetB led to the subsequent characterization of three pathogenicity loci (PAL) that are characteristic of NE isolates [8]. Two PAL (NELoc1, NELoc 3) are plasmid-encoded, usually on different plasmids [8]. Two plasmids on which these PAL are found have recently been fully sequenced [9]. NE isolates belong to two major lineages or clones [10], suggesting that these lineages have adapted to cause NE in chickens.

The intestinal number of *C. perfringens* in healthy and in NE-affected birds are different. The *C. perfringens*population is found to be normally less than 10^2 to 10^4 colony-forming units (CFU) per g of the intestinal contents in the small intestine of healthy chickens compared to 10^7 - 10^9 CFU/g in diseased birds [11].

NE occurs in broilers aged between two and six weeks [4,12]. Mortality can reach 1% per day with a total mortality of 10-40% [13]. Clinical signs include depression, dehydration, diarrhea, ruffled feathers and lower feed intake [4]. The gross lesions of the small intestine range from thin and friable walls to frank and extensive necrotic lesions [12]. Two forms of the disease are described, clinical and subclinical [4,7,14]. The clinical form appears with the clinical signs and mortality noted above. The subclinical form presents as poor performance (reduced growth, reduced feed efficiency) without mortality. This form of the disease can be diagnosed by reduced feed conversion, by gross lesions in the small intestine and by bacteriology [14]. Most of the economic losses due to NE are related to the subclinical form and the high cost of preventing the disease with antibiotics.

Antibacterial drugs are commonly used to prevent or control the disease. In recent years, the European Union has banned the use of in-feed antimicrobials or growth promoters, leading to an increase in disease outbreaks in broiler flocks in European countries [15,16]. Globally, the economical impact of the disease is estimated at US$ 2 billion year through mortalities and poor performance and the cost of prevention and treatment [15,17]. In EU countries, the profit of severely NE affected broiler flocks has been 33% less than flocks with low level of the disease [17]. The variables affected the significant economic cost of subclinical NE have been estimated [18].

In recent years there has been an explosion of interest in understanding the pathogenesis of NE and investigating how it can be prevented by approaches other than the use of antibiotics. Many of these studies necessitate experimental induction of the disease. However, published and anecdotal reports attest to the difficulty that some workers have experienced in reproduction of the disease [16,19,20]. It is the purpose of this review to summarize the different approaches used to reproduce NE, to identify factors that are critical to successful production of experimental disease, and to highlight areas of uncertainty that require further investigation. The purpose of the review is to assist researchers to understand NE so that their experimental procedures are based on an evidence-based and logical approach.

Necrotic enteritis is a complex and multi-factorial disease. The factors affecting development of the disease in the field were well summarized by Williams [21], unfortunately just before the discovery of NetB. Figure 1 is a simplified diagram, extending that of William's earlier figure, which summarizes some of the critical factors influencing the development of the disease.

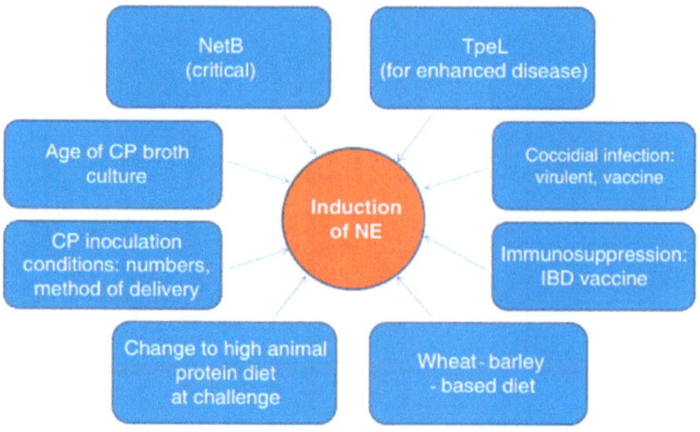

Figure 1: Critical factors influencing the development of necrotic enteritis. Summary of different factors important for the successful reproduction of necrotic enteritis; the most critical factor is presence of netB and the netB plasmid, but other factors summarized in the figure all affect the outcome of experimental infection. They can be manipulated by researchers to vary the severity of the disease produced and the outcome desired.

DIFFERENT REASONS TO REPRODUCE NECROTIC ENTERITIS

Different researchers have different reasons for reproducing necrotic enteritis, which will impact the design of studies as well as the severity of disease that they wish to produce. Reasons to reproduce the disease have included comparison of antimicrobial drugs [22-27], vaccines [28-31], assessment of virulence determinants [6,32], or assessment of pathological processes [19]. Others have studied the effect of different predisposing factors including nutritional components on the severity of NE [2,33-37], the effects of probiotics and prebiotics [23], or different experimental models of disease [38-41]. Design considerations will also include the need for control groups and the need for isolation facilities to ensure lack of spread of infection between control and infected birds. The novice researcher is advised to perform a small scale pilot study both to confirm their ability to reproduce the disease and to identify the different effects of variables discussed below that affect the severity of the disease that they wish to produce. It would be anticipated that production of severe experimental disease would mask some of the beneficial effects of interventions such as feed components or immunization.

POINTS TO BE CONSIDERED IN SUCCESSFUL REPRODUCTION OF NECROTIC ENTERITIS

Nutritional factors

Feeding indigestible non-starch polysaccharides

Several studies have shown that feeds (barley, rye, wheat) containing high amount of water-soluble indigestible non-starch polysaccharide (NSP), such as β-glucans or arabinoxylans, increase the viscosity of the digesta and predispose chickens to NE [13,14,42,43]. The higher viscosity of digesta in diets containing wheat or barley leads to prolonged transit time in the intestine, which may be responsible for the direct correlation between intestinal viscosity and clostridial counts [42]. However, equally or more importantly, NSP also interact with glycoproteins on the epithelial surface to increase mucin production [44]. *C. perfringens* has an "arsenal" of up to 56 glycoside hydrolases directed at the muco-oligosacharides prominent in the mucosal layers of the intestine [45,46]. The two prominent chitinase genes present on the major pathogenicity locus (NELoc1) of NE isolates are speculated to have mucin degradation functions [8].

In a *C. perfringens* challenge model, mortalities in birds fed a supernatant of digested maize ranged from 0-12%, whereas birds that received barley, rye or wheat showed mortality of 26-35% [47]. Mortality due to NE in coccidiosis-challenged chicks with a corn-based diet was also less than mortality in a wheat-based diet [48]. The number of *C. perfringens* in the intestine in corn-based diet fed broilers were 1.2-1.5 $\log_{10}$ colony-forming units/g lower than in the birds fed 50% rye in their feed [49]. Others have also reported the increased incidence of NE associated with wheat or barley diets [14,50]. Since NSPs are not well digested they reach the lower intestinal tract and alter its environment [51,52].

The size of the feed particles has been shown to affect the number of *C. perfringens* in the intestine. As expected, highly ground feed allows *C. perfringens* to proliferate faster and to larger numbers than coarse ground feed [48,53], and can predispose birds to NE [48,54].

Other nutritional factors can impact the severity of NE. For example, trypsin inhibitors in non-toasted soya bean based ration increased the severity of NE lesions, in direct proportion to the quantity of soya bean in the feed [55]. Trypsin inhibition is well established as a predisposing factor to enteric disease caused by *C. perfringens*, since trypsin in the small intestine destroys *C. perfringens* toxins [4].

Researchers should ensure that feed of experimental birds contains neither antibiotics nor anti-coccidials, recognizing that the latter may also have antibacterial properties.

Feeding large amounts of animal protein (fish meal)

A characteristic of *C. perfringens* identified through genome sequencing is the inability of this "anaerobic flesh eater" to synthesize the majority of amino acids; *C. perfringens* rapidly breakdown tissues through the extraordinary array of hydrolytic enzymes that it produces [56]. Large amounts of animal-origin protein in the diet predispose poultry to NE [21,50,57]. The presence of high crude protein concentration and some amino acids are related to commencement of *C. perfringens* overgrowth and production of alpha toxin [58]. Glycine is among the amino acids that stimulate growth and production of alpha toxin [59,60] and is positively correlated with the number of *C. perfringens*in the intestine [61]. Therefore the glycine content of the diet may be important to predispose birds to NE. The level of *C. perfringens* has been found highest with the greater amount of animal protein (40% crude protein/feed) and lowest in plant-source protein diets fed to chicks [19,62]. Large amounts of fish meal have been associated with *C. perfringens* proliferation and the occurrence of NE [63]. The amounts of glycine and methionine, which increase *C. perfringens* proliferation and alpha toxin concentrations in vitro, are higher than other amino acids in fish meal protein-based diets [60]. Although there has been no study of the effect of diet specifically on NetB toxin production, both the *netB* gene as well as the internalin gene adjacent to it on NELoc1 have VirR boxes [8,64], suggesting that, like alpha toxin, their expression is under control of the VirR-VirS regulatory system that controls virulence gene expression in this organism. It is therefore likely that conditions that increase alpha toxin also increase the critically important NetB.

Having a diet with, or changing the diet to one with high protein before the time of challenge seems to enhance the severity of NE although this effect has not been critically evaluated in detail, and comparisons are difficult because of use of different scoring systems. Changing the diet to a high protein diet before *C. perfringens* challenge increased the severity of induced NE, but mixing the diet with 30-50% fish meal has been done either on the same day [65], one day after [41], or seven [24,26,65,66] days before *C. perfringens*challenge. In one study, turkey feed (28% protein) was mixed with 50% fish meal and given to chicks from 1–13 days of age, which resulted in 12% mortality and 65% of the birds showing NE lesions when the chicks were challenged with *C. perfringens* at 14 days of age [22]. Consumption of diets containing lower energy: protein ratios not only leads to increased feed intake and higher nitrogen content of the digesta and feces [13] but can also lead to an enhanced substrate for *C. perfringens*[67,68]. It seems that feeding birds with a high protein diet for a longer period of time is better in reproducing more severe NE, but details of timing have not been determined. The high protein ration should be present at the time of challenge.

Role of coccidia

Coccidiosis is an enteric parasitic disease caused in poultry by various *Eimeria* spp. [21]. Some (*E. brunetti,E. maxima, E. necatrix, E. tenella*) produce more severe disease than others (*E. acervulina, E. mitis, E. praecox*) [21]. Damage to the epithelium caused by coccidia is a major predisposing factor for NE, allowing*C. perfringens* to replicate rapidly and produce toxin [69], probably because leakage of proteins including plasma into the lumen of the gut during *Eimeria* infection provides the protein-rich nutrient substrates favorable to *C. perfringens* proliferation and toxin production [16]. The mucogenesis induced by coccidial infection may also be important [70].

For these reasons, *Eimeria* spp. have often been used in conjunction with *C. perfringens* to induce NE experimentally. Since NE is a disease of small intestine, *E. acervulina, E. maxima* or *E. necatrix* are the most suitable species [2,15,23,40,71]. There are differences in opinion as to whether the more virulent *Eimeria*, such as *E. necatrix* are better than the less virulent *E. acervulina* choices for this purpose [2,72]. To obtain the effect of coccidial challenge, damage to the epithelium should occur before challenge with *C. perfringens*[43]. Table 1 summarizes the timing and the effect of different *Eimeria* spp. in conjunction with the timing of *C. perfringens* challenge. *Eimeria* vaccines have also been used to enhance the effect of *C. perfringens* challenge [20,41].

Table 1: Effect of coccidial challenge on severity of experimental necrotic enteritis

Researchers	*Eimeria* spp.	Age of coccidia challenge (day)	Age of *C. perfringens* challenge (day)	% Mortality	
				With coccidia	Without coccidia
[71]	*E. necatrix*	11	15	28.3	16
[71]	*E. acervulina*	13	15	53.3	16
[70]	*E. acervulina E. maxima*	14	18, 19, 20	7.6	2.8
[2]	*E. necatrix*	4	5, 6, 7, 8, 9	22.5	0
[41]	Paracox-8 (Vaccine)	19	18, 19, 20, 21	0[1]	0
[41]	*E. maxima*	20	19, 20, 21, 22	0[1]	0
[41]	Paracox-8 (Vaccine)	16	19, 20, 21, 22	0[1]	0
[20]	Paracox-5 (vaccine)	20	19, 20, 21, 22	0[1]	0
[84]	Paracox-8 (Vaccine)	10	9, 10, 11, 12	0[1]	0[1]
[84]	Paracox-8 (Vaccine)	18	17, 18, 19, 20	0[1]	0[1]

[1]Sub-clinical necrotic enteritis (No mortality).

The time of administration of the coccidial vaccine or of virulent *Eimeria* is critical, and should be not more than 4–5 days before the *C. perfringens* challenge so that the coccidia-induced intestinal damage coincides with bacterial challenge [21,40]. When the *C. perfringens* challenge lasted for 4 days, no significant difference was observed in the severity of lesions in birds receiving coccidial vaccine 3 days before or one day after the onset of *C. perfringens* challenge [20,41].

The dose of *Eimeria* is also important; successful NE disease has been induced by 2×10^4*E. necatrix* or $2–5 \times 10^4$*E. maxima*[2,41,70]. Numbers above these may be fatal. For less pathogenic species such as *E. acervulina*, higher doses (7.5×10^4 up to 5×10^5) have been used [70,71]. Attenuated coccidial vaccines, which as commercial products may be more accessible for some researchers, have been used at 10-times recommended vaccination doses [20,41], since lower doses of the vaccine may not be as efficacious.

When reproducing NE, the purpose of the study will determine which combination of the *C. perfringens* and *Eimeria* spp. or *Eimeria* vaccines should be used, for example whether the intention is to produce severe or mild disease, or whether the intention is to test *C. perfringens* vaccines. The studies should be designed to include controls of *Eimeria* alone, *C. perfringens* alone, and combined *Eimeri*a and *C. perfringens*. The dose and species or type of coccidal challenge should be chosen with care, depending on the purpose of reproducing NE, since use of coccidia can readily result in severe disease. For example, when testing a vaccine, or a specific drug against NE, it is probably better to reproduce the NE without the help of virulent coccidial challenge, or to use attenuated coccidial vaccines.

An unresolved question is whether, if coccidia are used to enhance the disease process, it is a requirement for the *C. perfringens* to contain *netB*; it seems highly likely, but requires to be demonstrated.

The role of immunosuppression in experimental necrotic enteritis

Immunosuppressed chickens are more likely to develop necrotic enteritis, so that some researchers have used methods to induce immunosuppression. These methods mostly use Infectious Bursal Disease vaccine (IBD) [20,33,34,41]. It has resulted in a significant increase in NE lesions [33]. This has been done by administering a usual dose of IBD vaccine with a medium pathogenicity (intermediate class) [20,41], or 10 times the dose of an IBD vaccine with relatively higher pathogenicity (intermediate plus) [73]. The lesion scores are higher when IBD vaccine is used, even with a normal dose of an intermediate class IBD vaccine [41].

Stressful conditions may decrease immunity and predispose to NE [13]. Increasing stocking density, as a "stressful" measure, combined with IBD vaccine, was used in an experimental model of NE [73], but was not evaluated independently of IBD. Welfare considerations preclude deliberately "stressing" chickens. As evident from this review, there are numerous other factors that can be used to induce disease reliably. Use of immunosuppression as part of the induction of NE is inappropriate if vaccines are being evaluated.

Bacteriological aspects

Critical virulence features of C. perfringens strains involved in NE in chickens, and in reproducing the disease

Clostridum perfringens is notorious for its ability to produce a wide variety of toxins. Although for many years alpha toxin, a chromosomally-encoded zinc metalloenzyme with lecithinase and sphingomyelinase activity [43], was thought to be the major virulence factor in NE [72,74], the early histological changes in NE are not consistent with the sphingomyelinase or phospholipase C activities of alpha-toxin [19]. A critical study by Keyburn et al. [32], showed that a *cpa* mutant, which was unable to produce alpha toxin, was still able to produce the disease. The final breakthrough in understanding NE was the demonstration by the same workers of a novel pore-forming toxin, NetB, which was shown to be essential in producing disease [6]. NetB has homology to the pore-forming beta toxin of *C. perfringens*, as well as to the alpha hemolysin and gamma toxin of *Staphylococcus aureus*[7]. The *netB* gene is mostly found in isolates from NE outbreaks, and is relatively uncommon in isolates from healthy birds [7,75-78]. In a chicken experimental model assessing the virulence of 10 *C. perfringens* isolates from several sources, including cattle, normal chickens, humans, soil and swine, Cooper et al. [79] found that only the *netB*-positive isolate from a field case of NE was able to cause disease.

The *netB* gene is associated with a 42 kb pathogenicity locus (NELoc-1), which is on a 85 kb plasmid, as well as with another possibly less important plasmid-associated locus, NELoc3, present on a separate plasmid, and with a chromosomally-located pathogenicity locus, NELoc2 [8,9]. It seems very likely that the difficulty that many workers have experienced in reproducing disease can be attributed to the loss of the entire virulence plasmid containing the *netB* pathogenicity locus. It is however insufficient simply to use *C. perfringens* isolated from NE lesions to try to reproduce NE, since not all these may contain *netB*[76]. Recent multilocus sequence typing (MLST) studies have also identified two prevalent clonal groups among NE-associated isolates [10,75], suggesting that not just the virulence plasmids but also specific chromosomal genes (i.e., the bacterial host background) may also be important in NE pathogenesis or possibly for maintenance of the plasmids.

TpeL, a member of Large Clostridial Toxins (LCT) family [80], is present in some type A NE isolates [75]. There is evidence that *netB*-positive strains that are also *tpeL*-positive cause more severe disease than strains that lack *tpeL*[81].

In summary, emerging understanding of NE is that the strain and particularly the virulence plasmids of NE isolates are critical in producing disease, with *netB* being the only virulence factor to date shown to be essential in producing disease. Severity of disease may vary with the presence of other virulence determinants, of which the best implicated accessory toxin is *tpeL*. Because of the complexity of virulence regulation in *C. perfringens*, spontaneous mutations in VirR-VirS or other regulatory genes may affect virulence. It would therefore be prudent before embarking on the expense of large-scale NE studies for researchers to compare and confirm the virulence of potential *netB*-positive challenge strains in a pilot study. If more severe disease is desired, it is recommended to obtain a strain possessing *tpeL*. Because of the danger of loss of virulence plasmids, researchers attempting to reproduce NE should continuously maintain a "paranoid" approach to confirming throughout their work (using PCR) that the experimental strain has not lost the *netB* gene (and therefore the *netB* plasmid). The PCR should be done on individual colonies, not as a "sweep" of a blood plate, since PCR is so sensitive that researchers may not recognize through "sweeps" of a plate that the strain is gradually losing plasmids as it is subcultured. Maintaining a frozen stock of the virulent strain will ensure against loss of plasmid during subculture. A specific strain designation should always be given to the challenge strain, which should be made available to other researchers on request.

Preparation of clostridium perfringens for challenge

Type of culture media

Several different anaerobic culture media and different incubation times have been used to reproduce NE. The choice depends on both convenience and cost, so that fluid thioglycolate medium (with dextrose) (FTG) is the most common culture medium used for challenge purposes [19,33-35,38,39,47]. Adding peptone and starch to this medium increased the level of alpha toxin production [72], although as noted it is NetB not alpha toxin that is critically important in NE. Others have used cooked meat medium (CMM) [36,60] or brain heart infusion broth (BHI) [82-84], but CMM is expensive and BHI does not have reducing agents in it, so that it needs to be cultured anaerobically which will likely be inconvenient. FTG broth has the advantage that it can be cultured aerobically. Many researchers cultured the *C. perfringens*challenge strain initially in fluid CMM and then subsequently inoculate this CMM "stock" into FTG [12,22,65,66,79,85-87]. This system is mostly used for convenience but partly for historical reasons. The FTG is used as the challenge inoculum.

Incubation time

Younger (15 h) FTG cultures produce more severe disease than 24 h cultures [28,38] probably because of greater production of toxin(s) at this time. For example, 15 h broth culture increased lesion scores by over 50% compared to 24 h cultures [28]. It is also likely that older, stationary, phase cultures will produce proteases that degrade NetB and other toxins. Logistically, however, for researchers who challenge birds twice a day with broth, it may be difficult to prepare a 15 h culture for the afternoon challenge since they would need to start FTG incubation of their challenge strain at midnight. If researchers want to produce less severe disease, then an afternoon feeding with a 24-h culture can be used.

Successful challenge using *C. perfringens* alone depends on initiating intestinal damage by preformed toxin rather than by toxin produced in the intestine [72]. Therefore whole broth cultures (which contain pre formed toxins) and not just vegetative *C. perfringens* cells should always be used.

3.4.2.3. Amount of bacteria for challenge

The amount of *C. perfringens* used for challenge is important for successful challenge. It is normally between 10^7 to 10^9 CFU/mL [33,34,60]. A 15-h overnight FTG broth culture inoculated with a 3% (v/v) overnight CMM culture and incubated at 37°C will contain over 10^8*C. perfringens*/mL.

Challenge methods

One successful approach that has commonly been used is to present the challenge strain to birds through feed, inoculated at a ratio of 1.25-1.5 fluid FTG: feed (v/w). Birds are usually initially starved overnight so that they will eat the first batch of infected feed ravenously. Feed is usually prepared fresh twice daily (morning and evening). The period of feeding contaminated feed has varied from 1–5 days, with birds being euthanized on the day of or after the final feed [22,79,86]. On average, researchers challenging birds through the feed will challenge for 3 or 4 days and euthanize on day 4 or 5 (the first day after the last challenge). The time of exposure is important, since 5 days of challenge induced more than twice the mortality of one day challenge [38]. Infected feed should always be available to birds. The advantage of challenging birds through feed is that it does not involve handling birds individually. The disadvantage is that it involves handling and incubating large volumes of media, which can smell unpleasant because of production of hydrogen sulfide, requires often large number of flasks which logistically may be difficult to autoclave, and is expensive.

An alternative to infecting birds through large volumes of feed is to infect birds individually by crop gavage with broth cultures. This has involved inoculation of 3 mL of 10^5-

10^7 colony-forming units twice daily for three consecutive days [33-35] or 1 mL of 1–4 × 10^8 CFU/mL for 4 days or 7 days [19,20,41]. The method is combined with some NE risk factors such as coccidial challenge or IBD vaccination. For example, no lesions were detected using oral *C. perfringens* challenge without coccidial challenge [41]. McReynolds et al. [33] used IBD vaccine as an immunosuppressant followed by oral *C. perfringens* challenge, and this resulted to a significant increase in NE lesions comparing to the birds that just received *C. perfringens* challenge alone. However, as noted earlier, numerous studies have successfully used broth culture mixed with feed without using coccidial or immunosuppressing predisposition. In conclusion, researchers need to decide on the approach (*C. perfringens* alone in feed; coccidial or IBD immunosuppression, followed by *C. perfringens*given by gavage or in feed) that best fits their facilities, ability to handle birds, the severity of the disease that they wish to produce, and other considerations. Small-scale pilot studies using different variables should establish the conditions best fitted for their study.

OTHER CONSIDERATIONS

Most studies use broiler chickens, usually of mixed sex. It is possible that male birds, which eat more, may be more susceptible, as are male turkeys in field cases [62]. Immunization of the parent flock has shown to reduce the NE lesions and mortality [88] so chicks should not be from hens vaccinated with *C. perfringens*vaccines. Challenge at 2–3 weeks of age should ensure low maternally-derived antibodies in chicks from unvaccinated hens.

LESION SCORING SYSTEMS

Gross lesions of necrotic enteritis

The gross small intestinal lesions of necrotic enteritis comprise a spectrum of mucosal erosion-to-ulceration that vary in both extent and in individual character and severity. In many animals, individual lesions of various characters may be identified. Normally, the mucosal surface of the intestinal tract should be smooth and shiny, reflecting an intact mucosal epithelial barrier (Figure 2a). With erosion and ulceration one may see a complex of subtle mucosal dullness (reflecting fibrin exudation; Figure 2b), cavitation/ulceration (Figures 2c-e), acute hemorrhage (seen as localized intense reddening, often co-localized to areas of cavitation/ulceration, occasionally with frank blood clots in the intestinal lumen; Figure 2c), subacute hemorrhage (seen as localized green-black mucosal pigmentation, often co-localized to areas of cavitation/ ulceration; Figure 2d), and the formation of individual mucosal fibrin plaques that cannot be removed with a finger (Figure 2f). The disease process progresses, with or without obvious cavitation, to produce the large-scale accumulation of fibrin, necrotic tissue debris, and inflammatory cells that coalesce to form the suffusive extensive mat of tenacious exudate on the mucosal surface (Figures 2g-h) that is typical of field cases of birds dying of necrotic enteritis.

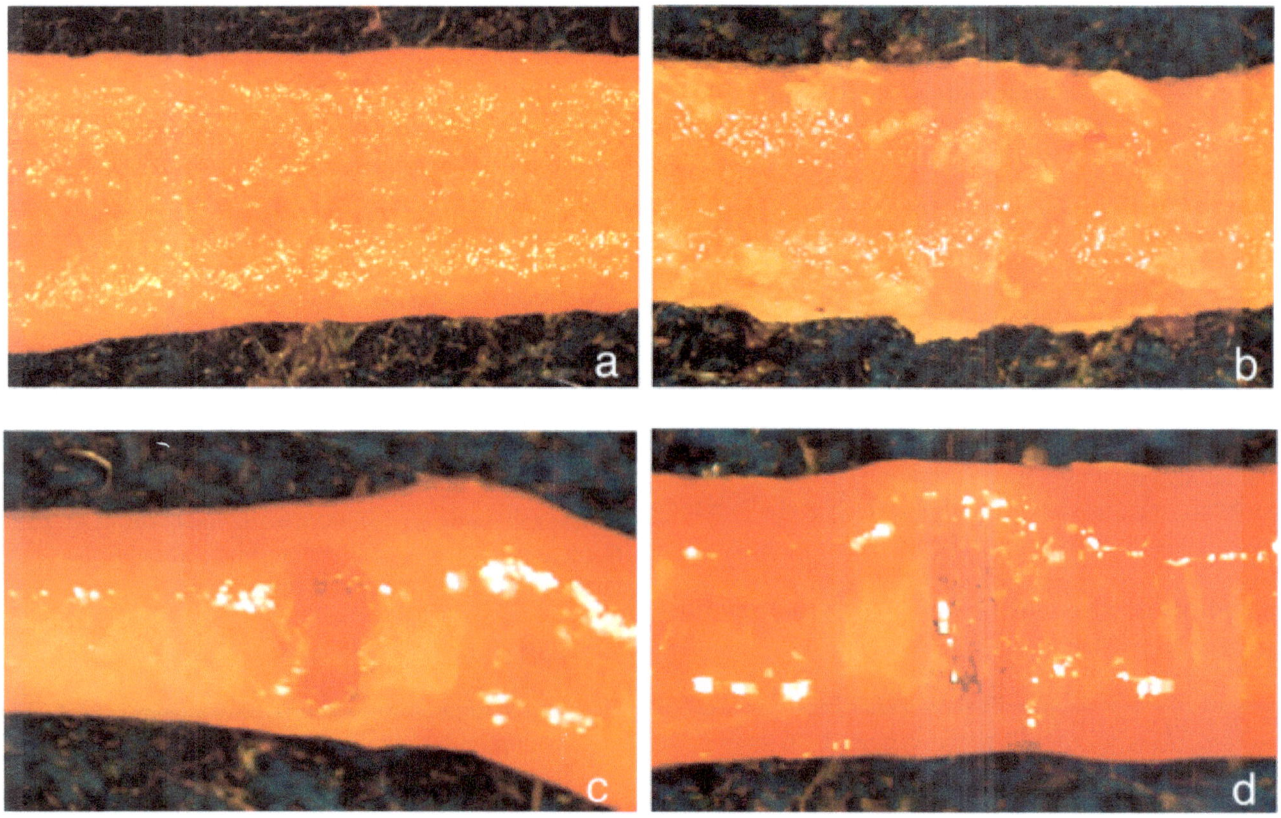

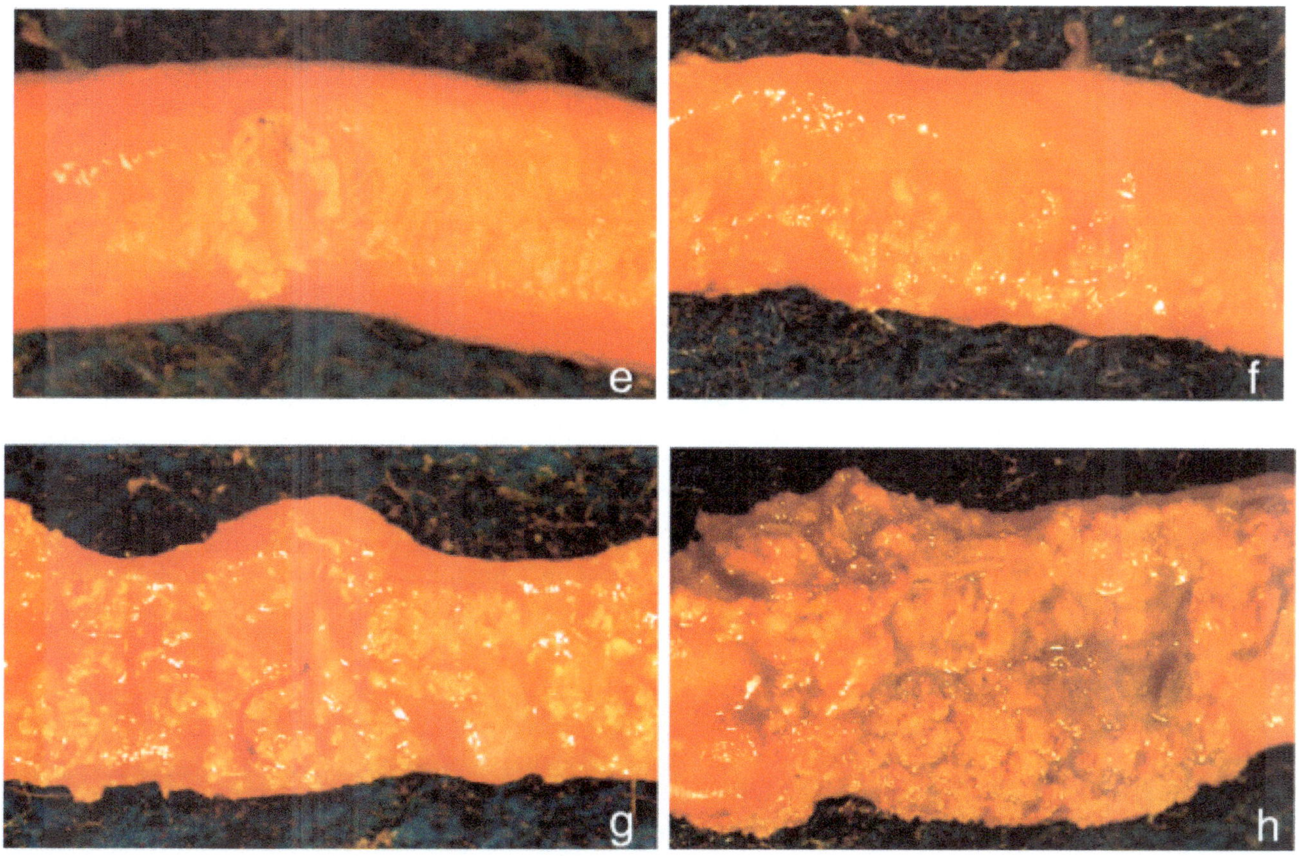

Figure 2: Different lesions of necrotic enteritis in chickens, used to illustrate the scoring system (Table 2). a: Necrotic enteritis score 0, everted jejunal segment. No gross lesions are present. b: Necrotic enteritis score 1, everted jejunal segment. There are no obvious ulcers in the mucosa, but the entire mucosal surface is covered with a layer of loosely adherent fibrin. c: Necrotic enteritis score 2–4, everted jejunal segment. There is an excavated ulcer of the mucosa with acute, bright red hemorrhage within the ulcer bed and scant crusting of fibrin around the periphery. d: Necrotic enteritis score 2–4, everted jejunal segment. There is an excavated ulcer of the mucosa with dark green-black pigment within the ulcer bed and scant crusting of fibrin over the surface. e-f: Necrotic enteritis score 2–4, everted jejunal segments. There are excavated ulcers of the mucosae, the periphery of which are covered by thick, tightly-adherent layers of fibrin, necrotic tissue, and inflammatory cells. g-h: Necrotic enteritis score 5–6, everted jejunal segment. The mucosae are covered by large, confluent plaques of fibrin, necrotic tissue, and inflammatory cells (g) to the point where they extend over broad regions of the intestinal mucosa (h).

Different scoring systems

Following humane euthanasia, for example by overdose of carbon dioxide, birds are necropsied and the small intestine examined for gross pathological lesions. It is important to assess the entire length of the small intestine, since lesions may be present in the upper duo denum that are not found elsewhere. Most lesions will however be in the jejunum. A variety of systems for scoring NE gross lesions have been used, using scales that have varied from 0–3 [31,41,70], 0–4 [12,22,26,33,79,87] to 0 – 6 [6,20,32,65]. A serious drawback of this variability, and of the different criteria used even within these scoring systems, is that it is impossible to compare studies that use different scoring systems. International adoption of a common standard system will considerably ease comparison between studies, including comparison of different control methods. One difficulty however of adopting a common scoring system is that there is variation in the gross lesions of NE, described above, which anecdotally may be exacerbated by the effects of different interventions, such as for example immunization of birds with different antigens.

An ideal scoring system should encompass the severity of the disease produced experimentally, have a reasonably wide range for purposes of statistical analysis, be simple so that large numbers of birds can be examined in a reasonable time, and be reproducible between observers. The scoring system that best approximates these criteria is the six-point system of Keyburn et al. [32]. We therefore propose that this system, with slight modification (Table 2), becomes the international standard for experimental NE studies. The modification proposed is that the "1" includes the presence of non-adherent fibrin in affected intestines (Figure 2b) as an additional alternative to "thin walled and friable intestine". It is recommended that researchers include an experienced pathologist in evaluating lesions of NE, that the lesions be scored "blind", and that at least two people work together to score the lesions. Figure 2 shows some of the variability in the gross lesions associated with NE, and the scores to which they would be assigned.

Table 2: Scoring system for experimental necrotic enteritis lesions (slightly modified from[32]) proposed for international adoption

Score	Lesion	Number of lesions
0	No gross lesions	-
1	Thin or friable walls, or diffuse superficial but removable fibrin	-
2	Focal necrosis or ulceration, or non-removable fibrin deposit	1 to 5 foci
3	Focal necrosis or ulceration, or non-removable fibrin deposit	6 to 15 foci
4	Focal necrosis or ulceration, or non-removable fibrin deposit	16 or more foci
5	Patches of necrosis 2 to 3 cm long	Variable
6	Diffuse necrosis typical of field cases	Variable, but extensive

Although some researchers have included histopathology as part of the scoring of lesions [19,41], this is both expensive and has considerable potential for bias, since lesions are usually pre-selected for histopathological examination. Our recommendation is therefore not to include histopathology as part of a routine scoring system, unless there are special reasons to do so.

REPRODUCTION OF CLINICAL AND SUB-CLINICAL NECROTIC ENTERITIS

Necrotic enteritis, can occur in two clinically different forms; clinical and subclinical [15]. The clinical form of the disease is associated with signs such as depression, ruffled feathers, diarrhea and even mortalities, while no clinical signs or mortality occur in the subclinical form [7,14,69,89,90]. Therefore if researchers are seeking to produce a mild form of the disease, for example to study the effect of interventions including prebiotics on production parameters over time, they may be interested to reproduce the less severe, subclinical, form of NE [41,90,91].

Factors determining outcome of the clinical form of NE with severe lesions and mortalities have been discussed; as noted, it is possible to vary parameters to determine the severity of the disease. To reproduce subclinical NE, the approach is to use approaches outlined to reduce the severity of the disease produced. For example, using even relatively large numbers of *C. perfringens* (10^8-10^{10} CFU/mL) when challenged by oral route, just once or twice or even 3 times a day for 4–5 days), when not combined with feed factors (high protein, NSP-rich grains) or use of coccidia or IBD vaccines, produced a subclinical form of the disease with no clinical signs [19,89,90]. Using *C. perfringens* strains that lack *tpeL*, or feeding birds 24-h cultures of FTG, will predictably reduce disease severity. Nevertheless, using strains that lack *netB* will almost certainly never produce subclinical NE [79].

Figure 1 summarizes important factors affecting successful induction of NE.

DETERMINING PERFORMANCE PARAMETERS (WEIGHT GAIN, FEED INTAKE, FEED CON-VERSION RATIO)

Since there is a correlation between performance parameters and lesion scores [87], measuring the performance of the birds, such as weight gain, feed intake and food conversion efficiency (FCR), can be used to evaluate the severity of the disease or the effect of interventions on disease [24-26,60]. This evaluation can be important in subclinical NE, when no clinical signs or mortalities occur. For this purpose, birds can be weighed every week, and at the time of interventions. Measuring feed consumption enables the researcher to determine the FCR. Groups will need to be appropriately large and randomized for performance parameters to be assessed for statistical significance.

WELFARE CONSIDERATIONS

Proposed studies on the reproduction of NE will require approval under national and local animal care legislation and regulations. It is important that the welfare of experimental birds be of the highest concern to researchers. An example of a score sheet and the criteria we use for humane euthanasia is given in Table3. It should be noted that birds with NE often appear normal until shortly before they die. We euthanize birds humanely using immersion in 100% CO_2 gas.

Table 3: An example of a scoring sheet used in a necrotic enteritis reproduction study

Date and Time dd/mm/yy and am-pm	Cage # or Group # as appears on the cage	Number of birds in the cage / group	General behaviour*: Score	Comments
			0 bright and alert;	
			1 reduced spontaneous activity	
			2 socially isolated but moves when approached	
			3 pronounced lethargy, only moves when stimulated	

*Actions to be taken.

CONCLUSIONS

This review has critically evaluated factors that affect the reproduction of NE in chickens. The reproduction of many infections experimentally is never guaranteed, but understanding the many variables that affect outcome and careful attention to these should allow researchers to reliably produce the disease. The use of small scale pilot studies should also identify the optimal way to produce the disease of desired severity.

AUTHORS' CONTRIBUTIONS

BS: Gathering information and papers, writing the outlines, writing the paper; JP: Proposing the subject, reviewing and editing the paper; AV: Preparation and interpretation of the pictures for the scoring system. All authors agreed on outlines and the final version of the paper.

ACKNOWLEDGEMENTS

The authors thanks the Ontario Ministry of Agriculture, Food and Rural Affairs, the Canadian Poultry Research Council,

Agriculture and Agri-Food Canada, the Poultry Industry Council and the Saskatchewan Chicken Industry Development Fund for support of research into necrotic enteritis.

REFERENCES

1. Parish WE. Necrotic enteritis in the fowl *Gallus gallus domesticus*. I. Histopathology of the disease and isolation of a strain of *Clostridium welchii*. J Comp Patho. 1961;71:377–393.
2. Baba E, Ikemoto T, Fukata T, Sasai K, Arakawa A, McDougald LR. Clostridial population and the intestinal lesions in chickens infected with *Clostridium perfringens* and *Eimeria necatrix*. Vet Microbiol. 1997;54:301–308. doi: 10.1016/S0378-1135(96)01289-8.
3. Songer JG, Meer RR. Genotyping of *Clostridium perfringens* by polymerase chain reaction is a useful adjunct to diagnosis of clostridial enteric disease in animals. Anaerobe. 1996;2:197–203. doi: 10.1006/anae.1996.0027.
4. Songer JG. Clostridial enteric diseases of domestic animals. Clin Microbiol Rev. 1996;9:216–234.
5. Engstrom BE, Fermer C, Lindberg A, Saarinen E, Baverud V, Gunnarsson A. Molecular typing of isolates of *Clostridium perfringens* from healthy and diseased poultry. Vet Microbiol. 2003;94:225–235. doi: 10.1016/S0378-1135(03)00106-8.
6. Keyburn AL, Boyce JD, Vaz P, Bannam TL, Ford ME, Parker D, Rubbo AD, Rood JI, Moore RJ. NetB, a new toxin that is associated with avian necrotic enteritis caused by *Clostridium perfringens*.PLoS Pathog. 2008;4:e26. doi: 10.1371/journal.ppat.0040026.
7. Keyburn AL, Bannam TL, Moore RJ, Rood JI. NetB, a pore forming toxin from necrotic enteritis strains of *Clostridium perfringens*. Toxins. 2010;2:1913–1927. doi: 10.3390/toxins2071913.
8. Lepp D, Roxas B, Parreira VR, Marri PR, Rosey EL, Gong J, Songer JG, Vedantam G, Prescott JF. Identification of novel pathogenicity loci in *Clostridium perfringens* strains that cause avian necrotic enteritis. PLoS One. 2010;5:e10795. doi: 10.1371/journal.pone.0010795.
9. Bannam TL, Yan XX, Harrison PF, Seeman T, Keyburn AL, Stubenrauch C, Weeramatri LH, Cheung JK, McClane BA, Boyce JD, Moore RJ, Rood JI. Necrotic enteritis-derived *Clostridium perfringens*strain with three closely related independently conjugative toxin and antibiotic resistance plasmids.MBio. 2011;2:e00190–e00211.
10. Hibberd MC, Neumann AP, Rehberger TG, Siragusa GR. Multilocus sequence typing subtypes of poultry *Clostridium perfringens* isolates demonstrate disease niche partitioning. J Clin Microbiol.2011;49:1556–1567. doi: 10.1128/JCM.01884-10.
11. Kondo F. *In vitro* lecithinase activity and sensitivity to 22 antimicrobial agents of *Clostridium perfringens* isolated from necrotic enteritis of broiler chickens. Res Vet Sci. 1988;45:337–340.
12. Cooper KK, Songer JG. Virulence of *Clostridium perfringens* in an experimental model of poultry necrotic enteritis. Vet Microbiol. 2010;142:323–328. doi: 10.1016/j.vetmic.2009.09.065.
13. McDevit RM, Brooker JD, Acamovic T, Sparks NHC. Necrotic enteritis; a continuing challenge for the poultry industry. World's Poult Sci J. 2006;62:221–247. doi: 10.1079/WPS200593.
14. Kaldhusdal M, Hofshagen M. Barley inclusion and avoparcin supplementation in broiler diets. 2. Clinical, pathological, and bacteriological findings in a mild form of necrotic enteritis. Poult Sci.1992;71:1145–1153. doi: 10.3382/ps.0711145.
15. Van Immerseel F, De Buck J, Pasmans F, Huyghebaert G, Haesebrouck F, Ducatelle R. *Clostridium perfringens* in poultry: an emerging threat for animal and public health. Avian Pathol. 2004;33:537–549. doi: 10.1080/03079450400013162.
16. Van der Sluis W. Clostridial enteritis is an often underestimated problem. World Poult. 2000;16:42–43.
17. Lovland A, Kaldhusdal M. Severely impaired production performance in broiler flocks with high incidence of *Clostridium perfringens*-associated hepatitis. Avian Pathol. 2001;30:73–81. doi: 10.1080/03079450020023230.
18. Skinner JT, Bauer S, Young Young V, Pauling G, Wilson J. An economic analysis of the impact of subclinical (mild) necrotic enteritis in broiler chickens. Avian Dis. 2010;54:1237–1240. doi: 10.1637/9399-052110-Reg.1.
19. Olkowski AA, Wojnarowicz C, Chirino-Trejo M, Drew MD. Responses of broiler chickens orally challenged with *Clostridium perfringens* isolated from field cases of necrotic enteritis. Res Vet Sci.2006;81:99–108. doi: 10.1016/j.rvsc.2005.10.006.
20. Timbermont L, Lanckriet A, Gholamiandehkordi AR, Pasmans F, Martel A, Haesebrouck F, Ducatelle R, Van Immerseel F. Origin of *Clostridium perfringens* isolates determines the ability to induce necrotic enteritis in broilers. Comp Immunol Microbiol Infect Dis. 2009;32:503–512. doi: 10.1016/j.cimid.2008.07.001.
21. Williams RB. Intercurrent coccidiosis and necrotic enteritis of chickens: rational, integrated disease management by maintenance of gut integrity. Avian Pathol. 2005;34:159–180. doi: 10.1080/03079450500112195.
22. Prescott JF, Sivendra R, Barnum DA. The use of bacitracin in the prevention and treatment of experimentally-induced necrotic enteritis in chickens. Can Vet J. 1978;19:181–183.
23. Hofacre CL, Froyman R, George B, Goodwin MA, Brown J. Use of Aviguard, virginiamycin, or bacitracin MD against *Clostridium perfringens*-associated necrotizing enteritis. J App Poult Res.1998;7:412–418.
24. Brennan J, Moore G, Poe SE, Zimmermann A, Vessie G, Barnum DA, Wilson J. Effect of in-feed tylosin phosphate for the treatment of necrotic enteritis in broiler chickens. Poult Sci. 2001;80:1451–1454.

25. Brennan J, Bagg R, Barnum D, Wilson J, Dick P. Effect of narasin in the prevention of necrotic enteritis in broiler chickens. Avian Dis. 2001;45:210–214. doi: 10.2307/1593030.

26. Brennan J, Skinner J, Barnum DA, Wilson J. The efficacy of bacitracin methylene disalicylate when fed in combination with narasin in the management of necrotic enteritis in broiler chickens. Poult Sci.2003;82:360–363.

27. Lanckriet A, Timbermont L, De Gussem M, Marien M, Vancraeynest D, Haesebrouck F, Ducatelle R, Van Immerseel F. The effect of commonly used anticoccidials and antibiotics in a subclinical necrotic enteritis model. Avian Pathol. 2010;39:63–68. doi: 10.1080/03079450903505771.

28. Thompson DR, Parreira VR, Kulkarni RR, Prescott JF. Live attenuated vaccine-based control of necrotic enteritis of broiler chickens. Vet Microbiol. 2005;113:25–34.

29. Kulkarni RR, Parreira VR, Sharif S, Prescott JF. Immunization of broiler chickens against *Clostridium perfringens*-induced necrotic enteritis. Clin Vaccine Immunol. 2007;14:1070–1077. doi: 10.1128/CVI.00162-07.

30. Kulkarni RR, Parreira VR, Sharif S, Prescott JF. Oral immunization of broiler chickens against necrotic enteritis with an attenuated *Salmonella* vaccine vector expressing *Clostridium perfringens*antigens. Vaccine. 2008;26:4194–4203. doi: 10.1016/j.vaccine.2008.05.079.

31. Lovland A, Kaldhusdal M, Redhead K, Skjerve E, Lillehaug A. Maternal vaccination against subclinical necrotic enteritis in broilers. Avian Pathol. 2004;33:81–90. doi: 10.1080/0379450310001636255.

32. Keyburn AL, Sheedy SA, Ford ME, Williamson MM, Awad MM, Rood JI, Moore RJ. Alpha toxin of*Chlostridium perfringens* is not an essential virulence factor in necrotic enteritis in chickens. Infect Immun. 2006;74:6496–6500. doi: 10.1128/IAI.00806-06.

33. McReynolds L, Byrd JA, Anderson RC, Moore RW, Edrington TS, Genovese KJ, Poole TL, Kubena LF, Nisbet DJ. Evaluation of Immunosuppressants and dietary mechanisms in an experimental disease model for necrotic enteritis. Poult Sci. 2004;83:1948–1952.

34. McReynolds JL, Byrd JA, Genovese KJ, Poole TL, Duke SE, Farnell MB, Nisbet DJ. Dietary lactose and its effect on the disease condition of necrotic enteritis. Poult Sci. 2007;86:1656–1661.

35. McReynolds J, Waneck C, Byrd J, Genovese K, Duke S, Nisbet D. Efficacy of multistrain direct–fed microbial and phytogenetic products in reducing necrotic enteritis in commercial broilers. Poult Sci.2009;88:2075–2080. doi: 10.3382/ps.2009-00106.

36. Baba E, Fuller AL, Gilbert JM, Thayer SG, McDougald LR. Effects of *Eimeria brunetti* infection and dietary zinc on experimental induction of necrotic enteritis in broiler chickens. Avian Dis. 1992;36:59–62. doi: 10.2307/1591716.

37. Branton SL, Lott BD, Deaton JW, Maslin WR, Austin FW, Pote LM, Keirs RW, Latour MA, Day EJ. The effect of added complex carbohydrates or added dietary fiber on necrotic enteritis lesions in broiler chickens. Poult Sci. 1997;76:24–28.

38. Long JR, Truscott RB. Necrotic enteritis in broiler chickens. III. Reproduction of the disease. Can J Comp Med. 1976;40:53–59.

39. Cowen BS, Schwartz LD, Wilson RA, Ambrus SI. Experimentally induced necrotic enteritis in chickens. Avian Dis. 1987;31:904–906. doi: 10.2307/1591050.

40. Williams RB, Marshal RN, La Ragione RM, Catchpole J. A new model for the experimental production of necrotic enteritis and its use for studies on the relationship between necrotic enteritis and anticoccidial vaccination of chickens. Parasitol Res. 2003;90:19–26.

41. Gholamiandehkordi AR, Timbermont L, Lanckriet A, Van Den Broeck W, Pedersen K, Dewulf J, Pasmans F, Haeesbrouck F, Ducatelle R, Van Immerseel F. Quantification of gut lesions in a subclinical necrotic enteritis model. Avian Pathol. 2007;36:375–382. doi: 10.1080/03079450701589118.

42. Annett CB, Viste JR, Chirino-Trejo M, Classen HL, Middleton DM, Simko E. Necrotic enteritis: effect of barley, wheat and corn diet on proliferation of *Clostridium perfringens* Type A. Avian Pathol.2002;31:599–602.

43. Dahiya JP, Wilkie DC, Van Kessel AG, Drew MD. Potential strategies for controlling necrotic enteritis in broiler chickens in post-antibiotic era. Anim Feed Sci Tech. 2006;129:60–88. doi: 10.1016/j.anifeedsci.2005.12.003.

44. Kleesen B, Hartmann L, Blaut M. Fructans in the diet cause alterations of intestinal mucosal architecture, released mucins and mucosa-associated bifidobacteria in gnotobiotic rats. Brit J Nutr.2003;89:597–606. doi: 10.1079/BJN2002827.

45. Ficko-Blean E, Stuart CP, Boraston AB. Structural analysis of CPF_2247, a novel a-amylase from*Clostridium perfringens*. Proteins. 2011;79:2771–2777. doi: 10.1002/prot.23116.

46. Ficko-Blean E, Stuart CP, Suits MD, Cid M, Tessier M, Woods RJ, Boraston AB. Carbohydrate recognition by an architecturally complex α-N-Acetylglucosaminidase from *Clostridiumperfringens*.PLoS One. 2012;7:e33524. doi: 10.1371/journal.pone.0033524.

47. Riddell C, Kong XM. The influence of diet on necrotic enteritis in broiler chicks. Avian Dis.1992;36:499–503. doi: 10.2307/1591740.

48. Branton SL, Reece FN, Hagler WM Jr. Influence of a wheat diet on mortality of broiler chicks associated with necrotic enteritis. Poultry Sci. 1987;66:1326–1330. doi: 10.3382/ps.0661326.

49. Craven SE. Colonization of the intestinal tract by *Clostridium perfringens* and fecal shedding in diet stressed and unstressed broiler chickens. Poult Sci. 2000;79:843–849.

50. Kaldhusdal M, Skjerve E. Association between cereal contents in the diet and incidence of necrotic enteritis in

broiler chickens in Norway. Prev Vet Med. 1996;28:1–16. doi: 10.1016/0167-5877(96)01021-5.

51. Reid CA, Hillman K. The effects of retrogradation and amylose/amylopectin ratio of starches on carbohydrate fermentation and microbial populations in the porcine colon. Anim Sci. 1999;68:503–510.

52. Weurding RE, Veldman A, Veen WAG, Van Der Aar PJ, Verstegen MWA. Starch digestion in the small intestine of chickens differs among feedstuffs. J Nutr. 2001;131:2329–2335.

53. Engberg RM, Hedemann MS, Jensen BB. The influence of grinding and pelleting of feed on the microbial composition and activity in the digestive tract of broiler chickens. Brit Poult Sci.2002;43:569–579. doi: 10.1080/0007166022000004480.

54. Branton SL, Reece FN, Hagler WM Jr. Influence of a wheat diet on mortality of broiler chickens associated with necrotic enteritis. Poult Sci. 1987;66:1326–1330. doi: 10.3382/ps.0661326.

55. Palliyeguru MWCD, Rose SP, Mackenzie AM. Effect of trypsin inhibitor activity in soya bean on growth performance, protein digestibility and incidence of sub-clinical necrotic enteritis in broiler chicken flocks. Brit Poult Sci. 2011;52:359–367. doi: 10.1080/00071668.2011.577054.

56. Shimizu T, Ohtani K, Hirakawa H, Ohshima K, Yamashita A, Shiba T, Ogasawara N, Hattori M, Kuhara S, Hayashi H. Complete genome sequence of *Clostridium perfringens*, an anaerobic flesh-eater. Proc Natl Acad Sci U S A. 2002;99:996–1001. doi: 10.1073/pnas.022493799.

57. Kaldhusdal MI. Necrotic enteritis as affected by dietary ingredients. World Poult. 2000;16:42–43.

58. Titball RW, Naylor CE, Basak AK. The *Clostridium perfringens* alpha toxin. Anaerobe. 1999;5:51–64. doi: 10.1006/anae.1999.0191.

59. Dahiya JP, Hoehler D, Wilkie DC, Van Kessel AG, Drew MD. Dietary glycine concentration affects intestinal *Clostridium perfringens* and Lactobacilli population in broiler chickens. Poult Sci.2005;84:1875–1885.

60. Dahiya JP, Hoehler D, Van Kessel AG, Drew MD. Dietary encapsulated glycine influences*Clostridium perfringens* and Lactobacilli growth in the gastrointestinal tract of broiler chickens. J Nutr.2007;137:1408–1414.

61. Wilkie DC, Van Kessel AG, White LJ, Laarveld B, Drew MD. Dietary amino acids affect intestinal*Clostridium perfringens* populations in broiler chickens. Can J Anim Sci. 2005;85:185–193. doi: 10.4141/A04-070.

62. Drew MD, Syed NA, Goldade BG, Van Larveld B, Kessel AG. Effect of dietary protein source and level on intestinal population of *Clostridium perfringens* in broiler chickens. Poult Sci. 2004;83:414–420.

63. Kocher A. Nutritional manipulation of necrotic enteritis outbreak in broilers. Recent Adv Anim Nutr.2003;14:111–116.

64. Cheung JK, Keyburn AL, Carter GP, Lanckriet AL, Van Immerseel F, Moore RJ, Rood JI. The VirSR two-component signal transduction system regulates NetB toxin production in *Clostridium perfringens*. Infect Immun. 2010;78:3064–3072. doi: 10.1128/IAI.00123-10.

65. Timbermont L, Lanckriet A, Dewulf J, Nollet N, Schwarzer K, Haesebrouk F, Ducattele R, Van Immerseel F. Control of *Clostridium perfringence*- induced necrotic enteritis in broilers by target-released butyric acid, fatty acids and essential oils. Avian Pathol. 2010;39:117–121. doi: 10.1080/03079451003610586.

66. Cooper KK, Songer JG. Necrotic enteritis in chickens: a paradigm of enteric infection by *Clostridium perfringens* type A. Anaerobe. 2009;15:55–60. doi: 10.1016/j.anaerobe.2009.01.006.

67. Williams BA, Martin WA, Verstegen ST. Fermentation in the large intestine of single-stomached animals and its relationship to animal health. Nutr Res Rev. 2001;14:207–227. doi: 10.1079/NRR200127.

68. Lan Y, Verstegen MWA, Tamminga S, Williams BA. The role of the commensal gut microbial community in broiler chickens. World's Poult Sci J. 2005;61:95–104. doi: 10.1079/WPS200445.

69. Van Immerseel F, Rood JI, Moore RJ, Titball RW. Rethinking our understanding of the pathogenesis of necrotic enteritis in chickens. Trends Microbiol. 2008;17:32–36.

70. Collier CT, Hofacre CL, Payne AM, Anderson DB, Kaiser P, Mackie RI, Gaskins HR. Coccidia-induced mucogenesis promotes the onset of necrotic enteritis by supporting *Clostridium perfringens*growth. Vet Immunol Immunopathol. 2008;122:104–115. doi: 10.1016/j.vetimm.2007.10.014.

71. Al-Sheikhly F, Al-Saieg A. Role of coccidia in the occurrence of necrotic enteritis of chickens. Avian Dis. 1980;24:324–333. doi: 10.2307/1589700.

72. Al-Sheikhly F, Truscott RB. The interaction of *Clostridium perfringens* and its toxins in the production of necrotic enteritis in chickens. Avian Dis. 1977;21:256–263. doi: 10.2307/1589345.

73. Nikpiran H, Shojadoost B, Peighambari SM. Experimental induction of necrotic enteritis in broiler chickens by *Clostridium perfringens* isolates from the outbreaks in Iran. J Vet Res. 2008;63:127–132.

74. Fukata T, Hadate Y, Baba E, Uemura T, Arakawa A. Influence of *Clostridium perfringens* and its toxin in germ-free chickens. Res Vet Sci. 1988;44:68–70.

75. Chalmers G, Bruce HL, Hunter DB, Parreira VR, Kulkarni RR, Jiang YF, Prescott JF, Boerlin P. Multi-locus sequence typing analysis of *Clostridium perfringens* isolates from necrotic enteritis outbreaks in broiler chickens populations. J Clin Microbiol. 2008;46:3957–3964. doi: 10.1128/JCM.01548-08.

76. Martin TG, Smyth JA. Prevalence of netB among some clinical isolates of *Clostridium perfringens*from animals in the United States. Vet Microbiol. 2009;136:202–205. doi: 10.1016/j.vetmic.2008.10.026.

77. Keyburn AL, Yan XX, Bannam TL, Van Immerseel F, Rood JI, Moore RJ. Association between avian necrotic

enteritis and *Clostridium perfringens* expressing NetB. Vet Res. 2010;41:21. doi: 10.1051/vetres/2009069.

78. Tolooe A, Shojadoost B, Peighambari SM, Tamaddon Y. Prevalence of netB gene among *Clostridium perfringens* isolates obtained from healthy and diseased chicks. J Anim Vet Adv. 2011;10:106–110.

79. Cooper KK, Theoret JR, Stewart A, Trinh HT, Glock RD, Songer JG. Virulence for chickens of*Clostridium perfringens* isolated from poultry and other sources. Anaerobe. 2010;16:289–292. doi: 10.1016/j.anaerobe.2010.02.006.

80. Amimoto K, Noro T, Oishi E, Shimizu M. A novel toxin homologous to large clostridial cytotoxins found in culture supernatant of *Clostridium perfringens* type C. Microbiol. 2007;153:1198–1206. doi: 10.1099/mic.0.2006/002287-0.

81. Coursodon CF, Glock RD, Moore KL, Cooper KK, Songer JG. TpeL-producing strains of*Clostridium perfringens* type A are highly virulent for broiler chicks. Anaerobe. 2012;18:117–121. doi: 10.1016/j.anaerobe.2011.10.001.

82. Kaldhusdal M, Hofshagen M, Lovland A, Langstrand H, Redhead K. Necrotic enteritis challenge models with broiler chickens raised on litter: evaluation of preconditions, *Clostridium perfringens*strains and outcome variables. Immun Med Microbiol. 1999;24:337–343. doi: 10.1111/j.1574-695X.1999.tb01303.x.

83. Pedersen K, Bjerrum L, Nauerby B, Madsen M. Experimental infection with rifampicin-resistant*Clostridiumperfringens*strainsinbroilerchickens using isolator facilities. Avian Pathol. 2003;32:401–408. doi: 10.1080/0307945031000121158.

84. Pedersen K, Bjerrum L, Eske Heuer O, Lo Fo Wong DMA, Nauerby B. Reproducible infection model for *Clostridium perfringens* in Broiler chickens. Avian Dis. 2008;52:34–39. doi: 10.1637/7955-022307-Reg.

85. Prescott JF. The prevention of experimentally induced necrotic enteritis in chickens by avoparcin.Avian Dis. 1979;23:1072–1074. doi: 10.2307/1589625.

86. Chalmers G, Bruce HL, Toole DL, Barnum DA, Boerlin P. Necrotic enteritis potential in a model system using *Clostridium perfringens* isolated from field outbreaks. Avian Dis. 2007;51:834–839. doi: 10.1637/7959-022807-REGR.1.

87. Cooper KK, Trinh HT, Songer G. Immunization with recombinant alpha toxin partially protects broiler chicks against experimental challenge with *Clostridium perfringens*. Vet Microbiol. 2009;133:92–97. doi: 10.1016/j.vetmic.2008.06.001.

88. Crouch CF, Withanage GSK, de Haas V, Etore F, Francis MJ. Safety and efficacy of a maternal vaccine for the passive protection of broiler chicks against necrotic enteritis. Avian Pathol.2010;39:489–497. doi: 10.1080/03079457.2010.517513.

89. Wilson J, Tice G, Brash ML, Hilaire SST. Manifestations of *Clostridium perfringens* and related bacterial enteritides in broiler chickens. World's Poult Sci J. 2005;61:435–449. doi: 10.1079/WPS200566.

90. Olkowski AA, Wojnarowicz C, Chirino-Trejo M, Laarveld B, Sawicki G. Sub-clinical necrotic enteritis in broiler chickens: Novel etiological consideration based on ultra-structural and molecular changes in the intestinal tissue. Res Vet Sci. 2008;85:543–553. doi: 10.1016/j.rvsc.2008.02.007.

91. Wu SB, Rodgers N, Choct M. Optimized necrotic enteritis model producing clinical and subclinical infection of *Clostridium perfringens* in broiler chickens. Avian Dis. 2010;54:1058–1065. doi: 10.1637/9338-032910-Reg.1.

CHAPTER 11

CHARACTERIZATION OF NEWCASTLE DISEASE VIRUS AND POULTRY-HANDLING PRACTICES IN LIVE POULTRY MARKETS, ETHIOPIA

Delesa Damena Mulisa[1], Menbere Kidane W/Kiros[1], Redeat Belaineh Alemu[1], Melaku Sombo Keno[1], Alice Furaso[2], Alireza Heidari[2], Tesfaye Rufael Chibsa[1] and Hassen Chaka Chunde[1]

[1] National Animal Health Diagnostic and Investigation Center, Sebeta, Ethiopia

[2] Research and Innovation Department, Istituto Zooprofilattico Sperimentale delle Venezie, OIE/FAO and National Reference Laboratory for Newcastle Disease and Avian Influenza,OIE collaborating Center for Diseases at the Human-Animal Interface, Legnaro, Padova, Italy

ABSTRACT

Newcastle disease represents the most severe poultry disease responsible for marked economic losses in Ethiopia. To provide a molecular characterization of Newcastle disease viruses circulating in this country, a cross sectional survey was conducted at five selected live poultry market sites in Addis Ababa. In addition, baseline data on the live poultry market system were acquired through a detailed questionnaire submitted to poultry traders. We identified 44/146 positive samples, 29 of which were virulent strains belonging to sub-genotype VIf. The very poor biosecurity practices, which have resulted from responses of the participants, suggest that they might have had a heavy impact in the spread of the disease. This study provides important information on epidemiology and control of NDV in Ethiopia and highlights the importance of implementing surveillances and biosecurity practices in live poultry markets.

INTRODUCTION

Poultry play an important economic, nutritional and socio-cultural role in the livelihoods of poor rural households in developing countries, including Ethiopia. The total poultry population in Ethiopia is estimated at 43 million, 97% of which are village chickens (Central Statistical Agency 2012). Poultry rearing is particularly important to women, who often own and manage chickens and the resulting income is often used to support education of children. Despite its role in raising incomes and reducing poverty in local communities of Ethiopia, poultry production is hampered by wide arrays of constraints among which infectious diseases, such as: Newcastle disease, Infectious Bursal Disease, Mycoplasmosis, Pasteurellosis and Salmonellosis, are the major ones (Chaka et al. 2012).

Newcastle disease(ND) is one of the major problems in village chickens in most parts of Ethiopia (Nasser 1998; Tadelle and Jobre 2004; Mazengia 2012). The disease has become endemic in poultry population and recurs every year inflicting heavy losses (Tadelle and Jobre 2004). The highest rate of ND outbreaks from March to May is suggested to be associated with high rate of chicken marketing for Easter (Spradbrow 1999). The main movement of chicken marketing is from periphery to the center (rural to towns) which favors the spread of diseases all over the country (Dessei and Ogle 2001). However, there is acute lack of information on bio-security situation and roles of poultry marketing practices in diseases dissemination in the country (Shewantasew et al. 2012).

ND is caused by virulent strains of Newcastle diseases virus (NDV) or avian paramyxovirus type 1 (APMV-1) that belongs to the genus *Avula* and family *Paramyxoviridae* (Mayo 2002). NDV has an enveloped, single-stranded negative sense RNA

Citation: Delesa Damena Mulisa, Menbere Kidane W/Kiros, Redeat Belaineh Alemu, Melaku Sombo Keno, Alice Furaso, Alireza Heidari, Tesfaye Rufael Chibsa and Hassen Chaka Chunde, Characterization of Newcastle Disease Virus and poultry-handling practices in live poultry markets, Ethiopia, DOI: 10.1186/2193-1801-3-459.

genome of approximately 15 kb that contains six genes encoding major structural proteins such as: nucleocapsid protein (NP), phosphoprotein(P), matrix protein(M), fusion protein(F), hemagglutinin-neuraminidase(HN), and the RNA-dependent RNA polymerase(L) (Kattenbelt et al. 2006) as well as two additional proteins, V and W from the P gene by a mechanism called RNA editing (Steward et al. 1993).

The key contributors to NDV pathogenicity are the formation of an active fusion protein upon cleavage of the F protein precursor (F0) as well as the presence of a number of basic residues in the fusion protein cleavage site (Toyoda et al. 1987; Glickman et al. 1988).

NDV that are virulent for chickens have a multibasic amino acid sequence ^{112}R/K-R-Q-K/R-R^{116} at the C–terminus of the F2 protein and F (phenylalanine) at residue 117, which is the N-terminus of the F1 protein, whereas the viruses of low virulence have a monobasic amino acid sequences in the same region of ^{112}G/E-K/R-Q-G/E-R^{116}and L (leucine) at residue 117 (Kim et al. 2008; Office of International Epizootes 2012).

Although ND represents the most severe poultry disease responsible for marked economic losses in Ethiopia, virological and epidemiological information concerning the virus strains circulating in the country especially in village chickens are extremely scarce. The aim of this study was therefore, to detect NDV and to perform a molecular characterization of the virulent strains currently circulating at five live poultry market sites in Addis Ababa. In addition, we investigated the biosecurity practices implemented at the market sites to identify the factors that can contribute to the spread of the virus.

MATERIALS AND METHODS

Sample origin

The study was conducted in December 2012 in five live poultry market sites in Addis Ababa namely: Kotebe, Merkato, Shola, Saris and Semen (Adisu gebeya) (Figure 1). These are among the biggest poultry market sites in Addis Ababa that host chickens originating from most parts of the country, mainly from places located within 300 kms radius such as: Sodo, Hosaina, Dessie, Shashemane, Jimma, and Ambo. All the markets are outdoor markets where chickens are kept in wire mesh cages, each housing up to 40 birds during the day and night.

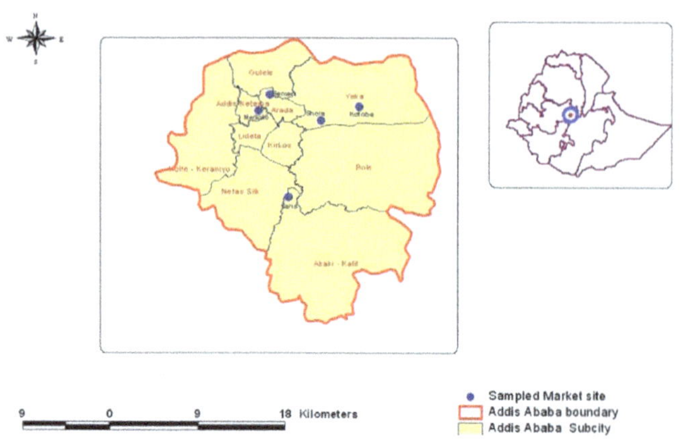

Figure 1: Map of Study area. Poultry market sites where samples were collected.

Sampling, data collection and virus isolation

A total of 365 chickens were sampled: From each market, 70 birds were sampled except Merkato from where 85 birds were sampled by considering its larger size compared to the others. Thus, 73 tracheal swabs (pool of five) and 73 cloacal (pool of five) were collected. In separate cryovial containing 2 ml of freshly prepared viral transport media (VTM).

The swabs were collected in pairs (Tracheal swab pools and Cloacal swab pools were always collected from the same chickens). After sampling, the specimens were transported to the National Animal Health Diagnostic and Investigation Center (NAHDIC) laboratory and stored at -80°C until processing. Besides, a standardized questionnaire was administered to the poultry traders in each market sites. A total of 100 volunteer traders were interviewed to assess the bio-security practices in live poultry markets. The questionnaire included questions about the source of the birds, means of transportation, the number of birds in each market site, cleaning practices at the market sites including the cages, health status of the birds and disposal of manures and dead chickens.

Viruses were isolated from the swab samples by standard virus isolation methods in embryonated chicken eggs. Three embryonated chicken eggs of 9 to 11-day-old per sample were used for inoculation (Alexander and Senne2008). The inoculated eggs were candled every 24 hours to check embryo vitality. Eggs containing dead embryo on each day and those remained at the end of incubation period, were removed from incubator and chilled at +4°C overnight. Allantoic fluids were harvested and tested by Haemagglutination (HA) test for its ability to haemagglutinate chicken RBCs.

Haemagglutination and Haemagglutination Inhibition tests

The HA assay was carried out in microtitre plate as outlined by the World Organization for Animal Health (Office of International Epizootes 2012). HA positive samples were tested by Heamaglutination Inhibition (HI) reaction to specifically determine the haemagglutinating agents. Inactivated antigen for HA test and positive and negative sera for HI controls were obtained from Istituto Zooprofilattico Spermentale delle Venezie (OIE/FAO Reference Laboratory for AI and ND), Padua, Italy.

Polymerase Chain Reaction tests

Forty four HA and HI positive allantoic fluids were analyzed by real- time reverse transcription (RT-PCR) tests. Viral RNA extraction from HI positive allantoic fluid was conducted using Qiagen® RNeasy Mini kit according to manufacturer's instruction. Real-time RT-PCR reactions were performed at National Animal Health Diagnostic Center, Sebeta using an Applied Biosystems 7500 Fast Real-Time PCR thermo cycler. A primer probe combination from conserved region of M gene APMV-1 F M+4100 5'-AGT GAT GTG CTC GGA CCT TC-3', APMV-1 R M-4220 5'-CCT GAG GAG AGG CAT TTG CTA-3' and Probe APMV-1 Probe M+4169 5'- FAM-TTC TCT AGC AGT GGG ACA GCC TGC BHQ-3' (Wise et al. 2004) was used to amplify and detect all NDV isolates. The M-gene positive samples were re-run by a second primer-probe set targeting the F gene Forward F+4829 5'-GGT

GAG TCT ATC CGG ARG ATA CAA G-3', Reverse Primer F- 4939 5'-AGC TGT TGC AAC CCC AAG-3' and Probe F+4894 5'-FAM-AAG CGT TTC TGT CTC CTT CCT CCA-BHQ-3' (Wise et al. 2004) to specifically amplify and detect only pathogenic strains of NDV. Twenty nine F gene Positive allantoic fluids were submitted to Instito Zooprofilattico Sperimentale delle Venezie (OIE/FAO Reference Laboratory for AI and ND), Padua,Italy for further analyses.

Nucleotide Sequencing and phylogenetic analysis

Total RNA was extracted from infective allantoic fluids using Qiagen® RNeasy Mini kit according to manufacturer's instruction. Amplification was performed with primers NOH-For (5'-TAC ACC TCA TCC CAG ACA GG-3') and NOH-Rev (5'-AGT CGG AGG ATG TGT TGG CAG C-3') which encompass 260 bp region of the fusion (F) gene. Amplicons were then purified with ExoSAP-IT (USB Corporation, Cleveland, OH). Sequencing was carried out by using Big Dye Terminator v 3.1 cycle sequencing kit (Applied Biosystems, Foster City, CA, USA) in a 16-cappilary ABI PRISM 3131x Genetic Analyzer (Applied Biosystems, Forster City, CA,USA).

For complete sequencing of F gene, RNA was reverse transcribed with the Superscript III Reverse Transcriptase kit (Invitrogen, Carsbad, CA, USA) and amplified using primer pairs described in Table 1. Sequence data were assembled and edited with Seq Scape software v2.5 (Applied Biosystems). To determine the phylogenetic relationships, the sequences of the F gene were compared to the corresponding region of representative viruses of class II available in GenBank. Alignment and comparison of the nucleotide and amino acid sequences were performed using Clustal W in MEGA 5.0. Maximum likelihood (ML) trees were estimated using best-fit general time-reversible(GTR) model of nucleotide substitution with gamma-distributed rate variation among sites, and a heuristic SPR branch-swapping search available in PhyML version 3.0 (Guindon and Gascuel 2003). A bootstrap resampling process (100 replications) was employed to assess the robustness of individual nodes of phylogeny.

Table 1: Primers set for amplification of complete F-gene

Primers	Sequence 5' to 3'
MF3710-F	TGA AAA CGA CGG CCA GTC AAA GCT GTA DGG TTG TG
MF4650-R	CAG GAA ACA GTA TGA CCA AGA GGC CTG CCR TCA A
F5100-F	TGA AAA CGA CGG CCA GTA TGC AGC ART TTG TYA AT
HF011-R	CAG GAA ACA GTA TGA CCT ARG TAA TRA GAG CRG ATG
HF005-F	TGA AAA CGA CGG CCA GTA GAC YGA AGG CGC ACT YAC
HH008-R	CAG GAA ACA GTA TGA CCA GRG CCA CYT GCT TRT ATA
F-4514-F	TGA AAA CGA CGG CCA GTG TAG AAG ADT YTG GAT CC
F-5218-R	CAG GAA ACA GTA TGA CCG AAT ACY GTA GTC AAY TCR G
HF009-R	CAG GAA ACA GTA TGA CCA GGT GGC ACG CAT ATT ATT
F-5757-F	TGA AAA CGA CGG CCA GTA GAT RAC AAC ATG TAG RTG
F-6449-R	CAG GAA ACA GTA TGA CCG GCT AAC YGC RCG GTC CAT

RESULTS

Marketing practices

Chickens present at each market were estimated to be 300–500 on the days of visit. They are originated from different districts across the country, most of which were collected by traders from big towns such as: Sodo, Dessie, Shashemane, Jimma, Ambo, Hosaina and transported on public transport (bus) to Addis Ababa. The majority (99%) of traders mentioned that there is no habit of cleaning buses before loading and after unloading chickens owing to the fact that no vehicles is designed for poultry transportation alone. After arrival at the market sites, chickens are sold to wholesalers in the biggest live bird market site (Merkato) where birds from different origins are placed in the same cages (mixed) and sold either to traders in other live poultry markets in the city or to the consumers on spot. Ninety nine percent of the traders clean the holding cages once a week with clean water and the remaining 1% clean every day. All the traders responded that they dispose manure and dead birds either within the markets or on roadside. None of them seek for veterinary services when chickens are sick.

Laboratory results

Out of the 146 pooled samples tested, 44 were positive for NDV by both HA/HI and M gene real-time RT-PCR tests. Out of these, 29 isolates were identified as virulent based on the real-time RT-PCR of F gene. Among these, 14 Tracheal swab pools (TS) were positive though the corresponding Cloacal swab pools (CS) were negative. Similarly, 3 CS were positive though the corresponding TS were negative. However, the remaining 12 swab pools have shown direct correlation (12 TS and the corresponding 12 CS were positive) and were not considered as separate entity to avoid double counting of the samples (Table 2). The identification, pathotyping and genotyping of the 29 isolates were confirmed by genetic sequencing of the 260 bp region of fusion (F) gene and the complete F gene sequence of two isolates (KJ958913_13VIR3936-1 and KJ958914_13VIR3936-27) collected from the market sites Saris and Kotebe. Since all the viruses showed a high similarity at the 260 bp region of the F gene (Table 2), the selection was based on the sequencing quality (i.e. absence of degenerate bases).

The isolates were identified as virulent as deduced amino acid sequence of the fusion protein cleavage site indicated the presence of motif [112] RRQKR[116]*F[117] typical of NDV virulent strains. Phylogenetic analysis of the 260 fragment of the F gene of all the 29 sequenced isolates and complete coding region of the F gene of two representative viruses (Figure 2) indicated that the viruses are clustered together (similarity ranged from 98% to 100%) within the new sub-genotype VIf.

Table 2: Origin of positive swab pools and their genetic identity with reference sequence

Market sites from where the samples were collected	Number of M-gene real time RT PCR positive swab pools	Number of F-gene(virulent) real time RT PCR positive swab pools				Genetic identity with the reference sequence at the 260 bp region of the F gene
		Total	Both TS &CS	Only TS	Only CS	
Shola	12	8	4	4	0	98 to 100%
Meri	9	5	4	1	0	98.7 to 100%
Saris	7	3	2	0	1	99.3 to 100%
Merkato	10	9	2	5	2	100%
Kotebe	6	4	0	4	0	100%

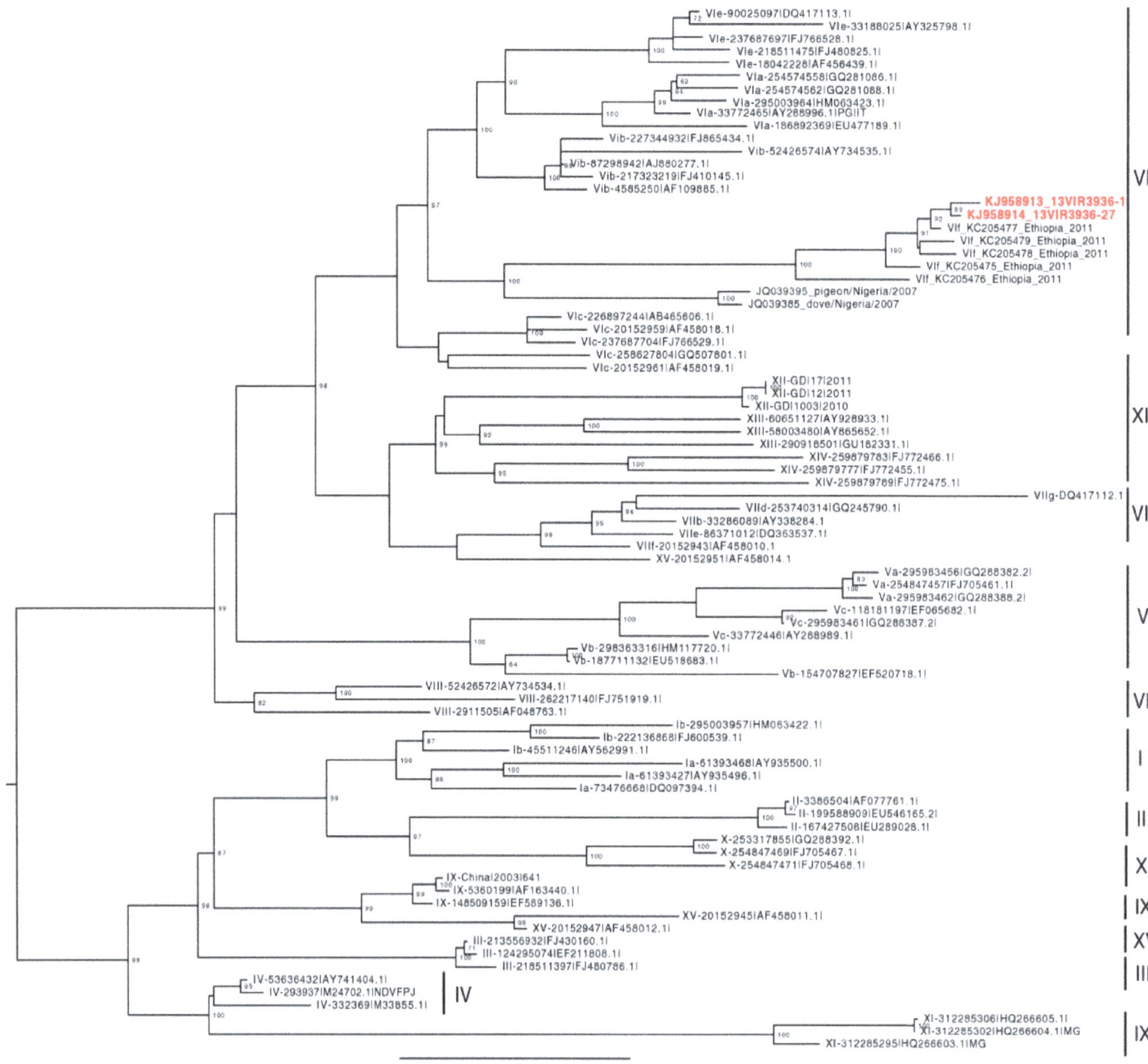

Figure 2: Phylogenetic tree of the complete nucleotide sequence of the F gene for two representative isolates. ML Phylogenetic tree of complete nucleotide sequence of Class II Newcastle diseases viruses. Ethiopian isolates included in this analysis (KJ958913_13VIR3936-1 and KJ958914_13VIR3936-27) are labeled in red. The Nomenclature system used in the phylogenetic tree is based on (Diel et al.2012). The numbers at branch points represent bootstrap values.

DISCUSSION

In this study, we assessed biosecurity practices in market sites in Addis Ababa that contribute to the spread of the diseases along market chain. We observed several practices that could promote Newcastle disease and other infectious diseases transmission among birds. These included limited cleaning and disinfection of the market places, holding cages, mixing of birds from different origins, inappropriate disposal of sick and dead birds and poor waste disposal mechanisms. Earlier reports indicated that marketing systems play a considerable role in the dissemination of diseases over wide geographical areas in a relatively short period of time in Ethiopia (Gebreab1995). Similar observation was reported from Addis Ababa live poultry market sites (Shewantasew et al. 2012). The current finding is also in agreement with a report from Nairobi live bird markets where poor biosecurity practices were suggested to play major roles for transmission of avian influenza viruses (Munyua et al. 2012). These factors were found to be associated with transmission of low pathogenic avain influenza viruses in markets in North America (Garber et al. 2007).

The current study showed that, virulent viruses with multiple basic amino acids at cleavage site of F protein ^{112}RRQKR^{116}*F^{117} are circulating in village chickens. The finding is in agreement with earlier studies which revealed that, the majority of the virus strains circulating in the village chickens in Ethiopia are virulent strains (Chaka et al. 2012). Virulent Newcastle disease virus (vNDV) is endemic in many countries of Africa, North, Central, and South America, and outbreaks of ND are frequently reported to the World Organization of Animal health (Office of International Epizootes 2011).

According to Diel et al. (2012) classification, our phylogenetic analysis of the 260 fragment of the fusion gene of all the 29 sequenced isolates indicated that the viruses are grouped in the new sub-genotype VIf class II viruses, and grouped with NDV identified in Ethiopia (de Almeida et al. 2013; Chaka et al.2013). The genotype was confirmed by analysis of complete coding region of the F gene of two representative viruses (Figure 2), which showed 95% to 99.3% similarity with the NDV isolated in 2011 suggesting the persistence of this sub-genotype in poultry in the country. While the 260 nucleotide sequences of samples collected from the market sites of Merkato and Kotebe were all identical, sequences of viruses from Saris, Shola and Meri showed a nucleotide identity ranging from 99.3% to 100%, from 98% to 100% and from 98.7% to 100%, respectively). Which revealed that, identical isolates are circulating in livebird markets in Addis Ababa. This could be associated with the poor biosecurity practices and the use of similar marketing channel in these market sites. However, Fentie et al. (2013) identified genotype VII viruses in the North western Ethiopia, indicating the co-circulation of different genotypes in Ethiopia. Genotype VI, include viruses that have been isolated from multiple avian species (Alexander2011; Czeglédi et al. 2006; Kim et al. 2008). Viruses of this group are important because of their frequent association with doves and pigeons and consequent risk for introduction in to poultry flocks (Alexander 2011; Kim et al. 2008). It is interesting to note that Ethiopian viruses analyzed here grouped with viruses collected in Nigeria from pigeon and doves (identity of about 90%), suggesting that this genotype may have emerged in Africa as a result of transmission from pigeon to poultry.

In conclusion, the current study revealed that village chicken flocks are endemically infected with virulent Newcastle disease virus, which could pose a threat to commercial poultry farms. This study highlights the importance of implementing surveillance and molecular investigations of Newcastle disease, in village chickens and wild birds, along with improved biosecurity measures in the live poultry markets in Ethiopia.

DECLARATIONS

Acknowledgements

This study was supported by National Animal Health Diagnostic center, Ethiopia. The authors would like to thank the molecular Biology Laboratory staff of NAHDIC, Ethiopia, and Istituto Zooprofilattico Sperimentale delle Venezie,Italy for their technical assistance and support in processing of the samples and genetic analysis of the isolates.

Authors' contributions

DD conceived and designed the study, participated in data collection, laboratory analysis and drafted the manuscript, MK participated in data collection, laboratory analysis and helped in drafting of the manuscript, RB and MS participated in data collection and laboratory analysis , AF carried out the sequencing, sequence alignment and phylogenetic reconstruction and revised the manuscript, AH participated in sequence alignment and phylogenetic reconstruction, TR participated in design and coordination of the work. HC participated in drafting and edition of the manuscript. All authors read and approved the final manuscript.

REFERENCES

1. Alexander DJ: Newcastle disease in the European Union 2000 to 2009. *Avian Pathol* 2011, 40(6):547-558. 10.1080/03079457.2011.618823
2. Alexander DJ, Senne DA: Newcastle disease, other avian paramyxoviruses, and pneumovirus infections. In *Diseases of Poultry*. 12th edition. Edited by: Saif YM, Fadly A, Glisson JR, Mc D, Larry R, Nolan LK, Swayne D. Ames, IA: Blackwell Publishing; 2008:750-798.
3. Central Statistical Agency: *Agricultural Sample Survey (2011/12) Volume II, Report on Livestock and Livestock characteristics, Statistical Bulletin, 505*. Addis Ababa, Ethiopia; 2012.
4. Chaka H, Goutard F, Bisschop SPR, Thompson PN: Seroprevalence of Newcastle disease and other infectious diseases in backyard chickens at markets in Eastern Shewa zone, Ethiopia. *Poult Sci* 2012, 91: 862-869. 10.3382/ps.2011-01906
5. Chaka H, Goutard F, Gil P, Abolnik C, Servan De Almeida R, Bisschop S, Thompson PN: Serological and molecular investigation of Newcastle disease in household chicken flocks and associated markets in Eastern Shewa zone, Ethiopia.*Tropl Anim Health Prod* 2013, 45(3):705-714. 10.1007/s11250-012-0278-y

6. Czeglédi A, Ujvári D, Somogyi E, Wehmann E, Werner O, Lomniczi B: Third genome size category of avian paramyxovirus serotype 1 (Newcastle disease virus) and evolutionary implications. *Virus Res* 2006, 120(1–2):36-48.

7. De Almeida RS, Hammoumi S, Gil P, Briand FX, Molia S, Gaidet N, Cappelle J, Chevalier V, Balanc G, Traore A, Grillet C, Maminiaina OF, Guendouz S, Dakouo M, Samake K, Bezeid OEM, Diarra A, Chaka H, Goutard F, Thompson P, Martinez D, Jestin V, Albina E: New avian paramyxoviruses type I strains identified in Africa provide new outcomes for phylogeny reconstruction and genotype classification. *PLoS One* 2013, 8(10):76413. 10.1371/journal.pone.0076413

8. Dessei T, Ogle B: Village poultry production system in the central highlands of Ethiopia. *Tropl Anim Health Prod* 2001, 33: 521-537. 10.1023/A:1012740832558

9. Diel DG, Da SLHA, LiuH WZ, Miller PJ, Afonso CL: Genetic diversity of avian paramyxovirus type 1: Proposal for a unified nomenclature and classification system of Newcastle disease virus genotypes Infection. *Genet Evol* 2012, 12: 1770-1779. 10.1016/j.meegid.2012.07.012

10. Fentie T, HeidariA AR, Kassa T, Capua I, Cattoli G, Sahle M: Molecular characterization of Newcastle disease viruses isolated from rural chicken in northwest Ethiopia reveals the circulation of three distinct genotypes in the country. *Tropl Anim Health Prod* 2013, 10: 11250-11263.

11. Garber L, Voelker L, Hill G: Description of live poultry markets in the United States and factors associated with repeated presence of H5 /H7 low-pathogenicity avian influenza virus. *Avian Dis* 2007, 51: 417-420. 10.1637/7571-033106R.1

12. Gebreab F: *Zoonotic diseases in Ethiopia. Ethiopian Society of Animal Production*. Addis Ababa, Ethiopia; 1995.

13. Glickman RL, Syddall RJ, Iorio RM, Sheehan JP, Bratt MA: Quantitative basic residue requirements in the cleavage-activation site of the fusion glycoprotein as a determinant of virulence for Newcastle disease virus. *J Virol* 1988, 62: 354-356.

14. Guindon S, Gascuel O: A simple, fast, and accurate algorithm to estimate large phylogenies by maximum likelihood. *Syst Biol* 2003, 52: 696-704. 10.1080/10635150390235520

15. Kattenbelt JA, Stevens MP, Gould AR: Sequence variation in the Newcastle disease virus genome. *Virus Res* 2006, 116(1–2):168-184.

16. Kim LM, King DJ, Guzman H, Tesh RB, Travassos DA, Rossa APA, Bueno R, Dennet JA, Afonso CL: Biological and phylogenetic characterization of pigeon paramyxovirus serotype 1 circulating in wild North American pigeons and doves. *J Clin Microbiol* 2008, 46(10):3303-3310. 10.1128/JCM.00644-08

17. Mayo: A summary of taxonomic changes recently approved by ICTV. *Arch Virol* 2002, 147: 1655-1656. 10.1007/s007050200039

18. Mazengia H: Review on major viral diseases of chickens reported in Ethiopia. *J Infect Dis Immun* 2012, 4(1):1-9.

19. Munyua MP, Githinji WJ, Waiboci WL, Njagi ML, Arunga G, Mwasi L, Mbabu MR, Macharia MJ, Breiman FR, Njenga KM, Katz AM: Detection of influenza A virus in live bird markets in Kenya, 2009–2011. *Influenza Other Respi Viruses* 2012, 10: 1750-2659.

20. Nasser M: *Oral Newcastle disease vaccination trial and studies of Newcastle disease in Ethiopia. (M.Sc. Thesis)*. AddisAbaba University and Freie Universitat, Addis Ababa, Ethiopia and Berlin, Germany; 1998.

21. Office of International Epizootes: *World Animal Health Information Database (WAHID) Interface*. 2011.http://web.oie.int/wahis/public.php?page_home&WAHIDPHPSESSID4d95e8777ff8b8a615b31617ac4c7835

22. Office of International Epizootes: *Newcastle Disease*. Manual of Diagnostic Tests and Vaccines for Terrestrial Animals, Paris, France; 2012. chapter 2.3.14

23. Shewantasew M, Melesse B, MesfinS MB: Assessment of Bio-security situation and practices in live poultry Markets of Addis Ababa, Ethiopia. *Asian J Anim Vet Adv* 2012, 7(5):421-433.

24. Spradbrow PB: Epidemiology of Newcastle Disease and the Economic of its control. In *Proceedings of international workshop on Poverty eradication and promotion of gender equality, held at Livestock Research Institute 26–26 March1999*. Denmark: Tune landboskole; 1999:165-173.

25. Steward M, Vipond IB, Millar NS, Emmersion PT: RNA editing in Newcastle disease virus. *Journal of General Virology* 1993, 74: 2539-2547. 10.1099/0022-1317-74-12-2539

26. Tadelle , Jobre Y: A review of the importance and control of Newcastle disease in Ethiopia. *Ethiop Vet J* 2004, 1: 71-81.

27. Toyoda T, Sakaguchi T, Imai K, Inocencio NM, Gotoh B, Hamaguchi , Nagai Y: Structural comparison of the cleavage-activation site of the fusion glycoprotein between virulent and avirulent strains of Newcastle disease virus. *Virology* 1987, 158: 242-247. 10.1016/0042-6822(87)90261-3

28. Wise MG, Suarez DL, Seal BS, Pedersen JC, Senne DA, King DJ, Kapczynski DR, Spackman E: Development of a real-time reverse-transcription PCR for detection of Newcastle disease virus RNA in clinical samples. *J Clin Microbiol* 2004, 42(1):329-338. 10.1128/JCM.42.1.329-338.2004

CHAPTER 12

NEWCASTLE DISEASE IN LOCAL CHICKENS OF LIVE BIRD MARKETS AND HOUSEHOLDS IN ZAMFARA STATE, NIGERIA

A. H. Jibril[1] J. U. Umoh[2] J. Kabir[2] L. Saidu[3] A. A. Magaji[1] M. B. Bello[1] and A. A. Raji[1]

[1]Department of Veterinary Physiology, Faculty of Veterinary Medicine, Usmanu Danfodiyo University, Sokoto P.M. B 2346, Nigeria

[2]Department of Veterinary Public Health and Preventive Medicine, Ahmadu Bello University, Zaria, Nigeria

[3]Ahmadu Bello University Veterinary Teaching Hospital, Zaria, Nigeria

ABSTRACT

Newcastle disease constitutes a major constraint to rural poultry production system in Nigeria. This study used serological method to estimate the level of circulating antibodies against ND in nonvaccinated village chickens, raised under traditional management system in Zamfara State, Nigeria. Competitive Enzyme Linked Immunosorbent Assay was used to analyze 504 chicken sera for Newcastle disease virus antibodies from randomly selected households and live bird markets. Higher seroprevalence rate of Newcastle disease virus antibodies was detected in both household and live bird markets. Overall, seropositive rate was found to be 32.5% (164/504). About 35.8% (115/321) sero-positive rate was obtained from live bird markets while 26.8% (49/183) seropositive rate was found in households. Comparison was made between the sero prevalence of house hold and live bird markets as well as between sexes. Live bird markets show a statistically significant higher prevalence rate ($P<0.05$) when compared with chickens sampled from households (OR 1.53; 95% CI, 1.024–2.275). The prevalence of ND indicated the presence of the virus amongst the population, and hence there should be an improvement in the vaccine campaign against ND for rural poultry especially the use of thermostable vaccine to reduce the chances of vaccine failure.

INTRODUCTION

Newcastle disease (ND) is a major viral disease of economic importance in poultry [1] and rated as one of the greatest constraints to the development of rural poultry production in Nigeria and in most developing countries, causing serious threats [2]. All ages of different species of birds are susceptible to ND, although being substantially less with advancement to maturity [3]. The acute and virulent form may result in 90% mortality or more in affected flocks [4]. It is an acute, rapidly spreading, contagious, nervous and respiratory disease of birds of all ages [5]. The clinical signs of ND are known to vary based on the virulence and tropism of the ND virus involved, species of the bird, age of the host, immune status, and environmental condition [6].

Nigeria poultry population is estimated to be 137.6 million, with backyard poultry population constituting 84% (115.8 million) and 16% (21.7 million) of exotic poultry, with a higher percentage of this poultry raised for subsistence production [7]. Village poultry production provides an important source of high quality protein, is reserved for times of celebrations, and is a good source of income for rural families [8]. This category of birds represents a significant part of the Nigerian rural economy in particular and of the national economy as a whole and is kept under the extensive management system

Citation: A. H. Jibril, J. U. Umoh, J. Kabir, et al., "Newcastle Disease in Local Chickens of Live Bird Markets and Households in Zamfara State, Nigeria," ISRN Epidemiology, vol. 2014, Article ID 513961, 4 pages, 2014. doi:10.1155/2014/513961.

[9]. The resources derivable from the chickens cannot be fully utilized unless the disease is controlled particularly in the village poultry flocks that are believed to keep the virus in circulation and act as reservoirs and carriers to themselves and the more susceptible exotic breeds in commercial farms [10].

MATERIALS AND METHODS

Study Area

The study was carried out in six local governments (Bungudu, Gusau, Talata-Mafara, Bakura, Kaura-Namoda, and Zurmi) of Zamfara State, Nigeria. Zamfara State is located between latitudes 10°50 N and 13°58 N and longitudes 4°16 E and 7°13 E. It has a warm tropical climate between March and May. The vegetation of the state consists of Sudan and Northern Guinea Savannah. It has a total human population of 3,278,873 [11] and an estimated poultry population of 5 845,508 [7]. The state has 14 local governments and has 3 senatorial districts.

Sera Collection

Multistage sampling procedure was applied to divide the state into three stages corresponding to three senatorial districts. Two local governments were then randomly selected from each district, making a total number of six local governments that were considered in this study. A total of 504 sera samples were collected from live bird markets and households from all the six selected local governments across the state. Two milliliter of chicken blood was collected through the brachial vein using a 21-gauge sterile hypodermic needle and 2 mL syringes. The syringes were labeled and kept in slanting position till clot formation. Sera were harvested, transferred into a sterile serum bottles, and stored at −20°C. All sera at the end of the sampling were taken to the viral zoonosis laboratory of the Department of Veterinary Public Health and Preventive Medicine, Ahmadu Bello University, Zaria, for serology.

Serology

Competitive ELISA diagnostic kit was obtained from ID Vet, Innovative Diagnostics, France. The kit procedure is based on blocking Enzyme Linked Immunosorbent Assay. 100 μL of positive control was added to positive control wells A1 and B1 and 100 μL of negative control to negative control wells C1 and D1 using micropipette. 80 μL of dilution buffer 2 was added to each of the wells. Using multichannel pipette, 20 μL of undiluted serum was then added to the remaining selected wells and mixed thoroughly with the buffer. The plates were then sealed and incubated at room temperature for 30 minutes. Anti-NDV conjugate 10x was prepared by diluting anti-NDV-HRP conjugate to 1/10 dilution buffer 5. After incubation the plates were washed 3 times with wash solution. Using multichannel pipette, 100 μL of anti-NDV conjugate 1x was added to each well. The plates were rinsed three times with wash solution. 100 μL of the substrate solution was added to each well. And this was incubated at room temperature for ten minutes in the dark. The reaction was stopped by adding 50 μL of stop solution to each well which is mixed thoroughly. Optical density was read at 450 nm by using microplate reader.

Data Analysis

The data obtained was subjected to SPSS package version 16. Categorical variables (sex, location) were evaluated using Chi-square to check for independence, and odds ratio at 95% confidence interval was used to measure the strength of association between variables and prevalence of Newcastle disease. Values of were considered significant.

RESULTS

The overall seroprevalence of Newcastle disease in the study area was 32.5%. The highest prevalence was found in Gusau local governments (56.0%) while the least was detected in Kaura-Namoda local governments (14.1%) (Table 1). Table 2 indicates that chickens from live bird markets show a higher prevalence rate (35.8%) when compared to those sampled from households (26.8%). Prevalence of 35.7% was recorded in male chickens while 28.9% was obtained from female chickens as indicated in Table 3.

Table 1: Prevalence of Newcastle disease from selected local governments of Zamfara State

S/N	Local governments	Number of samples	Number of positives	Number of negatives	Prevalence (%)
1	Gusau	100	56	44	56.0
2	Bungudu	70	34	36	48.5
3	Zurmi	75	26	49	34.7
4	Kaura-Namoda	99	14	85	14.1
5	Bakura	70	12	58	17.1
6	Talata-Mafara	90	22	68	24.4
	Total	504	164	340	32.5

Chi-square value = 58.94.
P value = 0.001.

Table 2: Prevalence of Newcastle based on location in Zamfara State

S/N	Location	Number of samples	Number of positives	Number of negatives	Prevalence (%)	Odds ratio	95% CI
1	LB markets	321	115	206	35.8	1.53*	1.024–2.275
2	Households	183	49	134	26.8	1.00	
	Total	504	164	340	32.5		

Chi-square value = 3.946.
P value = 0.0470.
*Statistical significance between variables when using odd ratio.

Table 3: Sex-specific prevalence of Newcastle disease in Zamfara State

S/N	Sex	Number of samples	Number of positives	Number of negatives	Prevalence (%)	Odds ratio	95% CI
1	Male	272	97	175	35.7	1.37	0.936–1.990
2	Female	232	67	165	28.9	1.0	

Chi-square value = 2.324.
P value = 0.1274.

DISCUSSION

The present serological study revealed the presence of circulating antibodies of Newcastle disease among sampled village chickens from selected local governments of Zamfara State. An overall seroprevalence of 32.5% from the six local governments of Zamfara State is an indication of endemicity. Antibodies detected may be a result of natural infection since vaccination of the village poultry is rarely undertaken in Nigeria [12]. In similar studies, [13] reported a variable sero prevalence of 25–81.5% in Tanzania, in Ethiopia, 43.68% seropositive rate of NDV was reported in the cool central highlands [14] while [15] reported 19.78%, [16] reported 14% sero prevalence in non-vaccinated village chickens in Niger. Reference [17] reported a prevalence of 63% in south eastern Nigeria. Reference [18] reported a prevalence of 46% in village chickens in Borno State and [19] reported an ND prevalence of 54.67% in Nasarawa State. This finding of NDV sero prevalence in these apparently healthy birds suggests that the birds have either recovered from clinical ND or are having subclinical infections [20]. A similar study was conducted in Ibadan using indirect ELISA and an overall prevalence rate of 73.3% was obtained [21]. Although there is a statistically significant ($P<0.05$) higher prevalence in Gusau compared to other local government areas (LGAs), the higher circulating antibodies in Gusau may be due to higher concentration of live bird markets in this LGA. The lower prevalence rate in Bakura, Talata-Mafara, and Kaura-Namoda may be due to vaccination activities of commercial poultry that may contribute to mild infection due to the spread of vaccine virus to local birds through commercial poultry workers [19].

Live bird markets show a statistically significant higher prevalence rate ($P<0.05$) when compared with chickens sampled from households (OR 1.53; 95%CI, 1.024–2.275). This may be due to the fact that live bird markets contribute to the persistence and spread of ND virus. These birds are exposed to birds from multiple sources having a higher tendency of circulating the virus and may serve as a source of infection to house hold chickens when introduced [22] Similar studies conducted by [23] show 25.5% prevalence in live bird markets of Kogi State, Nigeria.

This study also shows a higher prevalence rate among the male chickens. It was however observed that this difference is statistically insignificant ($P<0.05$). In a similar study conducted by [15] in Ethiopia, ND shows a higher prevalence rate among males (21.74%) than among females (19.16%). However, a slightly higher prevalence of 32.63% among female chickens was obtained by [24] when compared with a prevalence of 31.63 among male chickens.

ACKNOWLEDGMENTS

The authors would like to thank all the farmers that allowed them to take samples from their chickens and to all staff of the department of Veterinary Public Health and Preventive Medicine, Ahmadu Bello University, for their technical support.

REFERENCES

1. G. N. Anosa and D. F. Adene, "Comparative tissue reactivity of lentogenic strains of Newcastle disease vaccines in Nigeria," Nigerian Veterinary Journal, vol. 28, no. 3, pp. 6–10, 2007.
2. S. B. Oladele, P. Abdu, K. A. N. Esievo, A. J. Nok, and N. M. Useh, "Prevalence of Newcastle disease virus antibodies in chickens reared in Zaria," in Proceedings of the 28th Annual Conference of Nigerian Society of Animal Production, vol. 28, pp. 7–9, 2003.
3. F. R. Beaudette, "A review of literature on Newcastle disease," in Proceedings of the 4th Annual Meeting US Livestock Association, vol. 47, pp. 122–177, 1943.
4. D. J. Alexander and W. H. Allan, "Newcastle disease virus pathotypes," Avian Pathology, vol. 3, pp. 269–278, 1974.
5. E. N. Okeke and A. G. Lamorde, "Newcastle disease and its control in Nigeria," in Viral Disease of Animals in Africa, A. Olufemi Williams and W. N. Masiga, Eds., CTA/OAU/STRC/ Publication, Lagos, Nigeria, 1988.
6. R. Alders and P. B. Spradbrow, Controlling Newcastle Disease in Village Chickens, Monograph Australian Center for International Resources, Canberra, Australia, 2002.
7. Federal Ministry of Agriculture and Rural Development, Federal Department of Livestock and Pest Control Services, Highly Pathogenic Avian Influenza Standard Operating Procedures, February 2006.
8. M. B. Abubakar, A. D. El-yuguda, A. A. Yerima, and S. S. Baba, "Seroprevalence of active and passive immunity against egg drop syndrome 1976 (EDS 76) in village poultry in Nigeria," Asian Journal of Poultry Science, vol. 2, pp. 58–61, 2008.
9. M. K. Ajala, B. I. Nwagu, and C. U. Osuhor, "Socio-economic of free-range guinea fowl production among agro-pastoral Fulani women in Giwa L.G.A of Kaduna state, Nigeria," International Journal of Tropical Agriculture, vol. 15, pp. 37–44, 1997.
10. A. O. Olabode, A. G. Lamorde, N. N. Shidali, and A. A. Chukwuedo, "Village chickens and Newcastle disease in Nigeria," Australian Centre For International Agricultural Research Proceedings, no. 39, pp. 159–160, 1992.
11. National Population Commission, "Social Statistic in Nigeria," Beaureu of Statistics, Lagos, Nigeria, p. 300, 2009.

12. P. A. Abdu, S. U. Abdullahi, A. A. Adesiyun, and C. D. Ezeokoli, "Challenge study on infectious bursal disease in chicks derived from vaccinated hens," Tropical Animal Health and Production, vol. 19, no. 1, pp. 47–52, 1987. View at Publisher · ·
13. M. G. S. Yongolo, Epidemiology of Newcastle disease in village chickens in Tanzania [M.S. thesis], Sokoine University of Agriculture, Morogoro, Tanzania, 1996.
14. H. Ashenafi, Survey on identification of major diseases of local chickens in three selected agroclimatic zones in central Ethiopia [M.S. thesis], Faculty of Veterinary Medicine, Addis Ababa University, Debre Zeit, Ethiopia, 2000.
15. Z. Aschalew, S. Teshale, G. Esayas, and A. Gelegay, "Newcastle disease in village chickens in the southern and rift valley districts in Ethiopia," International Journal of Poultry Science, vol. 4, no. 7, pp. 507–510, 2005.
16. C. Courtecuisse, F. Japiot, N. Bloch, and I. Diallo, "Serological survey on Newcastle and Gumboro diseases, pasteurellosis and pullorosis in local hens in Niger," Revue d›Elevage et de Médecine Vétérinaire des pays Tropicaux, vol. 43, no. 1, pp. 27–29, 1990. ·
17. L. J. E. Orakaja, D. F. Adene, B. M. Anene, and E. A. Onuoha, "Seroprevalence of Newcastle disease in local chickens from south east derived Savannah zone of Nigeria," Revue d›Elevage et de Médecine Vétérinaire des pays Tropicaux, vol. 52, pp. 185–188, 1999.
18. A. D. EL-Yuguda, I. S. Ngulde, M. B. Abubakar, and S. S. Baba, "Village chicken health, management and production indices in selected villages of Borno State," Nigeria Family Poultry Journal, vol. 17, no. 1-2, 2007.
19. A. E. Salihu, A. A. Chukwuedo, G. O. N. Echeonwu et al., "Seroprevalence of Newcastle disease virus infection in rural household birds in Lafia, Akwanga and Keffi Metropolis, Nasarawa State Nigeria,"International Journal of Agricultural Sciences, vol. 2, no. 2, pp. 109–112, 2012.
20. J. G. Bell and S. Mouloudi, "A reservoir of virulent Newcastle disease virus in village chicken flocks,"Preventive Veterinary Medicine, vol. 6, no. 1, pp. 37–42, 1988. ·
21. O. G. Ohore, P. C. Ozegbe, B. O. Emikpe, and V. E. Okojie, "Survey of antibodies to Newcastle disease virus in apparently healthy adult Nigeria indigenous chickens (Gallus domesticus) in Ibadan using ELISA," African Journal of Clinical and Experimental Microbiology, vol. 3, no. 1, pp. 38–40, 2002.
22. M. L. Killian, "National veterinary services laboratories avian influenza and Newcastle disease diagnostics report," in Proceedings of the 113th Annual Meeting of the United States Animal Health Association, pp. 590–593, 2009.
23. O. N. Ameji, P. A. Abdu, and L. Saidu, "Seroprevalence of Avian influenza, Newcastle disease and Gumboro disease in chicken in Kogi State, Nigeria," Bulletin of Animal Health and Production African Journal, vol. 59, no. 4, 2011.
24. T. Sarkelm, A. Hagos, and A. Zeleke, "Seroprevalence study of Newcastle disease in local chickens in central Ethiopia," International Journal of Applied Research in Veterinary Medicine, vol. 3, no. 1, pp. 25–29, 2005.

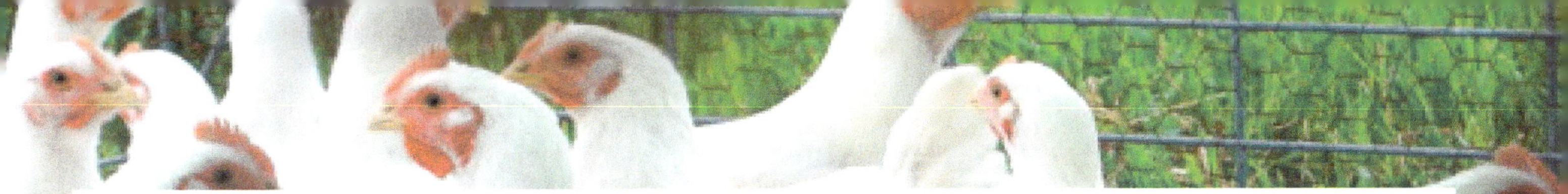

CHAPTER 13

CHARACTERIZATION OF A NOVEL CHICKEN MUSCLE DISORDER THROUGH DIFFERENTIAL GENE EXPRESSION AND PATHWAY ANALYSIS USING RNA-SEQUENCING

Marie F Mutryn[1], Erin M Brannick[1], Weixuan Fu[1], William R Lee[2] and Behnam Abasht[1]

[1] Department of Animal and Food Sciences, University of Delaware, 531 South College Ave, Newark, DE 19716, USA

[2] Maple Leaf Farms, Leesburg, IN, USA

ABSTRACT

Background

Improvements in poultry production within the past 50 years have led to increased muscle yield and growth rate, which may be contributing to an increased rate and development of new muscle disorders in chickens. Previously reported muscle disorders and conditions are generally associated with poor meat quality traits and have a significant negative economic impact on the poultry industry. Recently, a novel myopathy phenotype has emerged which is characterized by palpably "hard" or tough breast muscle. The objective of this study is to identify the underlying biological mechanisms that contribute to this emerging muscle disorder colloquially referred to as "Wooden Breast", through the use of RNA-sequencing technology.

Methods

We constructed cDNA libraries from five affected and six unaffected breast muscle samples from a line of commercial broiler chickens. After paired-end sequencing of samples using the Illumina Hiseq platform, we used Tophat to align the resulting sequence reads to the chicken reference genome and then used Cufflinks to find significant changes in gene transcript expression between each group. By comparing our gene list to previously published histology findings on this disorder and using Ingenuity Pathways Analysis (IPA®), we aim to develop a characteristic gene expression profile for this novel disorder through analyzing genes, gene families, and predicted biological pathways.

Results

Over 1500 genes were differentially expressed between affected and unaffected birds. There was an average of approximately 98 million reads per sample, across all samples. Results from the IPA analysis suggested "Diseases and Disorders" such

Citation: Marie F Mutryn, Erin M Brannick, Weixuan Fu, William R Lee and Behnam Abasht, Characterization of a novel chicken muscle disorder through differential gene expression and pathway analysis using RNA-sequencing, DOI 10.1186/s12864-015-1623-0.

as connective tissue disorders, "Molecular and Cellular Functions" such as cellular assembly and organization, cellular function and maintenance, and cellular movement, "Physiological System Development and Function" such as tissue development, and embryonic development, and "Top Canonical Pathways" such as, coagulation system, axonal guidance signaling, and acute phase response signaling, are associated with the Wooden Breast disease.

Conclusions

There is convincing evidence by RNA-seq analysis to support localized hypoxia, oxidative stress, increased intracellular calcium, as well as the possible presence of muscle fiber-type switching, as key features of Wooden Breast Disease, which are supported by reported microscopic lesions of the disease.

BACKGROUND

In terms of consumption, poultry meat is highly regarded as one of the most efficient food sources; it contains high quality nutrients such as protein, and is relatively inexpensive for purchase. However, muscle disorders of commercial chickens such as deep pectoral myopathy (DPM) [1-3] and white striping [4], as well as other conditions such as pale, soft, and exudative condition (PSE) or dry, firm, and dark condition (DFD) have had an increasing negative impact on worldwide chicken meat production and quality [5]. Recently, flocks of commercial broiler chickens in the United States have developed a myopathy affecting the pectoralis major, and occasionally minor, muscle. Previously described by Sihvo et al. 2014 [6], this disease is colloquially referred to as "woody" or "wooden" breast, due to clinical and microscopic changes to the muscle resulting overall in palpable severe hardness of the breast muscle. Hereafter this syndrome will be referred to as Wooden Breast. The superficial area of the pectoralis muscle tends to be more affected than deeper portions of the muscle. Lesions can be detected clinically through manual palpation of the breast muscle in live birds as early as 3 weeks in age. Owens (2014) [7] has recently reported that severe cases of Wooden Breast disease can likely affect about 10% of an entire flock; but it was also noted that some degree of Wooden Breast disease has been anecdotally reported to affect up to 50% of a flock. The disease is emerging on a global scale, already present in Finland [6] and to the authors' knowledge in several other countries.

Sihvo et al. 2014 [6] specifically studied the microscopic and histologic properties of the pectoralis muscle from chickens affected with Wooden Breast. Although histological evidence indicated multifocal degeneration and necrosis of muscle tissue with infiltration of inflammatory cells, the underlying etiology of this disorder was not apparent [6]. Wooden Breast has also previously been reported in the United States by Bilgili 2013 [8] at the University of Auburn in Alabama with the general phenotypic properties of the myopathy described being in agreement with Sihvo et al. 2014 [6]. Lesions associated with the myopathy appear to be aseptic, superficially-located, and include muscle fiber fragmentation, hyalinization, and swelling with replacement by fibrous connective tissue, as well as an influx of macrophages and other immune cells and the occurrence of irregular adipose tissue throughout the muscle. Bilgili 2013 [8] hypothesizes that these features may be associated with localized hypoxia due to a reduction in capillary supply.

Previously described muscle disorders in chickens, such as white striping and nutritional myopathy, have been shown to affect the integrity of the pectoralis major muscle in chickens. White striping is identified through the observation of white fatty lines on the breast muscle running in the same direction as the muscle fibers of the breast muscle [9]. It is speculated that white striping is caused from a mineralization of fat on myofibers, along with general necrosis of the muscle [9]. Interestingly, there may be a correlation between white striping and Wooden Breast, as birds affected by Wooden Breast are likely to show gross features of white striping [6]. It is also possible that the two disorders represent a disease spectrum, with white striping cases being the less severe form of the myopathy as compared to Wooden Breast.

Nutritional myopathy also affects the breast muscle of broiler chickens and is generally associated with low levels of vitamin E and selenium in diet [10]. The main clinical features of nutritional myopathy can be observed grossly as white striations in the skeletal muscle [11] and histologically as degradation, necrosis, mineralization, and regeneration of myofibers in the muscle [10]. Although some of the characteristics of white striping and nutritional myopathy overlap with lesions of Wooden Breast, the grossly palpable hardness of the pectoralis muscle remains unique to Wooden Breast. Additionally, unlike in nutritional myopathy, no lesions are observed in other muscle groups, such as the gizzard or heart, beyond the pectoralis major and minor in Wooden Breast.

The overall objective of this paper is to use RNA-sequencing to identify biological and molecular pathways that are involved in the underlying etiology and pathogenesis of this emerging muscle disorder of the pectoralis muscle in commercial broiler chickens. We used RNA-sequencing as this powerful technology provides comprehensive and accurate gene expression data, performing better than previous technologies such as microarrays [12]. Also, useful tools have been generated for RNA-sequencing data analyses that make for user-friendly and efficient analysis of the data.

METHODS

Chickens used in this study were all males from a high breast meat yield purebred line of broiler breeder chickens raised on the floor, in pens of 300, by Heritage Breeders in the Delmarva region of the United States. Birds were given free access to both feed and water, and were housed according to optimal industry growing standards. Birds were euthanized at 47 days of age by cervical dislocation. After euthanasia, pectoral muscle samples were collected at necropsy. Based upon clinical examination and manual palpation of pectoral muscle for evidence of palpable "hardening", eight affected and eight unaffected birds were identified; affected birds were those deemed to have "severe" to "moderately-severe" lesions, while unaffected birds showed no apparent gross lesions. Samples from the pectoralis major were taken from the caudal aspect of the right superficial pectoral muscle, perpendicular to myofibers and to the keel bone. Samples were taken with the Keyes biopsy punch (8 mm) manufactured by HNM. Roughly one to two grams of tissue was extracted from each sample location and immediately flash frozen in liquid nitrogen. The protocols were submitted to, and the use of the collected samples for research was approved by, the University of Delaware Agricultural Animal Care and Use Committee (protocol number: 44 12-15-13R).

Total RNA was extracted from the breast muscle tissue samples using the *mir*Vana™ miRNA Isolation Kit according to the manufacturer's protocol (Life Technologies®). Multiple quality checks were performed to assess the RNA quality and integrity using NanoDrop 1000 and Angilent Bioanalyzer 2100 to measure RNA concentrations following the established manufacturer protocol. The RNA integrity number of samples was larger than 8, which is considered acceptable for cDNA library preparation.

Eleven samples, five affected and six unaffected, were prepared to create cDNA libraries for RNA-sequencing. All samples used for RNA-sequencing were also strictly verified for correct identity. cDNA libraries were constructed following the TruSeq Stranded mRNA Sample Prep Kit following the protocol for low sample (LS). After construction, the 11 cDNA libraries were normalized as suggested by the manufacturer, to 10 nm/μl using Tris buffer (Tris-Cl 10 mM, 0.1 % Tween 20, pH 8.5). The 11 uniquely indexed, normalized libraries were pooled together in 2 tubes and submitted to the Delaware Biotechnology Institute (DBI) for 101 nucleotides paired-end sequencing on 2 lanes of a flow cell using the Illumina Hiseq 2000 system and on 1 lane of a flow cell using the Illumina Hiseq 2500 system.

The quality of the data received from DBI was checked with FastQC v0.10.1 [13]. RNA sequencing reads that passed this quality control measure were then mapped to the chicken reference genome (Galgal4.0 Nov 2011) using TopHat v2.0.4 [14]. Parameters of TopHat were set to only report read alignments if 1) both reads in a pair could be mapped, 2) there were no more than two mismatches per read, 3) concordant mapping occurred for both reads in a pair, 4) no more than one mismatch per segment (—segment-mismatches), and 5) mean inner distance between mate pairs set at 110. TopHat cut up input reads into smaller segments and mapped these segments independently. The default parameter (25 nucleotides) was used for segment length.

Cufflinks v2.1.1 [15] was used for the differential expression analysis: parameters of Cuffdiff were set to allow normalization of the number of fragments mapping to individual loci to improve the strength of differential expression analysis (change in default-- added –N/--upper-quartile-norm parameter). Cuffdiff labeled genes as significant or not significant based on whether the p-value of statistical test for differential expression was greater than the false discovery rate (FDR) after Benjamini-Hochberg correction for multiple testing [15]. Genes with a q-value or FDR-adjusted p-value of <0.05 and a fold change greater than 1.3 were considered statistically significant and submitted to Ingenuity Pathway Analysis (IPA®) [16] for functional annotation and identification of significant biological pathways and upstream regulatory factors. The fold change for each gene was provided by Cuffdiff as $\log_2$(fold change) and was then calculated as $2^{\log_2 \text{(fold change)}}$ for genes with a positive $\log_2$(fold change) and $-1/(2^{\log_2 \text{(fold change)}})$ for genes with a negative $\log_2$(fold change) before submission to IPA.

To verify the gene expression data we used NanoString nCounter® technology previously described by Geiss et al. 2008 [17]. We selected 192 target genes, along with 12 housekeeping genes across various RNA-sequencing projects within our lab to be measured. The 11 samples used in this paper were sent to NanoString Inc. (Seattle, WA, USA), where they custom designed 204 individual probes for target sequences. NanoString Inc. hybridized 100 ng of each RNA sample to the 204 designed probes. After incubation, the samples went through the nCounter® Prep Station and the Digital Analyzer for final transcript counting. Control factors and housekeeping genes were used to normalize the data for further analysis [17]. Finally, the $\log_2$(fold change) for gene expression between affected and unaffected birds were calculated from the NanoString results to be compared with the $\log_2$(fold change) of gene expression from the RNA-sequencing results.

RESULTS AND ANALYSIS

The total number of reads per sample provided from RNA-sequencing. The average number of reads across all 11 samples was 97,890,272.

Expression data for each gene within each sample was used to create a heatmap for cluster classification. The heatmap was generated using the R package "plots" (Fig. 1). This cluster analysis revealed a clear separation between affected and unaffected samples. It should be noted that one sample (Sample 51 unaffected) was seemingly clustered in the incorrect group. We believe that this inconsistency is likely due to the broad range of disease severity possible in Wooden Breast. It is reasonable to suspect that the syndrome was in fact developing in Sample 51, but not yet expressed in terms of the palpable muscle firmness. This suggests clinicopathological heterogeneity in the classification of this disease.

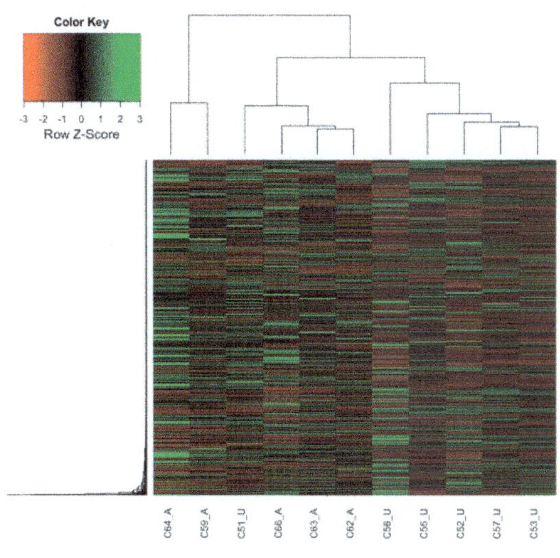

Figure 1: Heatmap gene cluster classification for Wooden Breast and unaffected muscle samples. Using the expression for each gene (in rows) and sample (in columns), the heatmap is generated by the R package "plots". The expression levels of each gene across samples are shown as Z-scores scaled by their FPKM from RNA-seq. The scaled expression values are color-coded according to the legend. The dendrogram depicting hierarchical clustering is based on the expression of all genes.

We verified our RNA-sequencing data using the Nanostring nCounter gene expression assay. Comparison of the log_2(fold change) for normalized NanoString count data against our RNA-sequencing data using the Pearson pair-wise correlation coefficient were very high, with a value of 0.861 across all overlapped genes tested in RNA-seq.

Ensembl ID of differentially-expressed (DE) genes, i.e., genes with a q-value <0.05 and a fold change higher than 1.3, were submitted to IPA® for functional annotation as well as mapping to canonical pathways and identifying upstream regulators. The differentially expressed genes with positive or negative fold change values are considered to be, respectively, upregulated or downregulated genes in affected birds relative to their expression in unaffected birds. Among the 1637 significant DE genes identified, IPA recognized 1390 of these genes for analysis. The Ingenuity Knowledge Base®, which supports the mapping of genes, relies on ortholog information for only human, mouse, and rat. Some genes went unmapped because there is no known ortholog with either of these species (human, mouse, rat). A summary of the top ten up-regulated and top ten down-regulated genes in the affected birds, along with the fold change for each gene is presented in Table 1.

Table 1: Top ten upregulated and downregulated genes with fold change for Wooden Breast myopathy-affected birds

Gene	Description	RNA-seq fold change	Nanostring fold change
ENSGAL00000009603	Prolactin-like protein precursor	43.9	N/A
CA3	Carbonic anhydrase III	28.5	25.5
CLEC3A	C-type lectin domain family 3, A	25.3	N/A
KPNA7	Karyopherin alpha 7	24.4	8.0
CSRP3	Cysteine and glycine-rich protein 3	23.2	27.3
CRISP1	Cysteine-rich secretory protein 1	21.5	N/A
FAM132A	Family sequence similarity 132, A	18.0	N/A
MB	Myoglobin	14.3	12.4
CRH	Corticotropin releasing hormone	14.3	13.3
PHGDH	Phosphoglycerate dehydrogenase	11.6	5.4
GC	Group Specific Component	−48.0	N/A
PIT54	PIT 54 protein precursor	−46.0	N/A
FGA	Fibrinogen alpha chain	−20.8	-3.0
FGG	Fibrinogen gamma chain	−18.1	-2.8
OGCHI	Orosomucoid 1	−16.9	N/A
ALB	Albumin	−16.8	-4.0
ENSGAL00000016859	Uncharacterized protein	−14.9	N/A
FGB	Fibrinogen beta chain	−13.3	-3.8
APOH	Apolipoprotein H	−13.1	N/A
YFV	MHC I antigen precursor	−12.9	N/A

This table provides a summary of both the top ten upregulated and downregulated genes found among affected chickens within the sample population. Positive and negative fold change values support, respectively, upregulation and downregulation of gene expression in affected birds relative to the gene expression in unaffected birds. The fold change for each gene is also presented along with the fold change for each gene that was tested using the NanoString nCounter® Technology to verify our expression data

A summary of the genes identified in the IPA® category of "Top Biological Functions" is presented in Table 2 and contains the subcategories of "Diseases and Disorders", "Molecular and Cellular Functions", "Physiological System Development and Function" and "Top Canonical Pathways". Also presented in Table 2 is the significance or P-value listed for each subcategory. IPA determines the P-value for each subcategory by dividing the number of DE genes (# of Genes) for each subcategory by the total number of known genes within that specific subcategory present in the IPA software database "Query Ingenuity Knowledge Base" (IPA website). The P-value for the top canonical pathways is also determined in the same manner. The "Genes" and "Ratio" columns in this subcategory were determined by dividing the number of observed DE genes by the total number of genes within that specific canonical pathway present within the IPA software database: "Query Ingenuity Knowledge Base" [16].

Table 2: Top biological functions of genes differentially expressed between Wooden Breast myopathy-affected and unaffected birds as presented by Ingenuity Pathway Analysis (IPA®)

Biological Functions	***P-value***		**# Molecules**
Diseases and disorders:			
Cancer	3.18E-31 – 4.08E-05		1208
Gastrointestinal Disease	9.84E-26 – 3.06E-05		890
Cardiovascular Disease	7.45E-21 – 4.06E-05		293
Hepatic System Disease	1.86E-20 – 3.06E-05		593
Neurological Disease	1.95E-17 – 3.92E-05		407
Molecular and Cellular Functions:			
Cellular Assembly and Organization	7.25E-19 – 1.14E-05		321
Cellular Function and Maintenance	7.25E-19 – 2.06E-05		402
Cellular Movement	1.80E-17 – 3.43E-05		322
Cell Morphology	1.51E-16 – 2.53E-05		387
Cellular Growth and Proliferation	2.81E-16 – 3.82E-05		476
Physiological System Development and Function:			
Nervous System Development/Function	9.74E-14 – 3.90E-05		195
Tissue Development	9.74E-14 – 3.82E-05		501
Cardiovascular System Dev./Function	2.75E-13 – 3.70E-05		237
Organismal Development	5.44E-13 – 3.63E-05		432
Embryonic Development	9.51E-13 – 3.10E-05		306
Top Canonical Pathways:	P-Value	Genes	Ratio
Hepatic Fibrosis/Stellate Cell Activation	2.83E-12	43/197	0.218
Epithelial Adherens Junction Signaling	2.39E-08	30/146	0.205
Actin Cytoskeleton Signaling	3.18E-07	36/217	0.166
Axonal Guidance Signaling	1.27E-06	56/433	0.129
Coagulation System	1.39E-06	12/35	0.343

Top Biological Functions of DE genes associated with affected chickens from the sample population within this study provided by Ingenuity Pathway Analysis (IPA®). The P-value provided by this table was determined by IPA by comparing the number of genes found within each category (# of Genes) with the number of known genes within the IPA software system. The P-value for the "Top Canonical Pathways" is also determined by IPA in the same manner

The resultant RNA-seq profile for Wooden Breast indicated by these analyses includes evidence of altered intracellular calcium, hypoxia, oxidative stress, potential fiber-type switching, and cellular repair within affected muscle. Additionally, there is direct correlation between RNA-sequencing data and the histologic lesions observed in the Wooden Breast myopathy.

DISCUSSION

Intracellular buildup of calcium

Through analysis of DE genes in this study, there is ample evidence to suggest that intracellular calcium overload with the potential to impact membrane integrity is occurring in the pectoralis major muscle of broilers affected with Wooden Breast. The ATPase, Ca++ transporting, cardiac muscle, slow twitch 2 (*ATP2A2)* gene, which is upregulated in birds affected with Wooden Breast, encodes for sarco(endo)-plasmic reticulum Ca^{2+} -ATPase isoform 2a and 2b (SERCA2a/SERCA2b) [18]. *SERCA2a* and *SERCA2b* differ in the location where they are generally expressed with *SERCA2a* showing high levels of expression in the heart and in slow-twitch skeletal and smooth muscle, whereas *SERCA2b* is expressed in all tissues [18]. SERCA2 is a critical component of the endoplasmic reticulum (ER) and sarcoplasmic reticulum (SR) and acts as a pump to sequester [19] and translocate Ca^{2+}[20]. SERCA pumps also have a role in contraction and relaxation of myofibrils, maintaining calcium homeostasis by sustaining the correct calcium levels required for relaxation and as well as maintaining "reloading" calcium levels needed for contraction [18, 20]. Increased expression of *SERCA2* leads to quicker calcium uptake and larger amounts of calcium loading within the ER [21]. Previously, a study in chickens showed that *SERCA*expression could be influenced by extrinsic factors such as disease [22]. The upregulation of *ATP2A2* in Wooden Breast birds may be occurring in response to increased amounts of intracellular calcium within muscle cells, potentially leading to up-take and loading calcium within the sarcoplasmic reticulum at faster than normal rates in affected birds.

Parvalbumin (*PVALB*), another upregulated gene in Wooden Breast birds, is essential to calcium buffering and regulating calcium concentrations within the cell [20]. PVALB acts to insure relaxation of the muscle through rapidly sequestering calcium from the sarcoplasm of the cell [20]. The upregulation of *PVALB* in birds affected within the current study may be compensatory to avoid a significant rise in intracellular calcium levels. This type of compensatory change has also been hypothesized in other muscle disorders such as Duchenne dystrophy in humans, in which excess calcium negatively impacts the muscle [23]. Therefore, it seems that increases in *PVALB*expression may act to stop hypercontraction of the muscle by inducing relaxation through calcium buffering and binding.

Abnormal accumulation of intracellular calcium can occur because of damaged cellular membranes of muscle cells or during episodes of metabolic imbalance between calcium and other ions [24]. The resultant damage to muscle cells can occur in various ways; it is hypothesized that extra calcium may activate proteases or lipases within the cell, which eventually leads to muscle fiber breakdown and an increase in calcium influx, initiating a "vicious cycle" of further muscle damage and calcium release [24]. It is also thought that excess calcium can impede mitochondrial performance ultimately decreasing the available energy supply when calcium cannot be effectively pumped out of the cell [24, 25]. Calcium overload can result in the activation of calpains and phospholipase A_2 (PLA_2), increase the overall production of ROS, and may also lead to excess mitochondrial calcium [25]. Damage to the sarcolemmal membrane occurs after activated PLA_2 disrupts mitochondrial function causing the formation of lysophospholipids [25] that in turn disrupt the sarcolemmal membrane [26]. In the current study, 2 membrane-associated phospholipase genes, the *PLA2G4A* gene, encoding cytosolic phospholipase A_2 (PLA2), and phospholipase B1 (*PLB1*) were upregulated in birds affected with Wooden Breast. *PLA2G4A* has previously been implicated in broad spectrum skeletal muscle myopathies in broiler chickens [27]. Overall, the upregulation of *PLA2G4A* and *PLB1*, and increased intercellular calcium may be causing changes in membrane integrity in Wooden Breast chickens.

Hypoxia

A number of significant differentially expressed genes in the present study have been found to be regulated by HIF-1 (Hypoxia-inducible factor- 1) (HIF-dependent expression), suggesting a hypoxic state in Wooden Breast. These genes include procollagen-lysine, 2-oxoglutarate 5-dioxygenase 2 (*PLOD2*), transforming growth factor beta 3 (*TGFB3*), asparagine synthetase (*ASNS*), matrix metallopeptidase 2 (*MMP2*), transient receptor potential cation channel, subfamily A, member 1 (*TRPA1*), muscle-specific carbonic anhydrase III (*CA3*), and 6-phosphofructo-2-kinase (*PFKFB3*). Hypoxia-inducible factor 1 (HIF-1) is an important transcription factor to consider when discussing hypoxia. HIF-1 regulates many genes involved in angiogenesis, energy metabolism, vasomotor regulation, and cell proliferation as well as cell survival, and it is critical in maintaining oxygen homeostasis within the cell [28-30]. Although genes encoding the two subunits of HIF-1, i.e., hypoxia-inducible factor 1-alpha (*HIF-1A*) and aryl hydrocarbon receptor nuclear translocator (*ARNT*), are not differentially expressed between normal birds and those affected by Wooden Breast, our significant gene list suggests the activation of this transcription factor in affected birds. It has been previously reported that in skeletal muscle *HIF-1A* is highly expressed in both hypoxic and normoxic conditions [31], which may give insight into why *HIF-1A* is not differentially expressed between affected and unaffected birds in the present study, though there is specific evidence for hypoxic conditions in the Wooden Breast profile.

For example, *PLOD2*, which is upregulated in wooden breast-affected birds, is an important gene associated with extracellular matrix composition, specifically extracellular matrix stiffening and collagen alignment, such as with fibrosis [32]. *PLOD2* expression is essential for correct collagen formation in response to hypoxic events [33]. HIF-1 increases *PLOD2* expression during hypoxia, which increases collagen content and impacts the extracellular matrix by increasing cell adhesion, elongation, and motility, creating a stiff cellular environment [33]. The upregulation of*PLOD2* in affected birds correlates with the histological characterization of fibrosis previously reported in chickens with Wooden Breast [6] and observed histologically in our laboratory (data not shown). Furthermore, this gene may play an integral role in the accompanying stiffness of Wooden Breast birds, possibly related to changes within the extracellular matrix surrounding muscle cells in the breast muscle.

TRPA1 is another HIF-dependent gene upregulated in affected birds in our study. Through the formation of calcium and zinc ion channels, *TRPA1* acts as a sensor to reactive compounds, such as oxidative and thiol compounds, which are mainly produced during oxidative stress [34]. *TRPA1* also mediates inflammation [35]. Hatano et al. 2012 [36] recently provided evidence for the upregulation of *TRPA1* by HIF. Their findings included the induced expression of *TRPA1* by TNF-alpha and IL1-alpha are primarily regulated through HIF. Although *TNF-alpha* is absent in chickens [37, 38], many *TNF* family members are differentially expressed between unaffected and affected birds in our study. Also, inflammation is a key characteristic of the breast muscle in Wooden Breast birds, which is critical as inflammatory cytokines and mediators induce *TRPA1* expression [36]. It should also be noted that within the current study, additional inflammatory cytokines IL-15, and IL-18 are both upregulated in affected birds.

Matrix Metallopeptidase-2 (*MMP2*), characterized as a HIF-dependent gene, is also upregulated in birds affected with Wooden Breast. MMP2 is a member of a large family of matrix metalloproteases and is typically associated with the degradation of cellular components such as the basement membrane and type IV collagen [39]. MMP2 also plays a role in regulating vascularization and response to inflammation [40]. Milkiewicz & Haas 2005 [41] observed that during instances of mechanical stretch to muscle, both the expression of *HIF-1A* and *MMP2* increased. More specifically, they detected increased gene expression of *MMP2* in capillary endothelium of muscle cells. Although the likely activation of HIF-1 within the current study may be the primary cause for the upregulation of HIF-dependent *MMP2*, it must also be considered that *MMP2* expression may be increased due to vascular smooth muscle stretch and remodeling secondary to venous damage or inflammation in birds affected with Wooden Breast.

Other differentially expressed genes within our study such as transforming growth factor, beta 3 (*TGFB3*), asparagine synthetase (*ASNS*), and muscle specific carbonic anhydrase III (*CA3*) were previously reported as regulated by HIF-1. *TGFB3*, which is upregulated in affected birds in our study, has been previously found to be upregulated in traumatized muscle during instances of chronic inflammation and regenerating muscle tissue, which is evident microscopically in this study (data not shown), and which stimulates a hypoxic microenvironment [42]. In the current study, *ASNS* is upregulated in affected chickens. Cui et al. 2007 [43] detail the impact that both hypoxic conditions and insufficient glucose levels have on *ASNS* in relation to tumor growth. They reported a significant increase in expression of *ASNS* in response to inadequate glucose levels. The upregulation of *ASNS*, possibly due to low glucose levels, also correlates with previous observations, such as the downregulation of *PFKFB3*, suggesting deficient glucose metabolism. *CA3* is also differentially expressed between the two groups of chickens in the present study, and is upregulated in affected birds. CA3 has previously been found to increase within the muscle tissue of human hypoxia-trained athletes [44]. It is suggested that the observed increase in CA3 may be a mechanism to increase the rate of H^+ ions delivery to the interstitial fluid of the cell in order to combat muscle fatigue [44]. However, as discussed under the "oxidative stress" section, the upregulation of *CA3* in affected muscle may be primarily associated with the antioxidant role of its protein product [45].

PFKFB3, a HIF-dependent gene, is found to be downregulated in birds affected with Wooden Breast in the current study. This is contrary to previous work, which demonstrated that under hypoxic conditions *PFKFB3* expression typically increases [46]. During hypoxic conditions, cells may switch from oxidative phosphorylation to glycolysis in order to maintain energetic homeostasis [46]; PFKFB3 plays a major role in this process as an activator and regulator of glycolysis and glucose consumption [47]. Since *PFKFB3* is downregulated in our study, it may be possible that glucose metabolism is regulated via a different mechanism under the hypoxic conditions associated with Wooden Breast in chickens. Further explanation for this finding remains to be studied.

Additionally, hypoxic conditions tend to stimulate satellite cell proliferation [31], which is extremely important for skeletal muscle regeneration [48], highlighting the significant role of oxygen concentrations and oxygen as a signaling molecule regulating satellite cells [49]. Hypoxic conditions can also influence the phenotype and differentiation ability of satellite cells [31]. Satellite cells constitute a supply of nuclei for muscle fibers during muscle growth and significantly contribute to compensatory muscle hypertrophy. Muscle growth in chickens, after hatch, can also largely be attributed to hypertrophy [50]. In broilers, satellite cells have high proliferation and differentiation rates just after hatch [51]. After this time, however, proliferation rates tend to drop off [52], but satellite cells continue to contribute to myofiber hypertrophy [51]. Myogenesis, or muscle formation, is regulated in part by the transcription factor paired-box 3 (PAX3), which is upregulated in birds affected with Wooden Breast in the present study. It has been suggested that PAX3 activates genes associated with myogenic regulatory factors and after muscle injury,*PAX3* expression increases within cells that express myogenic regulatory factors [53]. Overall, the stimulation of satellite cell expansion under hypoxic conditions has the ability to lead to muscle hypertrophy during myogenesis and myoregeneration, which has been observed microscopically in Wooden Breast muscle tissues in diagnostic cases analyzed in our laboratory (data not shown). Since all of the birds collected in this study were at the same developmental stage, it is likely that the upregulation of *Pax3* in affected birds is due to myoregeneration following muscle damage, rather than due to generalized muscle growth, though it is possible that this expression difference could also be linked with excessive muscle growth, characteristic of birds with Wooden Breast.

Oxidative stress

Oxidative stress caused by an increase in reactive oxygen species (ROS), may be a major contributor to the Wooden Breast phenotype. Many DE genes between the two groups of broilers being studied suggest an increase in ROS in birds affected with Wooden Breast. Increases in ROS within the skeletal muscle are typically generated as a response to increased contractile activity or after periods of major muscle disuse [54]. Increases in ROS can also occur following mitochondrial dysfunction as a result of oxidative phosphorylation [55]. A major increase in ROS is detrimental to muscle cells due to cytotoxicity and can impact cells by damaging or altering proteins and membrane lipids, thus altering cellular integrity [54]. It is also known that increased concentrations of ROS may impact calcium myofibril sensitivity and calcium release from the sarcoplasmic reticulum, resulting in damage to the contractile ability of muscle cells specifically [56]. Furthermore, increases in ROS also have the ability to impact and regulate cellular signaling pathways that are critical to gene expression and ultimately act on skeletal muscle remodeling and adaptation [54].

Oxidative stress can elicit high amounts of stress within the body and to specific tissues that undergo direct increases in ROS. Because of oxidative stress, the activation of stress response-related pathways and genes are appropriate reactions to prevent further damage. In the current study, the differential expression of many genes within the heat shock family and other stress response-related genes suggests the occurrence of oxidative stress within the breast muscle of affected chickens. The genes within the heat shock family that are upregulated in affected chickens include: heat shock transcription factor 2 (*HSF2*), heat shock 27 kDa protein family, member 7 (*HSPB7*), heat shock 70 kDa protein 4-like protein (*HSPA4L*), and heat shock 105 kDa/110 kDa protein 1 (*HSPH1*). Another gene within this family that is also differentially expressed but found to be downregulated in affected chickens is FK506 binding protein (*FKBP51*). Heat shock proteins are broadly regulated, and are a fairly large gene family, meaning that members respond to different stimuli [57]. This may explain why some heat shock protein family members in our study are upregulated while simultaneously another is downregulated. Heat shock proteins serve many functions such as molecular chaperones, guiding protein folding, and preventing protein buildup. During stressful events such as oxidative stress, the expression of heat shock proteins is known to increase greatly [58]. On the whole, the heat shock proteins are activated in order to stimulate a pro-survival response during oxidative damage [59]. Therefore, the upregulation of most heat shock proteins in affected birds, indicates the possibility of oxidative stress damages within muscle cells, and also confirms the likelihood of cellular stress in birds with Wooden Breast. In addition, corticotrophin-releasing hormone (*CRH*), a major factor important to stress response pathways, was identified as a top upregulated gene in affected birds (fold change = 14.31) in the current study. *CRH*expression has been previously found to aid in the protection of neurons against oxidative stress [60]. CRH is typically expressed in tissues outside the brain during inflammatory events [61]. The accumulation of immune cells in Wooden Breast birds may be a potential source of CRH, as some immune cells are known to secrete CRH [61].

Other well-known myopathies, such as Vitamin E/ Selenium deficiency-related (nutritional) myopathy, render skeletal muscle to be more susceptible to oxidative damages by depleting or overwhelming the antioxidant defense system [10, 62]. Such nutritional myopathies show overlapping microscopic lesions to Wooden Breast [6], such as muscle cell death, degradation and regeneration of myofibers [10], and white striations (adipose) within the musculature [11], vascular damage, and fibrosis [63]. These myopathies are frequently found in agricultural species, such as poultry, and negatively impact meat quality [10, 11, 64]. Most research surrounding nutritional myopathies, such as studies mentioned above, focus strongly on diet supplementation and feed intake [10, 62]. However, we can likely rule out nutritional deficiency as a major factor in Wooden Breast development because both affected and unaffected birds are exposed to the same diet. Additionally, unlike in nutritional myopathies, Wooden Breast appears to only affect the pectoral muscle rather than multiple muscles, gizzard, and heart, and myofiber mineralization is minimal to absent.

Nevertheless, selenoprotein-related deficiencies are strongly associated with oxidative stress damage, as selenoproteins are essential for counteracting oxidative stress [65]; the selenium-protein complex includes oxidative stress regulatory proteins such as glutathione peroxidase and thioredoxin reductase [65]. Within this study, selenoprotein O (*SELO*) is found to be downregulated in Wooden Breast affected broilers. SELO was recently characterized by Dudkiewicz et al. 2012 [66], and it is suggested that it has important roles in oxidative stress response and may be a factor in molecular transport and efflux systems [66]. Interestingly, gene expression for chickens with dietary selenium deficiency (i.e. nutritional myopathy or White Muscle Disease) shows a downregulation of *SELO*, along with other selenoprotein-related genes [67]. The downregulation of this gene within the context of this study may either indicate a deficiency in SELO among birds impacted with Wooden Breast or that seloprotein concentrations are locally diminished within breast muscle of affected birds. In contrast to the downregulation of *SELO*, another family of antioxidative enzymes glutathione peroxidase 7 and 8 (*GPX7*, *GPX8*) are observed to be upregulated in birds affected with Wooden Breast, potentially because of elevated ROS levels and also to compensate for changes to SELO. In past studies, GPX7 has been shown to provide antioxidant functions against high levels of ROS in order to combat oxidative damages in humans [68]. It was also suggested that the presence of GPX7 is needed in order to maintain low ROS levels in specific cell types like oesophageal cells found in the human throat [68]. Another gene that is upregulated in affected birds and likely serves an anti-oxidative function is carbonic anhydrase 3 (*CA3*). Within the current study, *CA3* is one of the top differentially expressed genes with a fold change of 28.47. It has been proposed that CA3 has the ability to serve as an anti-oxidizing agent against damaging molecules, has both regulatory and reparative functions, and is a critical player in the antioxidant defense system within skeletal muscle [45].

Fiber-type switching

In the current study, one of the most differentially expressed genes in affected samples was myoglobin (*MB*). Myoglobin is mainly distributed within Type I or aerobic muscle (slow twitch) fibers and serves to store oxygen. High myoglobin content is typically correlated with "red" meat, which has a high density of Type I fibers [69]. However, the pectoralis, a "white" muscle in chickens, consisting almost entirely of type II, or anaerobic (fast twitch) fibers, and in which myoglobin has previously either not been detectable [70] or observed at very low levels [71, 72]. In fact, the lack of myoglobin and increased glycogen content in Type II fibers account for the white color of pectoral meat [69]. Therefore high expression of myoglobin in the pectoralis muscle of broilers is unexpected and may possibly be explained by the phenomenon fiber-type switching, or a change from fast twitch to slow twitch fibers in response to myofiber degeneration and necrosis observed in the Wooden Breast myopathy. Muscle fibers are extremely dynamic and tend to adapt to environmental cues [73]. The phenotypic composition of muscle fibers can be altered by various stressors such as activity rate, mechanical stress, hormones, aging, response to muscle damage, and/or changes in muscle oxygenation [73]. These events have the capacity to modify the functional properties of a given muscle fiber, possibly leading to fiber-type switching [73].

Fiber type switching from fast-to-slow twitch fibers has also been suggested in turkeys exhibiting PSE muscle conditions [74]. Upregulation of troponin I type I, skeletal slow, (*TNNI1)* in the present study may support the hypothesis of fast-to-slow switch in Wooden Breast myopathy. *TNNI1* expression likewise differs by muscle type and, similar to *MB*, is also limited to expression in only slow skeletal fibers [75]. The *TNNI* subfamily has further been found to play a role in the mediation of skeletal muscle relaxation and contraction [76]. Other slow skeletal fiber-type isoforms upregulated in this study include myozenin 2 (*MYOZ2)* and myosin binding protein C, slow type (*MYBPC1). MYOZ2* expression has been reported in only cardiac and slow-twitch skeletal muscle, and acts to control for calcineurin, which is a positive regulator of slow-type fibers [77, 78]. Similarly, MyBPC1 is one of three MyBPC isoforms, and interacts with slow skeletal muscle to regulate muscle contraction [79]. In this study *TNNI1,MYOZ2*, and *MyBPC1* are upregulated in affected birds, potentially indicating fiber-type switching to type I fibers following myofiber damage in the Wooden Breast myopathy.

Jordan et al. 2004 [80] suggest that ryanodine receptor 1 (RyR1) in the pectoralis muscle in birds may act to suppress slow muscle specific genes. This is supported by high levels of reactive oxygen species (ROS) or nitric oxide (NO), which can irreversibly impact RyR1 subunits as a consequence of oxidation [81]. Consequently, the inhibition of RyR1 by ryanodine may lead to a fast-to-slow fiber type switch [80]. Mutation to the *RyR1* gene in pigs has been previously correlated with the occurrence of malignant hyperthermia, a skeletal muscle myopathy, which leads to defects in Ca^{2+} channel functioning

[82], PSE-type meat [82], and rigidity of the muscle caused by hypermetabolism [83]. It has also been suggested that inositol trisphosphate receptor 1 [84], protein kinase C alpha and theta [85] and muscarinic acetylcholine receptor (M1) [86], possess critical roles in fiber-type switching, although in the current study these genes remain insignificant. Fiber-type switching has also been characterized in the callipyge sheep muscle condition. This condition in sheep involves muscles within the pelvic region that exhibit an increase in muscle mass as well as leaner muscle and is associated with an increase in feed efficiency [87]. Callipyge sheep show some similar symptoms to birds affected with Wooden Breast such as hypertrophy of the affected muscle and localization to specific muscle regions; however, it is suggested that these sheep actually undergo a slow-to-fast fiber-type switch [88]. Thus, though there is indication that fiber-type switching may be occurring during Wooden Breast in chickens, the pathways altered for fiber-type switching are likely different in broiler chickens than those exhibited in myopathies of other species, such as the callipyge phenotype in sheep.

Cellular repair

Many genes involved in cellular repair and transport are differentially expressed within our dataset. It is highly probable that these genes are linked to the Wooden Breast myopathy in an effort to compensate for muscle damage in this degenerative muscle disease.

One of the top genes upregulated in affected chickens is cysteine and glycine-rich protein 3 (*CSRP3*) (fold change=23.17), which is also referred to as muscle LIM (Lin11, Isl-1, and Mec-3) protein within the literature [89, 90].*CSRP3* expression is present only in striated muscle, including skeletal muscle, and it plays a large role in myogenic differentiation [91]. The expression of *CSRP3* also correlates with myotube growth and formation [91], which is a key feature of muscle repair. Barash et al. 2005 [92] studied *CSRP3* knockout mice and found that deficient mice displayed an array of skeletal muscle defects such as shorter sarcomere length and muscle atrophy. They suggested that CSRP3 has a role in the maintenance of skeletal muscle and also supports skeletal muscle regeneration following injury through structural repair and gene regulation [92]. *CSRP3* may significantly increase in expression after periods of exercise in humans [93]. This may occur in order to promote muscle growth as CSRP3 has also been linked to involvement in muscle hypertrophy and regeneration through the calcineurin/NFAT signaling pathway and myogenic differentiation (MYOD) expression [91]. It is also interesting to note that *CSRP3* is mainly expressed in slow skeletal muscle, compared to its low expression in fast skeletal muscle [94]. Similar to this,*CSRP3* expression was upregulated during fast-to-slow fiber type switch in rats [94]. Therefore, as discussed above, fiber-type switching may be occurring in birds with Wooden Breast as a secondary response to the disease, acting as a mechanism of myofiber repair and/or regeneration under an altered redox homeostasis. Xu et al. 2009 [90] also suggest that the expression of *CSRP3* could impact meat quality since CSRP3 is involved in both myofiber generation and fiber-type switching.

Along a similar line, another highly upregulated gene in this study is nephroblastoma overexpressed (*NOV*) also referred to as *CCN3* [95] (fold change=7.33). NOV is a member of the CCN family of proteins, which contains cysteine-rich angiogenic protein 61 (CCN1), connective tissue growth factor (CCN2), and nephroblastoma overexpressed (CCN3) [96]. This protein family is an important role player for many biological functions such as cell migration, proliferation, differentiation, and extracellular modification [96]. It is also thought that the *CCN* gene family takes part in critical roles during cell development, wound healing, tissue homeostasis, and varying conditions including cancer and fibrosis [95]. Heath et al. 2008 [95] conclude from their results that *NOV* is necessary and required for normal muscle maintenance and use, showing that the over-expression of *NOV* leads to increased cell proliferation and promotes the survival of cells expressing myogenin. Myogenin is an essential regulator of myogenesis, and crucial to muscle maintenance, regeneration, and repair [97], and is overexpressed in musculoskeletal tumors [98]. *NOV* expression has also been previously linked with multiple components of cellular repair, as well as wound healing and endothelial adhesion and migration [99]. It is likely that NOV is involved in the Wooden Breast disease acting as a regulator of cellular and tissue repair through myoregeneration and cellular movement.

Other differentially expressed genes within the current study, such as musculoskeletal embryonic nuclear protein 1 (*MUSTN1*) also contribute to cellular repair and regeneration in skeletal muscle. In the current study *MUSTN1*, which is considered essential for skeletal muscle growth and regeneration [93, 100], is upregulated in affected birds. Increased expression of *MUSTN1* has also been reported in domestic chickens; its expression is higher in broiler chickens than it is in layer chickens. This observation supports the notion that *MUSTN1* may be involved in the regulation of muscle hypertrophy [101]. *MUSTN1* expression was also upregulated in correlation to exercise-induced muscle damage, supporting its possible involvement in muscle damage repair [93]. As both affected and unaffected birds in the present study were from the same genetic lineage of broiler chickens, upregulation of*MUSTN1* in affected birds likely indicates compensatory hypertrophy or muscle repair secondary to muscle damage rather than physiologic hypertrophy during bird growth.

Other key contributors to the actin cytoskeleton system, such as members of the Rho GTPase family, could also indicate cell differentiation or movement in the reparative phase of the disease. Within our dataset there are four members of this family that are upregulated. These include: Rho GTPase activating protein 10 (*ARHGAP10*), Rho GTPase activating protein 20 (*ARHGAP20*), and Rho GTPase activating protein 40 (*ARHGAP40*). Another significant member of this family that is downregulated is Rho-related BTB domain containing 3 (*RHOBTB3*). The Rho GTPase family are important regulators of the organization of the actin cytoskeleton [102]. Rho activation is necessary to maintain strong cellular and focal adhesion between cells [102], and Rho-GTPase proteins are involved in many general functions such as cell migration, cell proliferation, and cytoskeleton reorganization [103]. As an example, it is thought that the upregulation of *ARHGAP10* is essential to cell differentiation within the cytoskeleton [104]. Although some of the functions of Rho GTPase genes remain unknown, it is possible that the expression of these genes within the current study is due to disruption within the actin cytoskeleton and subsequent repair from the damage manifested by the Wooden Breast myopathy.

Results from IPA show that the canonical pathways "Actin Cytoskeleton Signaling" (p-value=3.18E-07) and "Axonal Guidance Signaling" (p-value=1.27E-06) have probable functions in tissue repair during Wooden Breast muscle disease. The "Actin Cytoskeleton Signaling" pathway contains 36 significant differentially expressed genes from our gene list. Most of the genes within this pathway relate to specific growth factors such as, epidermal growth factor (*EGF*) and fibroblast growth factor (*FGF*), and also include many cytoskeleton related genes such as, actin related protein complex (*ARPC*) and many member of the myosin heavy and light chain families (*MYH*/*MYL*). As shown in Fig. 1 the major endpoints of this pathway deal with the assembly, polymerization, and the stabilization of both actin and myosin. We hypothesize that the "Actin Cytoskeleton Signaling" pathway is mainly dealing with secondary response to injury in the form of cellular repair in affected muscle. It is important to point out the growth factors associated with this pathway include epidermal growth factor (*EGF*) and fibroblast growth factor 10 (*FGF10*) which are upregulated, and fibroblast growth factor 1 (*FGF1*) which is downregulated. It is more likely that growth factors are expressed differently in affected birds due to repair and regeneration occurring in the diseased muscle. The upregulation of *EGF* is important since *EGF* is previously known to promote myoblast proliferation to aid in muscle repair [105]. However, the downregulation of *FGF1* is unexpected, since it is known that FGF1 contributes greatly to skeletal muscle proliferation [106]. Mitchell et al. 1999 [107] also found a downregulation of *FGF1* when studying the response to muscle stretch, or stretch hypertrophy, in chickens. Mitchell et al. 1999 [107] were inconclusive as to why this phenomenon was occurring, but hypothesized that stretch itself may contribute to downregulation of FGF1. Also seven members of the myosin family are differentially expressed within the "Actin Cytoskeleton Signaling" pathway including three myosin heavy chain genes (*MYH2, MYH6, MYH10*), and four myosin light chain genes (*MYL1, MYL9, MYL12B, MYLK2*). Myosin is essential for muscle contraction and comprises most of the myofibrillar proteins within muscle cells [108]. Within this pathway myosin is functioning to create "actomyosin assembly contraction" (Fig. 1, IPA®). The assembly and contraction of the actomyosin complex is essential as both actin and myosin are responsible for muscle contraction [109].

The other canonical pathway related to cellular repair presented by IPA is "Axonal Guidance Signaling". This pathway contains 56 significant differentially expressed genes from our gene list. Some of the gene families within this pathway include the A Disintegrin and Metalloproteinase (ADAM) metallopeptidase family, myosin light chain family, and the SEMA (Semaphorins) domain family. Since the muscle and surrounding connective tissues are undergoing injury, inflammation, and edema in Wooden Breast, it is possible that there is a simultaneous disruption and repair in axons of nerve fibers within the muscle. As reported through IPA some of the possible functions of this pathway include, cytoskeleton reorganization, actin filament reorganization, axon outgrowth, and axon guidance. Several genes within this pathway are regulators of cellular repair and regeneration in the muscle and axon systems. For example, *ADAM12*, which is upregulated in affected birds, is most often expressed in adult muscle during regeneration, and may take part in reducing necrosis and inflammation [47]. Secondly, *SEMA3A*, which is upregulated in affected birds, acts to promote intramuscular re-innervation in damaged muscle fibers in order to restore muscle contraction [110]. It is also interesting to note that, clinically, birds with Wooden Breast typically display a drastic decrease in the amount of muscle fasciculations after death compared to normal birds (data not shown). Although this phenomenon remains to be studied more fully, it is possible that damage to either muscle or nerve fibers have led to loss of function within the muscle, though there is no significant histologic evidence of primary nerve damage within affected muscle. From the results given through IPA we postulate that both the "Actin Cytoskeleton Signaling" and "Axonal Guidance Signaling" canonical pathways are not likely primary causes of the Wooden Breast myopathy, but are secondary to the disease, differentially expressed during the repair phase of the illness.

Coagulation system pathway and related genes

The inflammation observed microscopically in birds affected with Wooden Breast suggests that genes involved in the coagulation system pathway would likely be upregulated due to vascular (venous) damage and inflammation. It is highly regarded that inflammation promotes the activation of coagulation [111]. However, our data supports the downregulation of genes within the coagulation system pathway in affected brids as given by IPA® (Fig. 2). It should be noted that the genes involved in the coagulation system pathway are mainly expressed in the liver, where most of the coagulation factors are synthesized, rather than in muscle. The DE genes involved within the coagulation pathway identified by the present study include: alpha-2-macroglobulin (*A2M)*, fibrinogen alpha chain *(FGA),*fibrinogen beta chain *(FGB),* and fibrinogen gamma chain (*FGG)*, kininogen 1 (*KNG1)*, plasminogen (*PLG)*, serpin peptidase inhibitor, clade A, member 1 (*SERPINC1)*, and von Willebrand factor (*VWF),* which are all found to be downregulated (Fig. 3). Other DE genes within this pathway which are upregulated include: coagulation factor V (*F5)*, coagulation factor X (*F10)*, coagulation factor II (*F2R)*, and protein S (alpha) (*PROS1)*. The reasons for the involvement of the coagulation pathway and its overall downregulation in Wooden Breast remain to be elucidated.

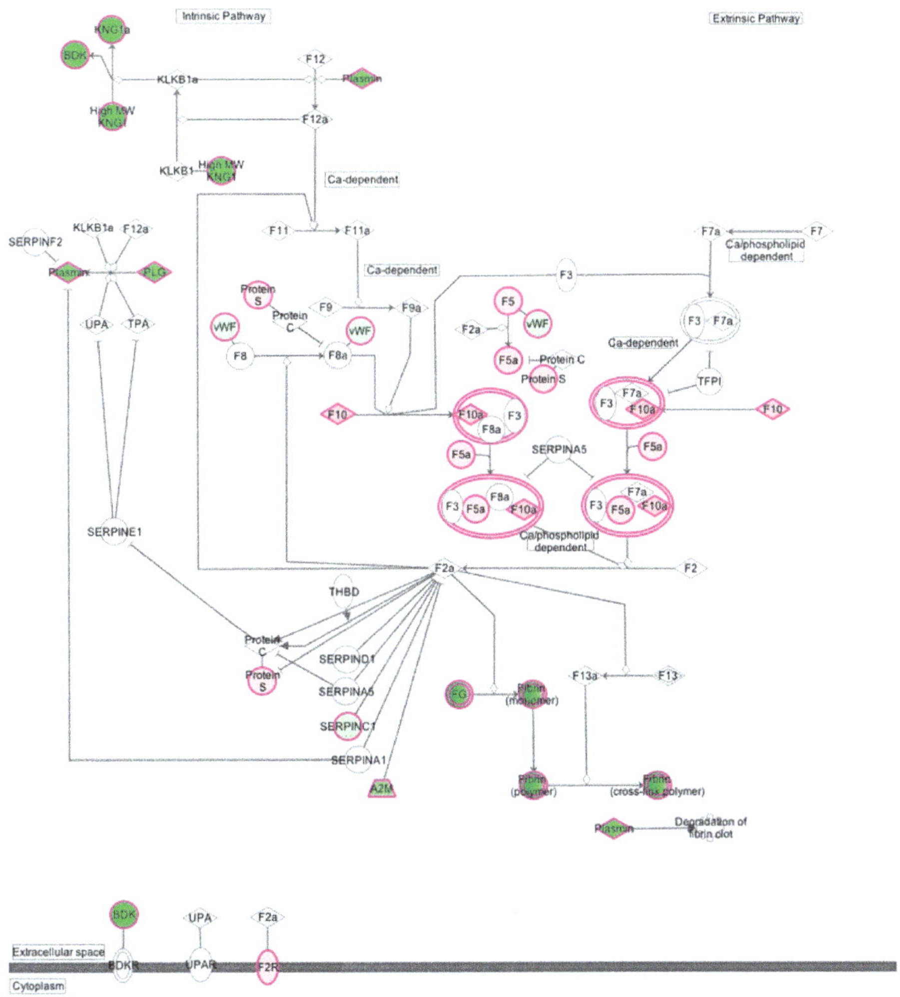

Figure 2: The "Coagulation System" pathway highlighting differentially expressed genes in birds affected with Wooden Breast myopathy. Canonical pathways were identified and depicted by Ingenuity Pathway Analysis (IPA®) software. This pathway shows the "Coagulation System" as related to significant DE genes in affected birds from the sample population. Genes that are highlighted in green are considered to be downregulated in affected birds. Genes that are highlighted in red are considered to be upregulated in affected birds.

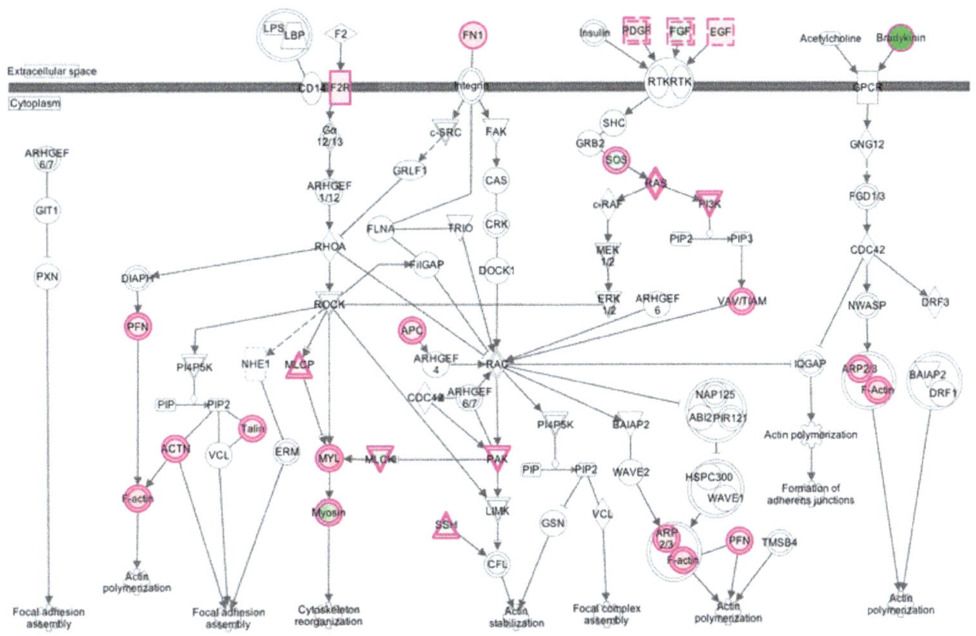

Figure 3: The "Actin Cytoskeleton Signaling" pathway highlighting differentially expressed genes of birds affected with Wooden Breast myopathy. Canonical pathways were identified and depicted by Ingenuity Pathway Analysis (IPA®) software. This pathway shows the "Actin Cytoskeleton Signaling" as related to significant differentially expressed genes in affected birds from the sample population. Genes that are highlighted in green are considered to be downregulated in affected birds. Genes that are highlighted in red are considered to be upregulated in affected birds.

Biological significance of gene expression profile

Features of the gene expression profile (increase in intracellular calcium, hypoxia, and oxidative stress, etc.) brought to light by this study have strong correlation to the histologic lesions reported previously by Sihvo et al. 2014 [6] and observed in diagnostic specimens evaluated by our laboratory (data not shown).

A major characteristic of increased intracellular calcium levels is myofiber hypercontraction. Hypercontraction associated with skeletal muscle degeneration has been previously identified across species [112, 113]. It is suggested that the accumulation of Ca^{2+} within the cell leads to hypercontraction either as a result of poor Ca^{2+} -ATPase performance [114] or because of interference with sarcolemma integrity [115]. Ultimately hypercontraction results in cell degeneration and necrosis [114]. Histologically hypercontraction can be established through the observation of irregular Z bands or as hyaline fibers, which form as a result of excess calcium [116, 117] and leads to the coagulation of the contractile proteins within the cells [117]. Although irregular Z bands have not been a prominent feature of Wooden Breast cases, swelling and hyalinization of fibers is the predominant myofiber lesion present in affected Delmarva poultry (data not shown) and has also been reported by Bilgili 2013 [8]. The "hypereosinophilic" nature of myofibers described by Sihvo et al. 2014 [6] would also correlate to hyaline degeneration of myofibers. Furthermore, it is highly likely that the microscopic swelling and coagulation of proteins observed to be widespread within affected muscle fibers may be contributing to clinically and grossly evident hardening of the pectoral muscle as a whole. These observations support the hypothesis of hypercontraction and/or contractile protein denaturation, potentially due to increased levels of intracellular calcium. It should also be noted that no significant mineralization within the muscle was observed grossly or microscopically to suggest dystrophic calcium deposition in degenerating or necrotic myofibers. As such, it appears that calcium overload, as supported by gene expression profiling results, mainly affects the contraction state of myofibers in Wooden Breast.

Birds affected with Wooden Breast also show characteristics of histologic changes and clinical symptoms associated with hypoxia [6, 8], potentially due to vascular damage or inadequacy [8]. From previous histologic reports [6, 8] it is unclear whether poor vasculature is the inciting cause of hypoxia or if there are other contributing factors, which establish a hypoxic environment. Hypoxia and oxidative stress have been continually linked in research, as in the present study. As mentioned, from RNA-seq results, it is likely that the pectoralis major muscle undergoes hypoxic events in Wooden Breast. Although vascular damage is present in affected birds, this is only seen on the venous side, rather than the arterial side of the vascular system; as such, there is little microscopic evidence to suggest impairment of oxygenated blood delivery to the tissues unless there is a subtle difference in vascular density between affected and unaffected birds. However, venous damage, supported by histologic evidence of the accumulation of immune cells surrounding and within veins in affected muscle, as reported by Sihvo et al., 2014 [6] and as observed in our laboratory (data not shown), could ultimately impair the removal of cellular metabolic waste products, leading to the build-up of oxidative metabolites, and triggering further damage to surrounding cells. Inflammation in the muscle may also be contributing to or responding to a hypoxic state in the tissue.

To study the impact of hypoxic environment in mice, Lopes-Ferreira et al. 2001 [48] investigated skeletal muscle degeneration using fish venom and reported histological outcomes associated with the hypoxic environment including, inflammation, infiltration of macrophages and leucocytes, fiber necrosis, variations in fiber size, hypercontracted fibers, as well as fibrosis. These microscopic findings are similar to those in Wooden Breast. Fibrosis in particular is a common sequela of muscle repair under hypoxic conditions, as the occurrence of fibrosis aims to replace lost muscle tissue with collagen and fibrocytes [48]. Fibrosis is evident microscopically in Wooden Breast muscle, and several genes within the collagen family have been determined to be upregulated in the present study, including: *COL3A1*, *COL4A3*, *COL4A4*, *COL4A5*, *COL5A1*, *COL5A2*, *COL6A1*, *COL6A2*, *COL6A3*, *COL8A1*,*COL8A2*, *COL11A1*, *COL12A1*, *COL14A1*, *COL16A1* ,*COL21A1*, *COL24A1*, *COL25A1*, and *COL27A1*. Furthermore, there is additional microscopic evidence to corroborate a hypoxic state; beyond fibrosis, the accumulation of lipid within affected muscle is also apparent histologically as variably-sized discrete vacuoles within the sarcoplasm of affected muscles (data not shown). Hypoxia has been previously linked with increases in lipid storage in cultured cells [118], cardiac muscle [119], and also in macrophages [120]. In support of the previous studies [6, 8], the present study revealed various differentially-expressed genes between affected and unaffected birds that may be correlated with a hypoxic state within the pectoralis major muscle of chickens with Wooden Breast. Hypoxia appears to be a critical factor in the Wooden Breast myopathy, though it is not apparent whether it is a primary cause for muscle lesions or is occurring secondary to inflammation and myofiber swelling from another cause.

Previous muscle disorders described in chickens, such as deep pectoral myopathy (DPM), have been associated with hypoxia resulting from restricted blood flow to the muscle as a predominant cause of muscle degeneration [1,121]. The incidence rate of DPM is typically associated with high-yield breast muscle birds with high growth rate [1]. In the authors' experience, Wooden Breast also has a high correlation with the growth rate and breast muscle weight of commercial broilers; most cases occur in breeding lines associated with fast growth, high feed efficiency, and high breast muscle yield. However, unlike in DPM, necrosis is limited to individual myofibers rather than widespread, and the superficial pectoral muscle is more affected than the deep pectoral muscle. Regardless, as Sihvo et al. 2014 [6] mention, it is highly likely that the high growth rate and increased breast muscle weight of modern-day broilers are key factors in myodegenerative disorders, including Wooden Breast and deep pectoral myopathy.

The gene expression profile brought to light within this study and previously reported histology of Wooden Breast suggests a pro-inflammatory response is taking place in affected birds, which involves the influx of immune cells. In the human muscular disease, Duchenne muscular dystrophy (DMD), cellular membrane damage caused by high intracellular calcium levels and inflammation leads to immune responses observed by a dramatic rise in inflammatory cell concentration within the affected area [122, 123]. Immune cells are known to generate ROS during inflammatory events in order to stimulate phagocytosis [124]; in mammals, ROS is formed by neutrophils and macrophages through NADPH-oxidase, a membrane-bound molecule [125]. ROS produced by immune cells has the ability to cause direct damage to muscle tissue or may act indirectly through the activation of catabolic signaling through immune molecule interaction with muscle receptors [126]. Histologic lesions for Wooden Breast suggest signs of oxidative stress because of observations such as fiber degeneration, variation in myofiber size, membrane and cellular rupture, inflammation, immune cell response, and replacement of myofibers with connective tissue and/or fat [6, 8]. Sihvo et al. 2014 [6] suggest that broiler selection for large breast muscle size coupled with an increased growth rate may cause broilers to be more vulnerable to oxidative stress.

Histologically, it is seen that tissue repair is occurring through mechanisms such as inflammation, myofiber regeneration, and fibrosis [6], as well as possibly through fiber-type switching. Canonical pathways reported by IPA such as "Actin Cytoskeleton Signaling" and "Axonal Guidance Signaling" also support attempted regeneration and repair of the muscle. The infiltration of immune cells to the area may support these efforts to repair damaged tissues. Macrophages are essential for removing damaged muscle proteins to allow regenerative fiber replacement; some macrophages have pro-regeneration qualities helping with muscle regeneration associated with their function [127]. Fibrosis and myofiber regeneration, both of which are also supported by the differentially expressed genes in our study, are other examples of microscopic observations that support a reparative phase is taking place. Ultimately, gene expression profiling undertaken in the present study has strong correlation to known microscopic lesions present in Wooden Breast.

CONCLUSION

Using RNA-sequencing and pathway analysis tools such as IPA, we were able to define possible primary and secondary factors affecting the breast muscle of affected chickens. We were further able to link RNA-sequencing data to histologic findings in our lab and previously published reports of Wooden Breast myopathy [6] to show potential biologic significance for the characteristic gene expression profile observed in Wooden Breast. Through the analyses of differentially expressed genes, significant differences were observed in genes associated with intracellular calcium, possible fiber-type switching, hypoxia, and oxidative stress (Table 3). Although it remains difficult to characterized if features of the disease are primary or secondary, it is likely that all play a significant role in the pathogenesis of this disease. Also, we were able to establish a trend of significant genes and pathways related to cellular repair, which are likely occurring secondary to tissue damage in the Wooden Breast myopathy.

Table 3: Summary of main categories of genes involved in Wooden Breast myopathy separated by category

Gene category	**Gene name**	**Symbol**	**RNA-seq fold change**	**Nanostring fold change**
Fiber-Type Switching:				
	Myoglobin	MB	14.3	12.4
	Myosin Binding Protein C, slow type	MYBPC1	9.1	16.2
	Myozenin 2	MYOZ2	7.8	7.7
	Troponin I type I, skeletal slow	TNNI1	4.0	N/A
Intracellular Calcium:				
	ATPase, Ca++ transporting, cardiac muscle, slow twitch 2	ATP2A2	2.1	N/A
	Cytosolic phospholipase A2	PLA2G4A	2.3	N/A
	Parvalbumin	PVALB	8.1	7.2
	Phospholipase B1	PLB1	3.4	N/A
Hypoxia:				
	6-phophofructo-2-kinase	PFKFB3	−4.1	N/A
	Arylhydrocarbon Receptor Nuclear Translocator 2	ARNT2	2.2	1.7
	Asparagine synthetase	ASNS	4.4	N/A
	Matrix metallopeptidase 2	MMP2	2.2	N/A

	Muscle-specific carbonic anhydrase III	CA3	28.5	25.5
	Procollagen-lysine, 2-oxoglutarate 5-dioxygenase 2	PLOD2	2.5	N/A
	Transforming growth factor beta 3	TGFB3	3.9	3.7
	Transient receptor potential cation channel, subfamily A	TRPA1	6.7	N/A
Oxidative Stress:				
	Corticotrophin-releasing hormone	CRH	14.3	13.3
	FK506 binding protein	FKBP51	−1.9	N/A
	Glutathione peroxidase 7	GPX7	2.3	N/A
	Glutathione peroxidase 8	GPX8	2.1	N/A
	Heat shock 27 kDa protein family, member 7	HSPB7	3.2	4.3
	Heat shock 70 kDa protein 4-like protein	HSPA4L	1.5	N/A
	Heat shock 105 kDa/110 kDa protein 1	HSPH1	2.2	N/A
	Heat shock transcription factor 2	HSF2	2.9	N/A
	Muscle-specific carbonic anhydrase III	CA3	28.5	25.5
	Selenoprotein O	SELO	−2.1	N/A
Cellular Repair:				
	ADAM metallopeptidase domain 12	ADAM12	2.2	N/A
	Cysteine and glycine-rich protein 3	CSRP3	23.2	27.3
	Epidermal growth factor	EGF	1.6	N/A
	Fibroblast growth factor 1	FGF1	−2.1	−1.9
	Fibroblast growth factor10	FGF10	2.4	1.3
	Musculoskeletal embryonic nuclear protein 1	MUSTN1	4.9	6.0
	Myosin, heavy chain 13, skeletal muscle	MYH13	−4.7	1.0
	Myosin, light chain 2, skeletal slow	MYL3	5.4	1.5
	Myosin, light chain 12A regulatory	MYL12A	1.9	N/A
	Myosin light chain kinase 2	MYLK2	−2.6	N/A
	Nephroblastoma Overexpressed	NOV	7.3	3.0
	Rho GTPase activating protein 10	ARHGAP10	2.2	N/A
	Rho GTPase activating protein 20	ARHGAP20	2.4	N/A
	Rho GTPase activating protein 40	ARHGAP40	3.0	2.8
	Rho-related BTB domain containing 3	RHOBTB3	−11.9	−5.1
	Sema domain, Ig, short basic domain, secreted, 3A	SEMA3A	1.6	N/A

For each gene category, the complete gene name, symbol, fold change from RNA-seq data, and fold change from Nanostring® data are provided. Positive and negative fold change values support respectively upregulation and downregulation of gene expression in birds affected by Wooden Breast myopathy relative to the gene expression in unaffected birds

The present work should be considered a first step towards elucidating the underlying genetic fingerprint of the Wooden Breast myopathy in commercial broilers. With the RNA-sequencing profile identified by this work, there is a potential to find specific genetic markers characteristic for this disease for use in diagnosis and detection of subclinical or carrier birds. Future work with RNA-sequencing across the time course of disease development would be beneficial. Since birds in the present study were all collected at market age, performing a time-series study using RNA-sequencing could help determine the specific age of onset of this disease and may help distinguish primary from secondary mechanisms contributing to Wooden Breast and associated gross and histologic lesions. Histochemical staining for specific fiber-type could further be implemented to confirm if a fiber-type switch is occurring in affected birds. Since it is also possible that a single gene or a few candidate genes are principle causal factors in this disorder, conducting a genome-wide association study (GWAS) could also be greatly beneficial.

To our knowledge, this is the first study on the Wooden Breast disease in commercial broiler chickens to focus on RNA-sequencing data and gene expression profiling. Although the underlying cause of this disease still remains unknown, this work has brought forward many factors associated with the pathogenesis of this muscle disease. This work further shows the importance of using RNA-sequencing in biologic correlation with gross and microscopic disease lesions to study and compare muscle disorders across species. While more research must be performed to gain insight into the specific origin of Wooden Breast myopathy in chickens, RNA-sequence profiling has the potential to directly contribute to disease diagnosis and research for myopathies across animal species, including humans.

Availability of supporting data

Samples used in this study were obtained from Heritage Breeders, LLC. The data supporting the results are included within the article and its additional files. Readers may contact the corresponding author for additional information.

DECLARATIONS

Acknowledgements

This work was supported and funded by Heritage Breeders, LLC and the Avian Biosciences Center at the University of Delaware. Thanks to Delaware Biotechnology Institute (DBI) for performing RNA-sequencing. Thanks to Nan Zhou, Zhu Zhuo, and Casey Spencer for help in preparing and creating cDNA libraries.

Authors' contributions

MM, BA, and EMB contributed to the preparation of the manuscript and to the scientific discussions. MM prepared cDNA libraries, performed quality checks on the data, conducted functional analyses and pathway analyses using Ingenuity Pathway Analysis (IPA), and wrote the first draft of the manuscript. BA secured funding for the project, obtained samples for the study, and conceived of the study. EMB provided gross and histologic characterization and clinicopathologic correlation of the disorder. WRL provided background knowledge to the study, managed the experimental birds, and sample collection. WF contributed to the bioinformatics analysis of the study. All authors read and approved the final manuscript.

REFERENCES

1. Bianchi M, Petracci M, Franchini A, Cavani C. The occurrence of deep pectoral myopathy in roaster chickens. Poult Sci. 2006;85:1843–6.
2. Bilgili SF, Hess JB. Green Muscle Disease in broilers increasing. World Poult. 2002;18:42–3.
3. Bilgili SF, Hess JB. Green Muscle Disease: Reducing the Incidence in Broiler Flocks. Ross Tech. 2008;8:48.
4. Kuttappan VA, Lee YS, Erf GF, Meullenet J-FC, McKee SR, Owens CM. Consumer acceptance of visual appearance of broiler breast meat with varying degrees of white striping. Poult Sci. 2012;1240–1247.
5. Lesiów T, Kijowski J. Impact of PSE and DFD Meat On Poultry Processing – A Review. Polish J Food Nutr Sci. 2003;12/53:3–8.
6. Sihvo H-K, Immonen K, Puolanne E. Myodegeneration with fibrosis and regeneration in the pectoralis major muscle of broilers. Vet Pathol. 2014;51:619–23.
7. Owens CM. Identifying quality defects in poultry processing. In: Watt Poult USA. 2014. p. 42–50. December.
8. Bilgili SF. Broiler Chicken Myopathies: II. Woody Breast? In: Worthw Oper Guidel Suggest. 2013. p. 1. April.
9. Kuttappan VA, Shivaprasad H, Shaw DP, Valentine BA, Hargis BM, Clark FD, et al. IMMUNOLOGY, HEALTH, AND DISEASE Pathological changes associated with white striping in broiler breast muscles. Poult Sci. 2013;92:331–8.
10. Guetchom B, Venne D, Chenier S, Chorfi Y: Effect of extra dietary vitamin E on preventing nutritional myopathy in broiler chickens. J Appl Poult Res. 2012;21(3):548–55.
11. Bains BS, Watson ARA. Nutritional Myopathy- A cause of ataxia in broiler chickens. N Z Vet J. 1978;26:31–2.
12. Wang Z, Gerstein M, Snyder M. RNA-Seq: a revolutionary tool for transcriptomics. Nat Rev Genet. 2009;10:57–63.
13. Fast QC [http://www.bioinformatics.babraham.ac.uk/projects/fastqc/]
14. Trapnell C, Roberts A, Goff L, Pertea G, Kim D, Kelley DR, et al. Differential gene and transcript expression

analysis of RNA-seq experiments with TopHat and Cufflinks. Nat Protoc. 2012;7:562–78.

15. Cufflinks [http://cole-trapnell-lab.github.io/cufflinks/]
16. Ingenuity Systems [http:/www.ingenuity.com]
17. Geiss GK, Bumgarner RE, Birditt B, Dahl T, Dowidar N, Dunaway DL, et al. Direct multiplexed measurement of gene expression with color-coded probe pairs. Nat Biotechnol. 2008;26:317–25.
18. Periasamy M, Reed TD, Liu LH, Ji Y, Loukianov E, Paul RJ, et al. Impaired cardiac performance in heterozygous mice with a null mutation in the sarco(endo)plasmic reticulum Ca2+−ATPase isoform 2 (SERCA2) gene. J Biol Chem. 1999;274:2556–62.
19. Prasad V, Boivin GP, Miller ML, Liu LH, Erwin CR, Warner BW, et al. Haploinsufficiency of Atp2a2, encoding the sarco(endo)plasmic reticulum Ca2+−ATPase isoform 2 Ca2+ pump, predisposes mice to squamous cell tumors via a novel mode of cancer susceptibility. Cancer Res. 2005;65:8655–61.
20. Mitchell MA. Muscle Abnormalities- Pathophysiological mechanisms. In: Richardson RI, Mead GC, editors. Poult Meat Sci. 25th ed. Oxon, UK: CAB International; 1999. p. 65–98.
21. Kuo TH, Kim HR, Zhu L, Yu Y, Lin HM, Tsang W. Modulation of endoplasmic reticulum calcium pump by Bcl-2. Oncogene. 1998;17:1903–10.
22. Kaprielian Z, Fambrough DM. Expression of fast and slow isoforms of the Ca2+−ATPase in developing chick skeletal muscle. Dev Biol. 1987;124:490–503.
23. Gailly P, Boland B, Himpens B, Casteels R, Gillis JM. Critical evaluation of cytosolic calcium determination in resting muscle fibres from normal and dystrophic (mdx) mice. Cell Calcium. 1993;14:473–83.
24. Mahon M. Muscle Abnormalities- Morphological Aspects. In: Richardson RI, Mead GC, editors. Poult Meat Sci. 25th ed. Oxon, UK: CAB International; 1999. p. 19–64.
25. Gissel H: The role of Ca2+ in muscle cell damage. Ann N Y Acad Sci. 2005;1066:166–80.
26. Jackson MJ, Jones DA, Edwards RH. Experimental skeletal muscle damage: the nature of the calcium-activated degenerative processes. Eur J Clin Invest. 1984;14:369–74.
27. Sandercock DA, Mitchell MA. Myopathy in broiler chickens: a role for Ca(2+)-activated phospholipase A2? Poult Sci. 2003;82:1307–12.
28. Shaw K. Environmental Cues Like Hypoxia Can Trigger Gene Expression and Cancer Development. Nat Educ. 2008;1:198.
29. Semenza GL. HIF-1: mediator of physiological and pathophysiological responses to hypoxia. J Appl Physiol. 2000;88:1474–80.
30. Brahimi-Horn MC, Bellot G, Pouysségur J. Hypoxia and energetic tumour metabolism. Curr Opin Genet Dev. 2011;21:67–72.
31. Urbani L, Piccoli M, Franzin C, Pozzobon M, de Coppi P. Hypoxia Increases Mouse Satellite Cell Clone Proliferation Maintaining both In Vitro and In Vivo Heterogeneity and Myogenic Potential. PLoS One. 2012;7.
32. Van der Slot AJ, Zuurmond A-M, Bardoel AFJ, Wijmenga C, Pruijs HEH, Sillence DO, et al. Identification of PLOD2 as telopeptide lysyl hydroxylase, an important enzyme in fibrosis. J Biol Chem. 2003;278:40967–72.
33. Gilkes DM, Bajpai S, Chaturvedi P, Wirtz D, Semenza GL. Hypoxia-inducible Factor 1 (HIF-1) Promotes Extracellular Matrix Remodeling under Hypoxic Conditions by Inducing P4HA1, P4HA2, and PLOD2 Expression in Fibroblasts. J Biol Chem. 2013;288:10819–29.
34. Macpherson LJ, Dubin AE, Evans MJ, Marr F, Schultz PG, Cravatt BF, et al. Noxious compounds activate TRPA1 ion channels through covalent modification of cysteines. Nature. 2007;445:541–5.
35. Bautista DM, Jordt SE, Nikai T, Tsuruda PR, Read AJ, Poblete J, et al. TRPA1 Mediates the Inflammatory Actions of Environmental Irritants and Proalgesic Agents. Cell. 2006;124:1269–82.
36. Hatano N, Itoh Y, Suzuki H, Muraki Y, Hayashi H, Onozaki K, Wood IC, Beech DJ, Muraki K: Hypoxia-inducible Factor-1 (HIF1) Switches on Transient Receptor Potential Ankyrin Repeat 1 (TRPA1) Gene Expression via a Hypoxia Response Element-like Motif to Modulate Cytokine Release. J Biol Chem. 2012;287(38):31962–72.
37. Ciraci C, Tuggle CK, Wannemuehler MJ, Nettleton D, Lamont SJ. Unique genome-wide transcriptome profiles of chicken macrophages exposed to Salmonella-derived endotoxin. BMC Genomics. 2010;11:545.
38. Tubak V, Határvölgyi E, Krenács L, Korpos E, Kúsz E, Duda E, et al. Expression of immunoregulatory tumor necrosis factor-like molecule TL1A in chicken chondrocyte differentiation. Can J Vet Res. 2009;73:34–8.
39. Sato H, Kida Y, Mai M, Endo Y, Sasaki T, Tanaka J, et al. Expression of genes encoding type IV collagen-degrading metalloproteinases and tissue inhibitors of metalloproteinases in various human tumor cells. Oncogene. 1992;7:77–83.
40. Ries C, Egea V, Karow M, Kolb H, Jochum M, Neth P. MMP-2, MT1-MMP, and TIMP-2 are essential for the invasive capacity of human mesenchymal stem cells: Differential regulation by inflammatory cytokines. Blood. 2007;109:4055–63.
41. Milkiewicz M, Haas TL. Effect of mechanical stretch on HIF-1{alpha} and MMP-2 expression in capillaries isolated from overloaded skeletal muscles: laser capture microdissection study. Am J Physiol Heart Circ Physiol. 2005;289:H1315–20.
42. Jackson WM, Aragon AB, Onodera J, Koehler SM, Ji Y, Bulken-Hoover JD, et al. Cytokine expression in muscle following traumatic injury. J Orthop Res. 2011;29:1613–20.
43. Cui H, Darmanin S, Natsuisaka M, Kondo T, Asaka M, Shindoh M, et al. Enhanced expression of asparagine synthetase under glucose-deprived conditions protects

pancreatic cancer cells from apoptosis induced by glucose deprivation and cisplatin. Cancer Res. 2007;67:3345–55.

44. Zoll J, Ponsot E, Dufour S, Doutreleau S, Ventura-Clapier R, Vogt M, et al. Exercise Training in Normobaric Hypoxia in Endurance Runners. III Muscular Adjustments of Selected Gene Transcripts Volume. 2006;100:1258–66.

45. Zimmerman U-J, Wang P, Zhang X, Bogdanovich S, Forster R. Anti-oxidative response of carbonic anhydrase III in skeletal muscle. IUBMB Life. 2004;56:343–7.

46. Minchenko A, Leshchinsky I, Opentanova I, Sang N, Srinivas V, Armstead V, et al. Hypoxia-inducible factor-1-mediated expression of the 6-phosphofructo-2-kinase/fructose-2,6-bisphosphatase-3 (PFKFB3) gene. Its possible role in the Warburg effect. J Biol Chem. 2002;277:6183–7.

47. Kronqvist P, Kawaguchi N, Albrechtsen R, Xu X, Schrøder HD, Moghadaszadeh B, et al. ADAM12 alleviates the skeletal muscle pathology in mdx dystrophic mice. Am J Pathol. 2002;161:1535–40.

48. Lopes-Ferreira M, Núñez J, Rucavado A, Farsky SHP, Lomonte B, Angulo Y, et al. Skeletal muscle necrosis and regeneration after injection of Thalassophryne nattereri (niquim) fish venom in mice. Int J Exp Pathol. 2001;82:55–64.

49. Rodrigues CAV, Diogo MM, da Silva CL, Cabral JMS. Hypoxia enhances proliferation of mouse embryonic stem cell-derived neural stem cells. Biotechnol Bioeng. 2010;106:260–70.

50. Yin H, Zhang S, Gilbert ER, Siegel PB, Zhu Q, Wong E a. Expression profiles of muscle genes in postnatal skeletal muscle in lines of chickens divergently selected for high and low body weight. Poult Sci. 2014;93:147–54.

51. Li Y, Yang X, Ni Y, Decuypere E, Buyse J, Everaert N, et al. Early-age feed restriction affects viability and gene expression of satellite cells isolated from the gastrocnemius muscle of broiler chicks. J Anim Sci Biotechnol. 2012;3:33.

52. Halevy O, Geyra A, Barak M, Uni Z, Sklan D. Early posthatch starvation decreases satellite cell proliferation and skeletal muscle growth in chicks. J Nutr. 2000;130:858–64.

53. Kuang S, Chargé SB, Seale P, Huh M, Rudnicki MA. Distinct roles for Pax7 and Pax3 in adult regenerative myogenesis. J Cell Biol. 2006;172:103–13.

54. Powers SK, Duarte J, Kavazis AN, Talbert EE. Reactive oxygen species are signalling molecules for skeletal muscle adaptation. Exp Physiol. 2010;95:1–9.

55. Balaban RS, Nemoto S, Finkel T: Mitochondria, oxidants, and aging. Cell. 2005;120(4):483–95.

56. Allen DG, Lamb GD, Westerblad H. Impaired calcium release during fatigue. J Appl Physiol. 2008;104:296–305.

57. Stephanou A, Latchman DS: Transcriptional modulation of heat-shock protein gene expression. Biochem Res Int. 2011;2011.

58. Kalmar B, Greensmith L: Induction of heat shock proteins for protection against oxidative stress. Adv Drug Deliv Rev. 2009;61(4):310–18.

59. Finkel T, Holbrook NJ. Oxidants, oxidative stress and the biology of ageing. Nature. 2000;408:239–47.

60. Lezoualc'h F, Engert S, Berning B, Behl C. Corticotropin-releasing hormone-mediated neuroprotection against oxidative stress is associated with the increased release of non-amyloidogenic amyloid beta precursor protein and with the suppression of nuclear factor-kappaB. Mol Endocrinol. 2000;14:147–59.

61. Karalis K, Muglia LJ, Bae D, Hilderbrand H, Majzoub JA. CRH and the immune system. In J Neuroimmunol Volume. 1997;72:131–6.

62. Fischer J, Bosse A, Pallauf J. Effect of selenium deficiency on the antioxidative status and muscle damage in growing turkeys. Arch Anim Nutr. 2008;62:485–97.

63. Brown RG, Sweeny PR, Moran ET. Collagen levels in tissues from selenium deficient ducks. Comp Biochem Physiol A Comp Physiol. 1982;72:383–9.

64. Lehnert SA, Byrne KA, Reverter A, Nattrass GS, Greenwood PL, Wang YH, et al. Gene Expression Profiling of Bovine Skeletal Muscle in Response to and during Recovery from Chronic and Severe Undernutrition. 2006. p. 3239–50. Volume 84.

65. Terrill JR, Radley-Crabb HG, Iwasaki T, Lemckert FA, Arthur PG, Grounds MD: Oxidative stress and pathology in muscular dystrophies: Focus on protein thiol oxidation and dysferlinopathies. FEBS J. 2013;280(17):4149–64.

66. Dudkiewicz M, Szczepińska T, Grynberg M, Pawłowski K. A novel protein kinase-like domain in a selenoprotein, widespread in the tree of life. PLoS One. 2012;7, e32138.

67. Huang J-Q, Li D-L, Zhao H, Sun L-H, Xia X-J, Wang K-N, et al. The selenium deficiency disease exudative diathesis in chicks is associated with downregulation of seven common selenoprotein genes in liver and muscle. J Nutr. 2011;141:1605–10.

68. Peng D, Belkhiri A, Hu T, Chaturvedi R, Asim M, Wilson KT, Zaika A, El-Rifai W: Glutathione peroxidase 7 protects against oxidative DNA damage in oesophageal cells. Gut. 2012;61(9):1250–60.

69. Young B, Lowe JS, Stevens A, Heath JW. Wheater's Functional Histology: A Text and Colour Atlas. Fifth. Philadelphia, PA: Elsevier; 2006.

70. Kranen RW, van Kuppevelt TH, Goedhart HA, Veerkamp CH, Lambooy E, Veerkamp JH. Hemoglobin and myoglobin content in muscles of broiler chickens. Poult Sci. 1999;78:467–76.

71. Blessing MH, Müller G. Myoglobin concentration in the chicken, especially in the gizzard (a biochemical, light and electron microscopic study). Comp Biochem Physiol A Comp Physiol. 1974;47:535–40.

72. Fleming BK, Froning GW, Yang TS. Heme Pigment Levels in Chicken Broilers Chilled in Ice Slush and Air 1. Poult Sci. 1991;70:2197–200.

73. Pette D, Staron RS. Transitions of muscle fiber phenotypic profiles. Histochem Cell Biol. 2001;115:359–72.

74. Malila Y, Tempelman RJ, Sporer KRB, Ernst CW, Velleman SG, Reed KM, et al. Differential gene expression between normal and pale, soft, and exudative turkey meat. Poult Sci. 2013;92:1621–33.

75. Mullen AJ, Barton PJR. Structural characterization of the human fast skeletal muscle troponin I gene (TNNI2). Gene. 2000;242:313–20.

76. Yang H, Xu ZY, Lei MG, Li FE, Deng CY, Xiong YZ, et al. Association of 3 polymorphisms in porcine troponin I genes (TNNI1 and TNNI2) with meat quality traits. J Appl Genet. 2010;51:51–7.

77. Frey N, Barrientos T, Shelton JM, Frank D, Rütten H, Gehring D, et al. Mice lacking calsarcin-1 are sensitized to calcineurin signaling and show accelerated cardiomyopathy in response to pathological biomechanical stress. Nat Med. 2004;10:1336–43.

78. Braun T, Gautel M. Transcriptional mechanisms regulating skeletal muscle differentiation, growth and homeostasis. Nat Rev Mol Cell Biol. 2011;12:349–61.

79. Chen Z, Zhao T-J, Li J, Gao Y-S, Meng F-G, Yan Y-B, et al. Slow skeletal muscle myosin-binding protein-C (MyBPC1) mediates recruitment of muscle-type creatine kinase (CK) to myosin. Biochem J. 2011;436:437–45.

80. Jordan T, Jiang H, Li H, DiMario JX. Inhibition of ryanodine receptor 1 in fast skeletal muscle fibers induces a fast-to-slow muscle fiber type transition. J Cell Sci. 2004;117:6175–83.

81. Fulle S, Protasi F, Di Tano G, Pietrangelo T, Beltramin A, Boncompagni S, et al. The contribution of reactive oxygen species to sarcopenia and muscle ageing. Exp Gerontol. 2004;39:17–24.

82. Fujii J, Otsu K, Zorzato F, de Leon S, Khanna V, Weiler J, et al. Identification of a mutation in porcine ryanodine receptor associated with malignant hyperthermia, Science (80-). 1991. p. 448–51.

83. Fiege M, Wappler F, Weisshorn R, Gerbershagen MU, Menge M, Schulte Am Esch J. Induction of malignant hyperthermia in susceptible swine by 3,4-methylenedioxymethamphetamine ("ecstasy"). Anesthesiology. 2003;99:1132–6.

84. Jordan T, Jiang H, Li H, DiMario JX. Regulation of skeletal muscle fiber type and slow myosin heavy chain 2 gene expression by inositol trisphosphate receptor 1. J Cell Sci. 2005;118:2295–302.

85. DiMario JX. Protein kinase C signaling controls skeletal muscle fiber types. Exp Cell Res. 2001;263:23–32.

86. Jordan T, Li J, Jiang H, DiMario JX. Repression of slow myosin heavy chain 2 gene expression in fast skeletal muscle fibers by muscarinic acetylcholine receptor and G(alpha)q signaling. J Cell Biol. 2003;162:843–50.

87. Jackson SP, Green RD, Miller MF. Phenotypic characterization of rambouillet sheep expressing the Callipyge gene.1. Inheritance of the condition and production characteristics. J Anim Sci. 1997;75:14–8.

88. Vuocolo T, Byrne K, White J, McWilliam S, Reverter A, Cockett NE, et al. Identification of a gene network contributing to hypertrophy in callipyge skeletal muscle. Physiol Genomics. 2007;28:253–72.

89. Hershberger RE, Parks SB, Kushner JD, Li D, Ludwigsen S, Jakobs P, et al. Coding sequence mutations identified in MYH7, TNNT2, SCN5A, CSRP3, LBD3, and TCAP from 313 patients with familial or idiopathic dilated cardiomyopathy. Clin Transl Sci. 2008;1:21–6.

90. Xu X, Qiu H, Du ZQ, Fan B, Rothschild MF, Yuan F, et al. Porcine CSRP3: Polymorphism and association analyses with meat quality traits and comparative analyses with CSRP1 and CSRP2. Mol Biol Rep. 2010;37:451–9.

91. Arber S, Halder G, Caroni P. Muscle LIM protein, a novel essential regulator of myogenesis, promotes myogenic differentiation. Cell. 1994;79:221–31.

92. Barash IA, Mathew L, Lahey M, Greaser ML, Lieber RL. Muscle LIM protein plays both structural and functional roles in skeletal muscle. Am J Physiol Cell Physiol. 2005;289:C1312–20.

93. Kostek MC, Chen Y-W, Cuthbertson DJ, Shi R, Fedele MJ, Esser KA, et al. Gene expression responses over 24 h to lengthening and shortening contractions in human muscle: major changes in CSRP3, MUSTN1, SIX1, and FBXO32. Physiol Genomics. 2007;31:42–52.

94. Schneider AG, Sultan KR, Pette D. Muscle LIM protein: expressed in slow muscle and induced in fast muscle by enhanced contractile activity. Am J Physiol. 1999;276:C900–6.

95. Heath E, Tahri D, Andermarcher E, Schofield P, Fleming S, Boulter CA. Abnormal skeletal and cardiac development, cardiomyopathy, muscle atrophy and cataracts in mice with a targeted disruption of the Nov (Ccn3) gene. BMC Dev Biol. 2008;8:18.

96. Chen CC, Lau LF: Functions and mechanisms of action of CCN matricellular proteins. Int J Biochem Cell Biol. 2009;41(4):771–83.

97. Sabourin LA, Rudnicki MA. The molecular regulation of myogenesis. Clin Genet. 2000;57:16–25.

98. Manara MC, Perbal B, Benini S, Strammiello R, Cerisano V, Perdichizzi S, et al. The expression of ccn3(nov) gene in musculoskeletal tumors. Am J Pathol. 2002;160:849–59.

99. Lin CG, Leu S-J, Chen N, Tebeau CM, Lin S-X, Yeung C-Y, et al. CCN3 (NOV) is a novel angiogenic regulator of the CCN protein family. J Biol Chem. 2003;278:24200–8.

100. Liu C, Gersch RP, Hawke TJ, Hadjiargyrou M. Silencing of Mustn1 inhibits myogenic fusion and differentiation. Am J Physiol Cell Physiol. 2010;298:C1100–8.

101. Zheng Q, Zhang Y, Chen Y, Yang N, Wang X-J, Zhu D. Systematic identification of genes involved in divergent skeletal muscle growth rates of broiler and layer chickens. BMC Genomics. 2009;10:87.

102. Hall A. Rho GTPases and the Actin Cytoskeleton, Science (80-). 1998. p. 509–14.

103. Bishop AL, Hall A. Rho GTPases and their effector proteins. Biochem J. 2000;348(Pt 2):241–55.

104. Bassères DS, Tizzei EV, Duarte AAS, Costa FF, Saad STO. ARHGAP10, a novel human gene coding for a potentially cytoskeletal Rho-GTPase activating protein. Biochem Biophys Res Commun. 2002;294:579–85.

105. Huard J, Li Y, Fu FH. Muscle injuries and repair: current trends in research. J Bone Joint Surg Am. 2002;84-A:822–32.

106. Sheehan SM, Allen RE. Skeletal muscle satellite cell proliferation in response to members of the fibroblast growth factor family and hepatocyte growth factor. J Cell Physiol. 1999;181:499–506.

107. Mitchell P, Steenstrup T, Hannon K. Expression of fibroblast growth factor family during postnatal skeletal muscle hypertrophy. J Appl Physiol. 1999;86:313–9.

108. Smyth AB, O' Neill E, Smith DM. Functional properties of muscle proteins in processes poultry products. In: Richardson RI, Mead GC, editors. Poult Meat Sci. 25th ed. Oxon, UK: CAB International; 1999. p. 377–96.

109. Rayment I, Holden HM, Whittaker M, Yohn CB, Lorenz M, Holmes KC, et al. Structure of the actin-myosin complex and its implications for muscle contraction. Science. 1993;261:58–65.

110. Do M-KQ, Sato Y, Shimizu N, Suzuki T, Shono J -i., Mizunoya W, Nakamura M, Ikeuchi Y, Anderson JE, Tatsumi R: Growth factor regulation of neural chemorepellent Sema3A expression in satellite cell cultures. AJP Cell Physiol. 2011;301(5)C1270–C1279.

111. Levi M, Keller TT, Van Gorp E, Ten Cate H: Infection and inflammation and the coagulation system. Cardiovasc Res. 2003;60(1):26–39.

112. Emery AE, Burt D. Intracellular calcium and pathogenesis and antenatal diagnosis of Duchenne muscular dystrophy. Br Med J. 1980;280:355–7.

113. Byrd SK. Alterations in the sarcoplasmic reticulum: a possible link to exercise-induced muscle damage. Med Sci Sport Exerc. 1992;24:531–6.

114. Tay JS, Lai PS, Low PS, Lee WL, Gan GC. Pathogenesis of Duchenne muscular dystrophy: the calcium hypothesis revisited. J Paediatr Child Health. 1992;28:291–3.

115. Oberc MA, Engel WK. Ultrastructural localization of calcium in normal and abnormal skeletal muscle. Lab Invest. 1977;36:566–77.

116. MacRae VE, Mahon M, Gilpin S, Sandercock DA, Hunter RR, Mitchell MA. A comparison of breast muscle characteristics in three broiler great-grandparent lines. Poult Sci. 2007;86:382–5.

117. VanVleet JF, Valentine BA. Muscles and Tendons. In: Maxie G, Saunders L, editors. Jubb, Kennedy, Palmer's Pathol Domest Anim. 5th ed. 2007.

118. Gordon GB, Barcza MA, Bush ME. Lipid Accumulation in Hypoxic Tissue Culture Cells. Am J Pathol. 1977;88:663–78.

119. Chabowski A, Górski J, Calles-Escandon J, Tandon NN, Bonen A. Hypoxia-induced fatty acid transporter translocation increases fatty acid transport and contributes to lipid accumulation in the heart. FEBS Lett. 2006;580:3617–23.

120. Boström P, Magnusson B, Svensson P-A, Wiklund O, Borén J, Carlsson LMS, et al. Hypoxia converts human macrophages into triglyceride-loaded foam cells. Arterioscler Thromb Vasc Biol. 2006;26:1871–6.

121. Lien RJ, Bilgili SF, Hess JB, Joiner KS. Induction of deep pectoral myopathy in broiler chickens via encouraged wing flapping. J Appl Poult Res. 2012;21:556–62.

122. Whitehead NP, Yeung EW, Allen DG. Muscle damage in mdx (dystrophic) mice: role of calcium and reactive oxygen species. Clin Exp Pharmacol Physiol. 2006;33:657–62.

123. Han R. Muscle membrane repair and inflammatory attack in dysferlinopathy. Skelet Muscle. 2011;1:10.

124. Tidball JG. Inflammatory processes in muscle injury and repair. Am J Physiol Regul Integr Comp Physiol. 2005;288:R345–53.

125. Brown NS, Bicknell R. Hypoxia and oxidative stress in breast cancer. Oxidative stress: its effects on the growth, metastatic potential and response to therapy of breast cancer. Breast Cancer Res. 2001;3:323–7.

126. Li YP, Atkins CM, Sweatt JD, Reid MB. Mitochondria mediate tumor necrosis factor-alpha/NF-kappaB signaling in skeletal muscle myotubes. Antioxid Redox Signal. 1999;1:97–104.

127. Tidball JG, Rinaldi C: Immunological Response to Muscle Injury. In Muscle Fundam Biol Mech Dis Vol 2. Edited by Griendling KK, Kitsis RN, Stull JT. London: Academic Press; 2012:899–920.

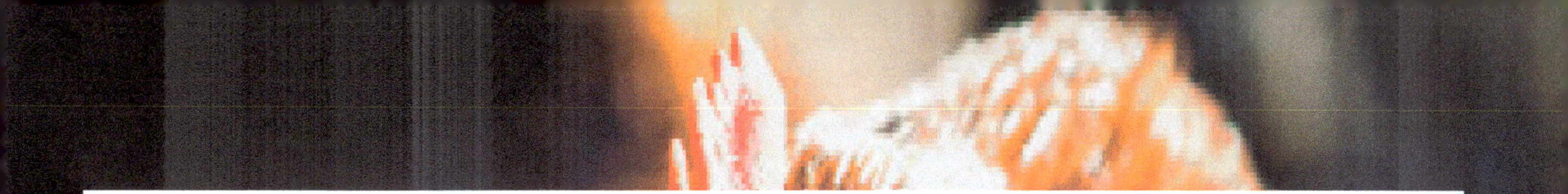

CHAPTER 14

LEG DISORDERS IN BROILER CHICKENS: PREVALENCE, RISK FACTORS AND PREVENTION

Toby G. Knowles[1], Steve C. Kestin[1], Susan M. Haslam[1], Steven N. Brown[1], Laura E. Green[2], Andrew Butterworth[1], Stuart J. Pope[1], Dirk Pfeiffer[3], Christine J. Nicol[1]

[1] School of Veterinary Science, University of Bristol, Langford, Bristol, United Kingdom

[2] Ecology and Epidemiology Group, Biological Sciences, University of Warwick, Coventry, United Kingdom

[3] The Royal Veterinary College, Royal College Street, London, United Kingdom

ABSTRACT

Broiler (meat) chickens have been subjected to intense genetic selection. In the past 50 years, broiler growth rates have increased by over 300% (from 25 g per day to 100 g per day). There is growing societal concern that many broiler chickens have impaired locomotion or are even unable to walk. Here we present the results of a comprehensive survey of commercial flocks which quantifies the risk factors for poor locomotion in broiler chickens. We assessed the walking ability of 51,000 birds, representing 4.8 million birds within 176 flocks. We also obtained information on approximately 150 different management factors associated with each flock. At a mean age of 40 days, over 27.6% of birds in our study showed poor locomotion and 3.3% were almost unable to walk. The high prevalence of poor locomotion occurred despite culling policies designed to remove severely lame birds from flocks. We show that the primary risk factors associated with impaired locomotion and poor leg health are those specifically associated with rate of growth. Factors significantly associated with high gait score included the age of the bird (older birds), visit (second visit to same flock), bird genotype, not feeding whole wheat, a shorter dark period during the day, higher stocking density at the time of assessment, no use of antibiotic, and the use of intact feed pellets. The welfare implications are profound. Worldwide approximately 2×10^{10} broilers are reared within similar husbandry systems. We identify a range of management factors that could be altered to reduce leg health problems, but implementation of these changes would be likely to reduce growth rate and production. A debate on the sustainability of current practice in the production of this important food source is required.

INTRODUCTION

Due to their short reproductive cycle and their worldwide popularity as a food, poultry represent the most highly selected livestock. Selection of broiler chickens (chickens grown for their meat) has been primarily directed at economic traits which have reduced costs of production[1]–[3]. Throughout the world the majority of broilers are reared using very similar, modern, intensive systems of production where birds are confined for their lifetime within high density housing [4] and reared from hatch to slaughter weight within approximately 40 days. However, there is evidence that in optimising traits for production the resulting birds, whilst producing meat at a low cost, have a reduced viability and reduced welfare [5]–[7], with poor walking ability, or locomotion, a primary concern.

Previous research has highlighted associations between management practices and levels of leg disorders. Most attention has focussed on the partially effective practices of reducing feed quantity or the nutrient density of feed [e.g.

Citation: Knowles TG, Kestin SC, Haslam SM, Brown SN, Green LE, Butterworth A, et al. (2008) Leg Disorders in Broiler Chickens: Prevalence, Risk Factors and Prevention. PLoS ONE 3(2): e1545. doi:10.1371/journal.pone.0001545.

8], [9], on providing more than 1-hour of darkness each 24-hour period [10], and on attempts to increase bird activity [11], [12]. There are also known genetic effects, with genotype influences on many traits associated with leg health [7],[13]–[15]. Despite a large body of work investigating the effects of specific risk factors[reviewed in 16], there has been little previous work to examine how these practices interact on real commercial farms to determine the overall level of leg disorders in particular flocks. There are also many management practices, with potential influences on leg disorders, which have not been looked at quantitatively. This study was therefore commissioned by the UK Department for Environment, Food and Rural Affairs to investigate the extent of variation of leg disorders within UK flocks and to identify methods by which these disorders could possibly be controlled.

MATERIALS AND METHODS

We studied broiler flocks belonging to five major UK producers who together accounted for over 50 per cent of UK production. Two other relatively large companies were invited to participate but declined. We obtained data from each producer in proportion to their respective annual broiler production. Visits were randomised to farm and flock and were made by veterinarians who had completed a five-day training course to evaluate broiler walking ability with a standardised gait scoring method [7]. Eighteen veterinarians with postgraduate qualifications in poultry medicine and production, or in welfare science, acted as flock assessors and were trained to categorise gait scores within a range from 0 (completely normal) to 5 (unable to stand). The scoring system primarily assesses walking ability rather than exhaustion, with assessors trained to identify rolling gaits, limping, jerky and unsteady movements and problems with manoeuvrability. The scoring system is also known to correlate well with other methods of assessing leg disorders that do not involve active movement, such as the latency-to-lie test [17]. Throughout the study the uniformity of the assessors' scoring was monitored and by the end of the course, average scores for each category were all within half a score. During the subsequent 18 month study, assessors were sent at approximately six and 12 months, a tape containing new video sequences covering a range of gait scores. The scoring of these tapes was monitored to ensure that the assessors remained in agreement. Reference movies of birds' walking ability for each of the six categories are given in the supplementary information. Each of 176 flocks was visited approximately three days before the flock was depopulated for slaughter and at least 250 birds from each flock were gait-scored from ten, pre-selected, randomised sites within a house.

Fifty seven of the 176 flocks in our study were not 'depopulated' for slaughter simultaneously. Instead, one of more groups of birds were removed sequentially over a period of days or weeks in a process known as 'thinning'. This process involved the removal of a portion of the flock, usually the female birds, to allow the remaining birds more room to grow on to a greater weight. To account for the effects of 'thinning' practices, an additional 30 visits were made as second visits approximately three days prior to a later depopulation of one of the original 176 flocks. The flocks visited a second time were also chosen at random from the initial set of flocks.

A primary aim of the study was to investigate possible risk factors associated with the wide inter-flock variation in leg disorders. Of particular interest were risk factors associated with bird husbandry which could possibly be altered when rearing future flocks. Information on these aspects was obtained for each flock by a direct interview with a farm representative. The same questionnaire was used for each visit and comprised 134 questions initially about the breeding flock that had supplied the farm, the facilities where the eggs had been hatched, the distance and time the chicks had been transported, and hatchery vaccination policies. Information was then obtained about the number, weight, sex and time of chicks placed, and their date of arrival. The largest section of the questionnaire sought information on husbandry practices including stocking density and thinning practices, nutritional information, layout and construction of the house, and background information on health, growth rates, mortality and culling policies. Finally, information about the personnel working with the flock, the farm, biosecurity measures and company policies was obtained. After conducting the direct interview, each veterinary assessor collected direct information relating to air quality, temperature, general cleanliness and feed quality.

Statistical Analysis

Statistical models were built to identify between-flock variables that were associated with the differences in average flock walking ability. The multilevel modelling software package MLwiN v2.01 (http://www.cmm.bristol.ac.uk/MLwiN/index.shtml) was used as it allowed us to create linear models within the hierarchical structure of the data of repeated measurements on flocks and flocks within companies.

RESULTS

The overall results of the survey, showing the distribution of gait scores prior to slaughter, are given in Table 1. The figures in Table 1 were calculated using the gait scores of a flock, weighted by the size of the flock as given by the number of birds placed as chicks. The minimum and maximum values in Table 1 show that there was considerable variation in walking ability between flocks, but overall, 27.6 per cent of birds represented by this survey had a gait score of 3 or above.

Table 1: The estimated percentage of birds in the survey population within each gait score category

	Gait Score					
	0	1	2	3	4	5
Mean	2.2	26.6	43.5	24.3	3.1	0.2
SD	4.8	21.1	15.9	21.3	7.0	0.5
Min	0.0	0.0	1.6	0.0	0.0	0.0
Max	34.7	82.7	74.6	83.7	45.9	3.2

Mean, SD, minimum and maximum for flocks are shown. The values are calculated from flock averages weighted by birds placed and include first and second visits. Total birds placed n = 4,845,962. Total birds gait scored-206 flocks × minimum of 250 birds per flock-n is approximately 51,000.
doi:10.1371/journal.pone.0001545.t001

Table 2 shows the percentage of birds within each gait score category broken down by the five companies and by the first and second visits. There was a large amount of variation in the distribution of gait score in flocks between the different companies. Company 4 notably produced only 8.5 per cent of birds with gait scores of 3 and above at the first visit compared with 22.7 to 29.7 per cent for the other companies, and only 0.6 per cent of birds with gait scores of 4 and above compared with 1.3 to 4.2 per cent for the other companies. Table 2 also shows the deterioration of gait over time for companies 1, 4 and 5 where a minimum of four second visits were made, the figures for the second visit to company 3 representing only one flock.

Table 2: The percentage of birds in each gait score category by producer and by first and second visit

			Gait Score								
			0	1	2	3	4	5	Mean GS	Birds Placed (n)	Flocks (n)
First Visit	Company	1	2.8	27.0	47.4	20.4	3.1	0.2	1.93	1,484,893	71
		2	1.0	21.9	48.1	25.3	2.2	0.5	2.07	191,285	18
		3	1.0	21.5	48.0	28.4	1.2	0.1	2.08	496,758	39
		4	4.7	44.1	46.6	7.8	0.5	0.1	1.58	378,145	36
		5	1.5	29.0	41.2	24.3	3.9	0.5	2.01	1,225,915	49
			0	1	2	3	4	5	Mean GS	Birds Placed (n)	
Second Visit	Company	1	3.2	8.3	48.3	40.6	0.0	0.7	2.46	206,360	11
		3	1.5	51.2	48.1	3.2	0.0	0.0	1.48	34,008	1
		4	4.5	26.6	57.5	11.1	1.2	0.1	2.08	118,180	4
		5	0.5	4.2	23.7	59.4	11.5	0.4	2.80	325,037	14

The table also shows the mean gait score and the number of birds represented in terms of birds placed.
doi:10.1371/journal.pone.0001545.t002

The average gait score for a flock was modelled in terms of the levels of the risk factors recorded by the veterinary assessors. In addition to the assessment of husbandry variables as linear predictors of average flock gait score, the age at which the birds were assessed, and a seasonal effect, were included in the model. It was necessary to correct for both age and season at the time of assessment, before the effects of different husbandry practices could be properly investigated. The seasonal effect was expected to be cyclical, so was modelled as a sinusoidal curve to identify any cyclical variation in average gait score over a 12 month cycle. Both Sine and Cosine terms for month (January=1, February=2, etc) were used in the modelling process allowing us to look for an annual maximum and a minimum effect of season on gait score. A number of variables in the model were centred by subtracting the mean of the variable from each of its measurements.

The most parsimonious multilevel model we obtained of the relationship between the average gait score of a flock, and the risk factors that were recorded within the survey, is shown inTable 3. When company was included as a fixed effect, rather than a random effect, in the model the parameter estimates shown in Table 3 were not meaningfully altered and there were no significant variable/company interactions. Similarly, when the veterinary assessors were included in the model as fixed effects the parameter estimates were not substantively altered. The parameter estimates in the final model are shown and also details of which of the variables are centred. The mean, minimum and maximum of the predictor variables are shown in Table 4, including all those variables which were centred.

Table 3: The parameter estimates, their standard error and significance for the model of average flock gait score

Variable	Variable Type	Parameter Estimate	SE	P
Constant		2.52	0.158	0.000
Season (Sin)	Continuous	−0.099	0.0408	0.016
Season (Cos)	Continuous	−0.035	0.0442	0.463
Age assessed (day)	Continuous (Centred)	0.048	0.0049	0.000
Second visit	Binary	0.25	0.089	0.005
Breed A (% in flock)	Continuous	−0.0024	0.00108	0.025
Dietary wheat (wk 3) %	Continuous	−0.017	0.0078	0.027
Average dark (hr/day)	Continuous (Centred)	−0.079	0.0283	0.005
Stocking density (kg/m^2)	Continuous (Centred)	0.013	0.0057	0.024
Antibiotic	Binary	−0.17	0.069	0.011
Dusty/broken feed pellets	Binary	−0.15	0.063	0.017

The parameter estimates give the amount of change in average flock gait score for a unit change in each variable. Note, as explained in the text, factors are not and cannot be arranged in order of importance. Positive parameter estimates mean that an increase in the value of a variable is associated with an increase in flock average gait score and negative parameter estimate, a decrease.
doi:10.1371/journal.pone.0001545.t003

Table 4: Mean, minimum and maximum values of the continuous predictor variables in the model of average flock gait score

Variable	Mean	Min	Max
Age assessed (day)	39.8	28	56
Breed A (% in flock)	85.6	0	100
Dietary wheat (wk 3) %	9.2	0	30
Average dark (hr/day)	2.9	0	8.5
Stocking density (kg/m^2)	31.3	15.9	44.8

doi:10.1371/journal.pone.0001545.t004

When all other variables were held constant, there was a seasonal pattern to the average gait score of the flocks (Table 3 and Figure 1) with the lowest (best) gait scores occurring in March and the highest (worst) in September. The age at which the birds were assessed was important in determining gait score, with every extra day, across the range of 28 to 56 days, leading to an average daily deterioration in score of 0.048. Although each flock was visited close to slaughter when gait is known to be poorest, within the survey as a whole we were able to evaluate the effect of age on locomotion problems throughout the growth period because of the wide range of age at slaughter. A post-thinning visit was associated with an increased average gait score of 0.25 over and above that due to the age at which the birds were assessed, probably due to the effect of the stress of the first thin, and/or the preponderance of larger, faster-growing male birds remaining in the flock after thinning.

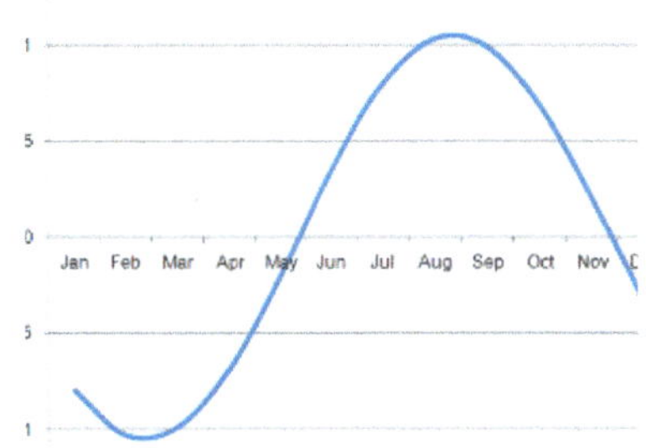

Figure 1: The modelled seasonal change in average flock gait score.

We found that a number of fundamental husbandry practices were significantly associated with average flock gait score and these are detailed below.

A major influence was bird genotype. Broilers worldwide are predominantly of two types, from either one of two major international breeder companies, labelled here A and B. Birds from both genotypes are sometimes reared together within one flock. For every percentage increase in Breed A birds in a flock, from between 0 to 100 per cent, there was a 0.0024 improvement in flock gait score.

Whole wheat is sometimes fed to broilers as part of their diet, predominantly to improve digestive function. For every percentage increase in dietary wheat fed, from 0 to 30 per cent, as measured during their third week of life, there was a 0.017 per cent improvement in flock gait score.

Broilers are reared under a wide variety of artificial lighting regimes. For every 1 hour increase in the daily period of darkness, across the range of 0 to 8.5 hours, there was a 0.079 improvement in flock gait score.

There has been debate about the importance of stocking density as an influence on bird welfare and locomotion [18]. Within limits, putting as many birds in a house as possible for each rearing cycle will improve profitability. For every 1 kg/m^2 increase in stocking density as measured at the time of the flock assessment, across a range from 15.9 to 44.8 kg/m^2, there was a 0.013 deterioration in flock gait score.

Antibiotics are routinely used during different stages of broiler rearing and their use can be quite difficult to quantify accurately. In our study farmers were simply asked if a flock had received antibiotic. A reply of 'yes' in this context meant that a flock had received an extra antibiotic treatment in addition to that which would be part of normal rearing practice. For the flocks for which the farmer had answered 'yes' flock gait score was reduced by 0.17.

Broiler feed is pelleted to minimise wastage and to increase the amount of feed that a bird can consume within a given time. In our study, veterinary assessors made a subjective judgement of whether the quality of the pelleting was good or poor (dusty/broken). For flocks with poor pelleting, gait score was on average 0.15 improved.

The magnitude of a parameter estimate given in Table 3 is not an indicator of the importance of the association of a variable with an increase or a reduction in gait score. This is because the magnitude of the parameter estimate is dependent upon the measurement scale used (e.g. kg or g, hour or day). Further, it is not possible to rank objectively the variables in terms of importance as subjective considerations such as practicality and the perceived cost of altering the husbandry practice have to be considered. For example, the results show that using 100% Breed A birds compared with 100% Breed B birds would reduce average flock gait score by 0.24. To achieve a similar reduction in average gait score by manipulating stocking density alone would require a *reduction* in stocking density of 18.5 kg/m^2. Despite these considerations there is value in using our model in a predictive capacity to show the improvement in average flock gait score that might be achieved on a hypothetical farm if each relevant variable attained the 'best' value actually recorded within the survey. Figure 2 shows the potential improvement from a baseline flock average gait score of 2.5, the middle of the range of possible scores. The Figure shows that no, one variable was associated with a large shift in average flock gait towards the score of 0, a perfect gait, but that the age at which birds are slaughtered appears to be of primary importance, followed by the hours of darkness that the birds are allowed.

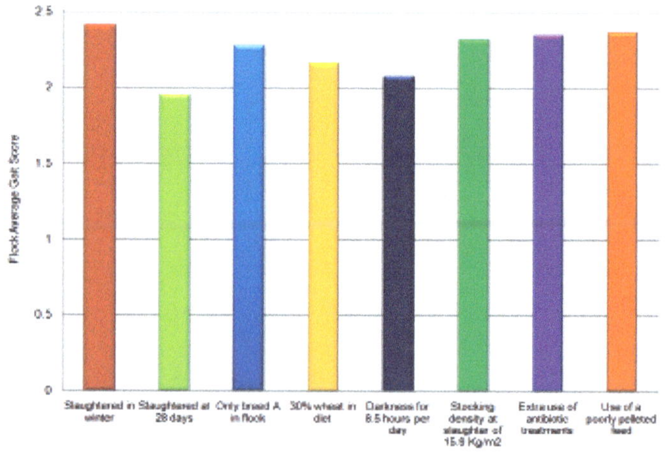

Figure 2: A modelling exercise reveals the extent to which average flock gait score might be improved (i.e. lowered from a notional average score of 2.5) by adoption of the 'best' management practice for each variable that we recorded within our study.

DISCUSSION

For comparison with previous surveys we draw attention to the prevalence of birds in our survey that had gait scores of 3 or above. This cut-off point is important because there is evidence from studies of the effects of analgesic drugs that birds in these categories can be in pain [19]–[22], Other surveys have reported between 14.1% and 30.1% of birds with gait scores of 3 or above in different European countries, although it is not always clear whether weighted or unweighted estimates have been used [7], [23], [24]. Our survey presents a conservative estimate of UK prevalence of leg disorders in meat chickens because the national proportion of birds slaughtered at second, and subsequent thinnings, when gait score tends to deteriorate, is higher than in our sample, and because we present results only from companies that volunteered to participate.

All companies had a policy of culling broilers and some farms separately identified "leg culls" conducted because of leg disorders. If a flock within the survey were to be heavily culled because of leg disorders it would be expected that the overall flock gait score would be improved. However, we found no association between the flock average gait score and the percentage of birds culled as "leg culls". However, the lack of a relationship may reflect the difficulties farmers have in recording these data in a standardised manner across the survey as a whole. Companies themselves report that these records are inconsistent between farms.

Despite examining a fuller range of husbandry and management practices than previous surveys, we did not identify many novel or previously unreported risks. An effect of season has been noted before in the US, where a higher percentage of leg abnormalities was reported in the summer [25]. The strong genotype effect that we found, confirms the important genetic component to leg disorders, and many of the husbandry effects detected most likely alter levels of leg disorder through direct or indirect effects on growth rate. Thus, we consider the effect of feeding whole wheat is probably due to the slower rate of digestion for whole wheat resulting in reduced growth rate, whilst providing broken or dusty pellets, rather than whole pellets, probably reduced overall consumption rates.

Birds reduce or cease their feed intake during periods of darkness, with associated reductions in growth rate. This is the most likely explanation for the beneficial effect of longer dark periods on the prevalence of leg disorders. The detrimental effect of higher stocking densities may be more complex, reflecting not only a lack of room available for birds to move and exercise, but also the extra environmental loading from increased biomass (e.g. additional ammonia and litter moisture) [18]. Finally, the improvement in leg health observed when antibiotics were used, was probably due to a reduction in the infectious disorders which can cause some types of leg problem.

The study indicates that modern husbandry and genotypes, biased towards economics of production, have been detrimental to poultry welfare in compromising the ability of chickens to walk. However, we demonstrate that within the current framework there is variation in the magnitude of the problem between different flocks, and so some scope to improve walking ability through alterations in husbandry practice. Work needs to be carried out on the predictability of these risks, and the economics of improved welfare practices, for them to gain industry acceptance. An informed balance could then be drawn between profitability and our moral obligation to maintain good standards of animal welfare. The agreement, in May 2007, within the EU of new regulations governing the conditions under which broilers may be reared[26] is a recognition of the problems associated with modern broiler production and is an attempt at a first step towards remedying the situation. The new measures will include the introduction of a maximum stocking density limit, data collection and scientific monitoring of impacts on chicken welfare. The new Directive will not come into force until 2010 but it will prevent farms from stocking birds at densities over 39 kg/m^2 in subsequent flocks where mortality levels in the past seven flocks have exceeded a set level. The animal welfare implications of monitoring mortality and culling rates are potentially complex. In the short-term, the new Directive could lead to less rigorous culling of birds with leg problems and thereby increase suffering. However, in the longer term, the Directive could act as a stimulus to breeding companies to produce more robust genotypes, with a reduced susceptibility to leg disorders.

Research shows that consumers currently know little about how broiler chickens are reared but can be shocked when presented with information about current commercial practices [27]. Since the sustainability of intensive broiler production depends on continued consumer acceptance of the farming practices involved, the broiler industry will need to work with the scientific community to develop more robust and healthier genotypes and to ensure that optimal husbandry and management practices are fully implemented.

ACKNOWLEDGMENTS

We are most grateful to the broiler companies and farmers who helped with the work and to the members of the expert steering committee, drawn from government, the broiler industry and academia, who gave their time to guide and support the study.

AUTHOR CONTRIBUTIONS

Conceived and designed the experiments: DP CN TK SK SB AB LG. Performed the experiments: TK SK SH SB AB SP. Analyzed the data: DP CN TK SK SH SB LG. Wrote the paper: DP CN TK SK SH LG.

REFERENCES

1. Emmans GC, Kyriazakis I (2000) Issues arising from genetic selection for growth and body composition characteristics in poultry and pigs. Occ Publi Br Soc Anim Sc 27: 39.
2. Farm Animal Welfare Council (1992) Report on the Welfare of Broiler Chickens: PB 0910. Tolworth, UK: FAWC.
3. Compassion in World Farming (2005) The welfare of Broiler Chickens in the European Union. CIWF Report, Petersfield, UK. ISBN 1 900156 35 0. Available:http://www.ciwf.org.uk/publications/reports/Welfare_of_Broiler_Chickens_in_the_EU_2005.pdf.
4. FAO–PPLPI Research Report. Industrial Livestock Production and Global Health Risks (June 2007). Available: http://www.fao.org/ag/AGAinfo/projects/en/pplpi/docarc/rep-hpai_industrialisationrisks.pdf.
5. Bessei W (2006) Welfare of broilers: a review. World Poultry Sci J 62: 455–466.
6. Butterworth A, Weeks CA, Crea PR, Kestin SC (2002) Dehydration and lameness in a broiler flock. Animal Welfare 11: 89–94.
7. Kestin SC, Knowles TG, Tinch AE, Gregory NE (1992) The prevalence of leg weakness in broiler chickens assessed by gait scoring and its relationship to genotype. Vet Rec 131: 190–194.
8. Su G, Sorensen P, Kestin SC (1999) Meal feeding is more effective than early feed restriction at reducing the prevalence of leg weakness in broiler chickens. Poult Sci 78: 949–955.
9. Brickett KE, Dahiya JP, Classen HL, Annett CB, Gomis S (2007) The impact of nutrient density, feed form, and photoperiod on the walking ability and skeletal quality of broiler chickens. Poult Sci 86: 2117–2125.
10. Moller AP, Sanotra GS, Vestergaard KS (1999) Developmental instability and light regime in chickens. Appl Anim Behav Sci 62: 57–71.
11. Classen HL, Riddell C (1989) Photoperiodic effects on performance and leg abnormalities in broiler chickens. Poult Sci 68: 873–879.
12. Reiter K (2006) Behaviour and welfare of broiler chicken. Archiv. fur Geflugelkunde 70: 208–215.
13. Kestin SC, Su G, Sorensen P (1999) Different commercial broiler crosses have different susceptibilities to leg weakness. Poult Sci 78: 1085–1090.
14. Kestin SC, Gorden S, Su G, Sorensen P (2001) Relationships in broiler chickens between lameness, live weight, growth rate and age. Vet Rec 148: 195–197.

15. Reiter K, Kutritz B (2001) Behaviour and leg weakness in different broiler breeds. Archiv fur Geflugelkunde 65: 137–141.
16. Bradshaw RH, Kirkden RD, Broom DM (2002) A review of the aetiology and pathology of leg weakness in broilers in relation to welfare. Avian and Poultry Biol Rev 13: 45–103.
17. Weeks CA, Knowles TG, Gordon RG, Kerr AE, Peyton ST, et al. (2002) A novel technique for objectively assessing lameness in broiler chickens. Vet Rec 151: 762–764.
18. Dawkins MS, Donnelly CA, Jones TA (2004) Chicken welfare is influenced more by housing conditions than by stocking density. Nature 427: 342–344.
19. Weeks CA, Danbury TD, Davies HC, Hunt P, Kestin SC (2000) The behaviour of broiler chickens and its modification by lameness. Appl Anim Behav Sci 67: 111–125.
20. Scientific Committee on Animal Health and Animal Welfare (2000) The Welfare of Chickens Kept for Meat Production (Broilers). European Commission. Available:http://ec.europa.eu/food/fs/sc/scah/out39_en.pdf.
21. Danbury TC, Weeks CA, Chambers JP, Waterman-Pearson AE, Kestin SC (2000) Self selection of the analgesic drug carprofen by lame broiler chickens. Vet Rec 146: 307–311.
22. McGeown D, Danbury TC, Waterman-Pearson AE, Kestin SC (1999) Effect of carprofen on lameness in broiler chickens. Vet Rec 144: 668–671.
23. Sanotra GS, Lund JD, Ersboll AK, Petersen JS, Vestergaard KS (2001) Monitoring leg problems in broilers: a survey of commercial broiler production in Denmark. World Poultry Sci J 57: 55–69.
24. Sanotra GS, Berg C, Lund JD (2003) A comparison between leg problems in Danish and Swedish broiler production. Animal Welfare 12: 677–683.
25. Laster CP, Hoerr FJ, Bilgili SF, Kincaid SA (1999) Effects of dietary roxarsone supplementation, lighting program, and season on the incidence of leg abnormalities in broiler chickens. Poult Sci 78: 197–203.
26. EU Press Release IP/07/630. Brussels 7th May 2007. Available:http://europa.eu/rapid/pressReleasesAction.doreferenceIP/07/630formatHTMLaged0languageEN.
27. Hall C, Sandilands V (2007) Public attitudes to the welfare of broiler chickens. Animal Welfare 16: 499–512.

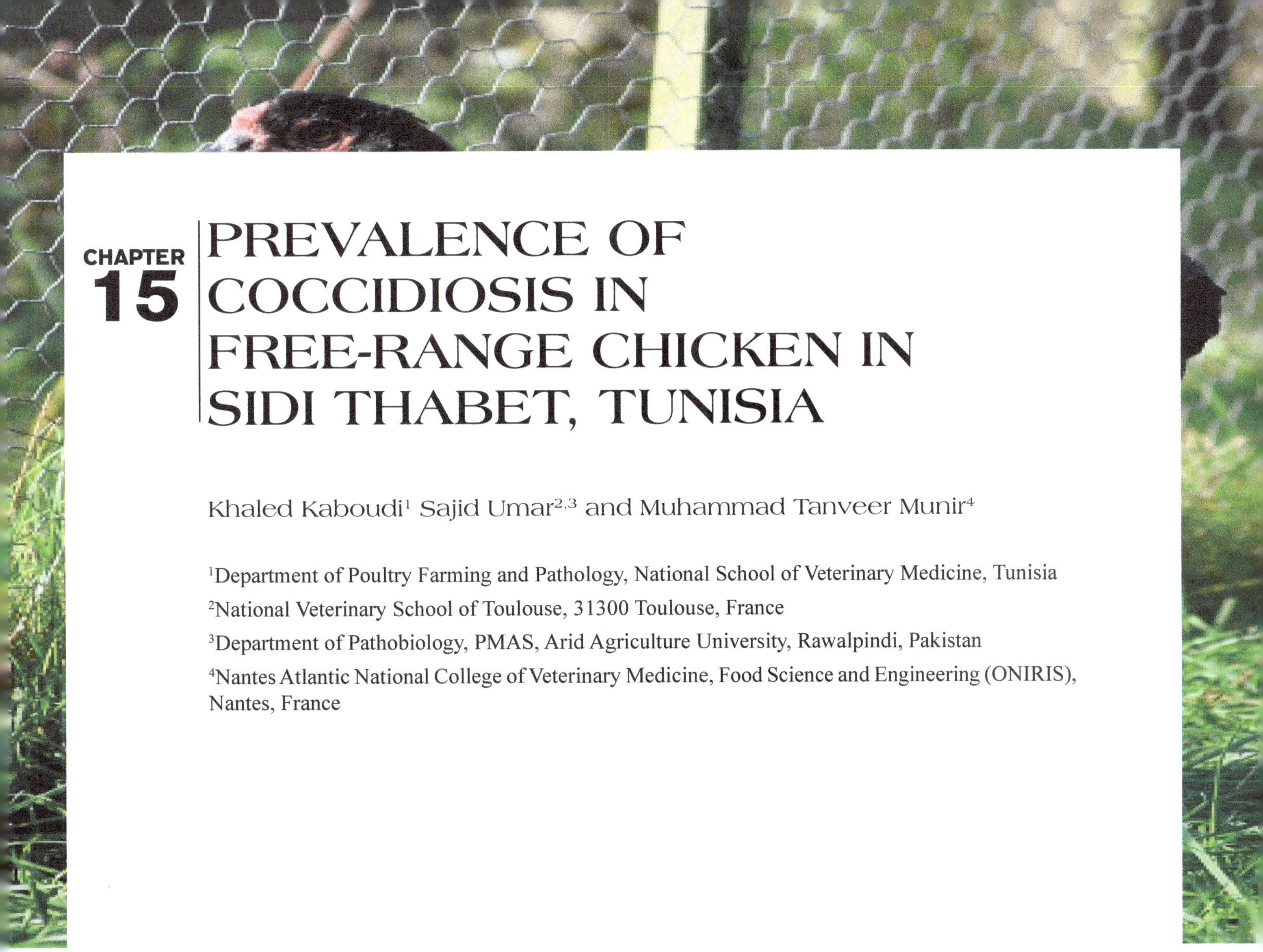

CHAPTER 15

PREVALENCE OF COCCIDIOSIS IN FREE-RANGE CHICKEN IN SIDI THABET, TUNISIA

Khaled Kaboudi[1] Sajid Umar[2,3] and Muhammad Tanveer Munir[4]

[1]Department of Poultry Farming and Pathology, National School of Veterinary Medicine, Tunisia

[2]National Veterinary School of Toulouse, 31300 Toulouse, France

[3]Department of Pathobiology, PMAS, Arid Agriculture University, Rawalpindi, Pakistan

[4]Nantes Atlantic National College of Veterinary Medicine, Food Science and Engineering (ONIRIS), Nantes, France

ABSTRACT

Background. Enteric diseases are an important concern to the poultry industry and coccidiosis is imposing a significant economic burden worldwide. Objectives. The main goal of the present study was to investigate the prevalence of coccidiosis in free-range chicken in Sidi Thabet, northeast Tunisia. Methods. Six hundred and thirty free-range chickens along with fecal samples were collected from 15 flocks in this region and two hundred chickens were found positive for oocysts of Eimeria spp. Intestines were dissected and examined for macroscopic lesions. The mucosa of small intestine and the caeca were examined for the presence and identification of parasitic forms using parasitology methods. The mean lesion scores were usually low (<2+) in different intestinal portions of different types of chicken and high scores (>2+) were attributed mainly to the caeca. Results. The overall rate of coccidiosis was 31.8%: E. tenella (61.5%), E. maxima (12%), and E. acervulina(1.5%). Mixed Eimeria species infection was observed with overall prevalence 26.5%. There was a statistically significant difference (P<0.05) among infection rates, age groups, season, diarrhea, and type of chicken. Conclusion. This is the first report of coccidiosis rate in free-range chicken in this region. Further additional studies are needed to develop better preventive measures against coccidiosis in the country.

INTRODUCTION

Enteric diseases are an important concern to the poultry industry because of production losses, increased mortality, reduced welfare of birds and increased risk of contamination of poultry products for human consumption. Avian coccidiosis is an enteric parasitic disease caused by multiple species of the protozoan parasite of the genus Eimeria. It is one of the most common and economically most important diseases of poultry worldwide [1, 2]. The disease occurs only after ingestion of sporulated oocysts in susceptible hosts and is characterized by diarrhea, enteritis, emaciation, drooping wings, poor growth, and increased morbidity and mortality. Poor management practices, such as wet litter and high stocking density, can exacerbate the clinical signs [3]. There are seven species of Eimeria as causative agents of coccidiosis in chickens, of which E. tenella, E. maxima, E. necatrix, and E. brunetti are highly pathogenic. Others, like E. acervulina, E. mitis, and E. praecox, are less pathogenic [4–6]. Species of the genus Eimeria are predominately host-specific; each species occurs in a single host species or a group of closely related hosts. Most Eimeria spp. affect birds between 3 and 18 weeks of age and can cause high mortality in young chicks. Mixed infections are commonly found under field conditions [5]. Coccidiosis is still a major problem worldwide possibly due to poor diagnosis

Citation: Khaled Kaboudi, Sajid Umar, and Muhammad Tanveer Munir, "Prevalence of Coccidiosis in Free-Range Chicken in Sidi Thabet, Tunisia," Scientifica, vol. 2016, Article ID 7075195, 6 pages, 2016. doi:10.1155/2016/7075195.

and biosecurity measures. Identification of different species based on morphology of oocysts is very challenging and requires expertise. Differential identification of each species is dependent upon the following characteristics: zone of intestine parasitized, the gross appearance of the lesion, oocyst morphology, minimum sporulation time, minimum prepatent time, schizont size, location of parasite in the host intestinal epithelium, and cross-immunization tests [7].

Poultry sector in Tunisia plays a vital role in income and employment generation as well as being a source of protein. Coccidiosis is a common important disease in commercial and free-range chicken in Tunisia. Mortality and morbidity are usually high and production performances are altered (feed conversion, body weight). Prevention of the disease is based on the hygienic measures, on chemoprevention, and on vaccination. In free-range flocks, coccidiosis is a major cause of mortality of birds because there are no preventive measures. The role of coccidiosis in economic losses of poultry is not clearly recognized in Tunisia. To the best of our knowledge, not a single report has been published on the epidemiological studies on coccidiosis in free-range chicken in Tunisia. This is first report on prevalence rate of coccidiosis in free-range chicken in Tunisia.

MATERIALS AND METHODS

Study Area and Sampling

This cross-sectional study was conducted on free-range chickens between September 2010 and August 2015. The total number of birds per flock varied from 30 to 1000 and birds ages were from 4 weeks to 32 weeks. All flocks were situated in and surrounding the village of Sidi Thabet in the Ariana Governorate, Tunisia. The flocks were visited on the basis of abnormal mortality associated with lameness, diarrhea, decreased feed intake, and low body weight. All of the flocks had no history of vaccination against coccidiosis. The chicks and fecal samples were brought to the laboratory for necropsy and parasitology examination, respectively. Information regarding the age, history of diarrhea, and type of chicken and other general information about farms and flocks were taken from farmers.

Sample Examination

The chickens (630) were subjected to routine postmortem examination. All viscera were examined for gross pathological changes at the Avian Pathology Clinical Service of the National Veterinary School of Tunisia. After a general examination of all systems, intestines of each bird were dissected and examined rigorously. Mucosal scrapings of small intestine and the caeca were made and examined microscopically for the presence and identification of oocyst and asexual forms of Eimeria. The presence of oocyst in the fecal samples was examined by the flotation method using saturated solution of sugar [3, 4]. The modified McMaster technique was used to quantify the oocyst. For sporulation, positive samples were placed in Petri dishes, conditioned with a solution of 2.5% potassium dichromate at room temperature, and aired daily for up to two days [8]. The Eimeria spp. were determined based on morphology of oocysts and sporocysts (shape, color, form index, micropyle, and presence or absence of residual) and time of sporulation [9]. For positive samples, the intensity of the infection was categorized as described by [10] (Table 1).

Table 1: Prevalence rate of coccidiosis in free-range chicken in Sidi Thabet, Tunisia

	Age groups			Birds type			History of diarrhea
	<10 wks	10–20 wks	<20 wks	Broiler	Pullet	Layer	
Number of birds examined (%)	210 (33.33)	210 (33.33)	210 (33.33)	210 (33.33)	210 (33.33)	210 (33.33)	200 (31.7)
Number of positive samples (%)	37 (17.6)	26 (12.38)	4 (1.9)	26 (12.54)	37 (17.30)	4 (1.90)	124 (62)
Number of negative samples (%)	173 (82.3)	184 (87.6)	206 (98.09)	184 (87.6)	173 (82.3)	206 (98.09)	76 (38)

Statistical Analysis

Statistical analysis was performed by using the software package SPSS version 16.0 for Windows. The differences among variables were evaluated by chi-square test. A P value <0.05 was considered statistically significant.

RESULTS AND DISCUSSION

Sidi Thabet is located at the northeast of Tunis city center, around 36°51′45″N 10°11′44″E with hot-summer Mediterranean climate, where winters are mild with moderate rainfall and summers are hot and dry. Temperatures in July and August can exceed 40°C (104°F). Winters are mild with temperatures rarely exceeding 20°C (68°F). The Coccidia infection rate in backyard chicken was determined to be 31.8% (Table 1); this rate is low compared to investigations in Iran but higher than studies in Nigeria [11] and Ethiopia [8]. Similarly, Sharma et al. [3] also observed higher prevalence rate (39.58%) of coccidiosis than present study. In previous studies, the infection rate was reported to be 54.3% in Turkey [12], 20.6% and 70.9% in Ethiopia [8, 13], 31.7% and 39.6% in India [3, 14], 36.7% and 52.9% in Nigeria [15], 71.9% in Pakistan [16], 78% in Jordan [17], 88.4% in Argentina [18], and 92% in Romania [19].

Significantly higher ($P<0.05$) prevalence of clinical coccidiosis was observed in pullets (13%) and broilers (12.5%) than layer (0%). Moreover, Pullet (12.5%) showed significantly higher prevalence of subclinical coccidiosis than layer (3.5%) and broiler (5%) (Table 2). The highest rate of Eimeria spp. was determined by E.tenella (61.5%), followed by E. maxima (12%) and E. acervulina (1.5%) (Table 3). These findings are in agreement with Hadipour et al. [20], who reported E. tenella as the most prevalent species in Iran. However, findings of current study are not in line with the findings of previous studies [21–24]. Our findings are in parallel with reports from Sweden, France, Argentina, and Jordan suggesting that detected species of Eimeriaare widespread in most countries [17, 18, 25, 26]. Mixed infections with two Eimeria spp. were observed in some of the positive farms, with highest frequency of E. tenella and E. maxima coinfections (25%) followed by coinfections of E. tenella and E. acervulina (1.5%).

Table 2: Prevalence of subclinical and clinical coccidiosis in free-range chicken in Sidi Thabet, Tunisia

	Broiler		Pullet		Layer	
Infection grade	Number of positive samples	% positive	Number of positive samples	% positive	Number of positive samples	% positive
Subclinical coccidiosis	10	5	25	12.5	7	3.5
Clinical coccidiosis	25	12.5	26	13	0	0

Table 3: Prevalence rate of different Eimeria species in free-range chicken in Sidi Thabet, Tunisia

Bird type	Broilers		Pullet		Layer		Prevalence
Eimeria spp.	Number of positive samples	% positive	Number of positive samples	% positive	Number of positive samples	% positive	%
E. tenella	50	25	71	35.5	2	1	61.5
E. maxima	11	5.5	7	3.5	6	3	12
E. tenella + E. maxima	17	8.5	29	14.5	4	2	25
E. tenella + E. acervulina	1	0.5	2	1	0	0	1.5

E. acervulina was only determined in mixed infections with E. tenella; mixed Eimeria infection (26.5%), with highest frequency of the coinfection by E. tenella and E. maxima (25%). This may be attributed to the bad management conditions where birds are exposed to a high-risk infection by different pathogens at the same time. In clinical coccidiosis positive samples, the number of oocysts was found to be between 11644 and 38251 per gram (Table 4).

Table 4: Seasonwise prevalence of coccidiosis in free-range chicken in Sidi Thabet, Tunisia

Season	Number of samples examined	Number of positive samples	Prevalence (%)	OPG (Mean ± SE)
Autumn (September, October, and November)	157	80	50.9	38251.33 ± 1488.2
Winter (December, January, and February)	157	58	36.9	18241.68 ± 756.99
Spring (March, April, and May)	157	57	36.3	15761.27 ± 1245.22
Summer (June, July, and August)	157	5	3.1	11644.23 ± 1987.3

OPG: oocyst per gram.

In current investigation, there was a statistical difference among coccidiosis rate, chicken type (χ^2 = 108.315; df = 2; P < 0.05), age groups (χ^2 = 38.344; df = 2; P < 0.05), diarrhea (χ^2 = 42.884; df = 1; P < 0.05), intensity of infection (χ^2 = 15.510; df = 4; P < 0.05), and season (χ^2 = 22.884; df

, and season (χ^2 = 22.884; df = 3; P < 0.05). Prevalence of infected birds is influenced by the type of chickens (P < 0.05) as described in Table 1. It was highest in pullets (17.30%), followed by broilers (12.54%) and layers (1.90%). This finding may be due to the physiognomy of the free-range poultry farming, which was based on the preservation of females, in order to enlarge the flock and increase the egg production. However, males are usually sold in live bird market for consumption as protein source. Similarly, Gharekhani et al. [4] showed higher prevalence of coccidiosis in young chicken (37.5%) of 4–6 wks of age in Iran. Olrija et al. [13] reported higher prevalence of coccidiosis (25.10%) in Bovans breed of chicken in Ethiopia. However, Olanrewaju and Agbor [1] reported higher prevalence of coccidiosis in cockerels (80%) in Nigeria.

The infection was observed all around the year (Table 4) but the prevalence was significantly higher (P < 0.05) in the autumn (50.9%) followed by winter (36.9%), spring (36.3%), and summer (3.1%). Our results are in line with Sharma et al. [3] and Khan et al. [16]. This high prevalence in the rainy period in Tunisia could be attributed to increase in humidity and drops in temperature, which is conducive for sporulation of oocysts for easy dispersion and transmission.

Age is one of the most principal factors in coccidiosis. Eimeria spp. can cause infection in all ages of chicken. However, rate of coccidiosis is usually higher in chicken of young ages and the lower rate of coccidiosis of older birds was due to immunity developed by the infection when they were young. In our study, the higher rate of coccidiosis was determined in >10 weeks age groups (17.6%; Table 1); the significant relationship was observed in agreement with other researchers [1, 4, 13, 15, 16, 23]. Sharma et al. [27] reported higher prevalence of coccidiosis in the age group of 31–45 days in broilers. This might be associated with the presence of high number of oocysts in the litter. A possible reason for this may be that during the period between 31 and 45 days of age the birds have not attained immunity against coccidiosis, resulting in the increased incidence of the disease, while the birds of age group 0–15 days were protected by the maternal immunity. Older birds are less susceptible possibly due to enhanced immunity with passage of age. Muazu et al. [15] suggested that all ages of poultry are susceptible to infection but it usually resolves itself around 6–8 weeks of age. It seems that the relationship between age and prevalence rate of coccidiosis is direct due to complete life cycle and the increase of oocysts consumption. Our findings are in accordance with the findings of many authors [28]. Similarly, McDougald and Fitz-Coy [5] reported that coccidiosis is more prevalent in chicken of 3–6 weeks of age.

Diarrhea is a serious sign in clinical coccidiosis [4]. In the present study, 62% of chicks with diarrhea were positive (Table 1). Our results taken with previous investigations are consistent with the idea that the coccidiosis rate correlated with diarrhea. However, our findings do not agree with the findings of Jatau et al. [11] who concluded that local chickens exhibit usually subclinical coccidiosis.

Necropsy investigation in clinical coccidiosis showed dehydrated and pale carcasses (possibly due to anemia) along with ballooning and hemorrhages in intestines and caeca (Figure 1(a)). Moreover, clotted blood and fibrino-caseous materials in the intestinal lumen were observed in the caeca of broilers and pullets (Figure1(b)). However, no gross lesions were observed in all free-range chickens with subclinical infection. However, subclinical coccidiosis has been reported to have negative effect on the performance of infected birds [29, 30]. Examination of intestines revealed that high gross lesions were attributed essentially to the caeca followed by duodenum, jejunum/ileum, and colon/rectum segments in broilers and pullets. However, gross lesion scores were significantly higher in jejunum/ileum than duodenum in layers (Table 5). Similar findings have been reported previously by Gari et al. [8] and Raman et al. [31]. Moreover, coccidiosis is a major predisposing factor in the occurrence of necrotic enteritis. Epithelium damage caused by Eimeria species allows Clostridium perfringens to replicate rapidly and produce toxin, probably because leakage of proteins-rich fluids into the lumen of the gut is favorable to Clostridium perfringens proliferation and toxin production [4].

Table 5: Gross lesions attributed to different intestinal segments of infected birds in free-range chicken in Sidi Thabet, Tunisia

Intestine	Broiler (<10 wks)		Pullet (10–20 wks)		Layer (>20 wks)	
	Number of birds examined	Number of positive samples (%)	Number of birds examined	Number of positive samples (%)	Number of birds examined	Number of positive samples (%)
Duodenum	210	58 (27.6)	210	63 (30)	210	41 (19.5)
Jejunum/ileum	210	30 (14.2)	210	44 (20.9)	210	78 (37.1)
Colon/rectum	210	8 (3.8)	210	11 (5.2)	210	9 (4.2)
Ceca	210	102 (48.5)	210	92 (43.8)	210	82 (39.04)

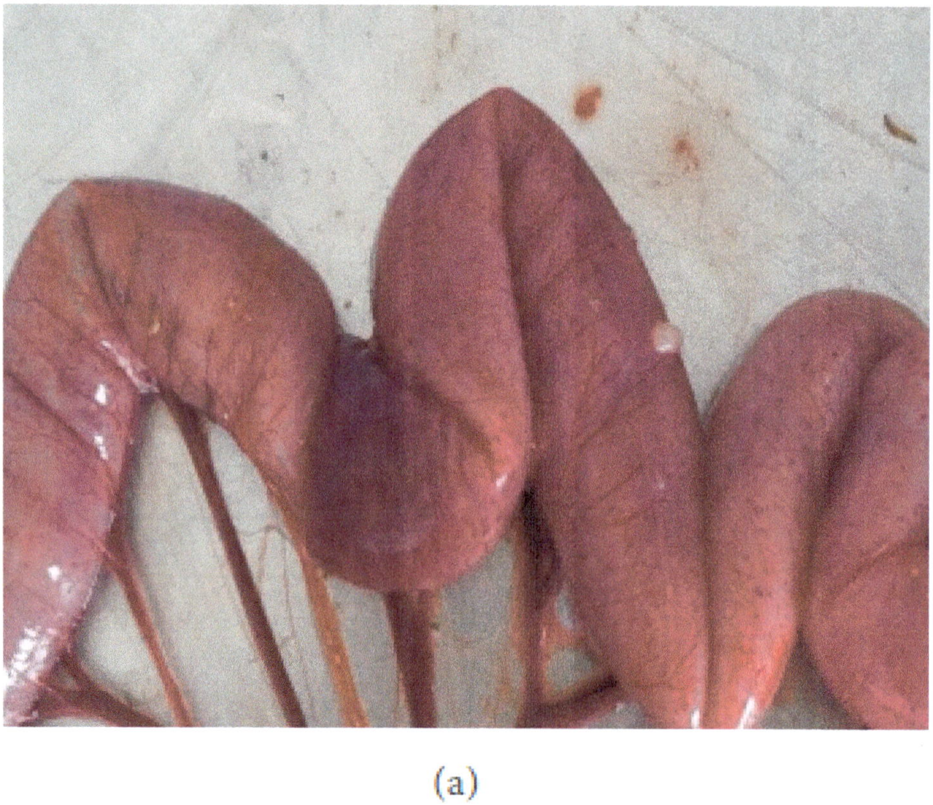

(a)

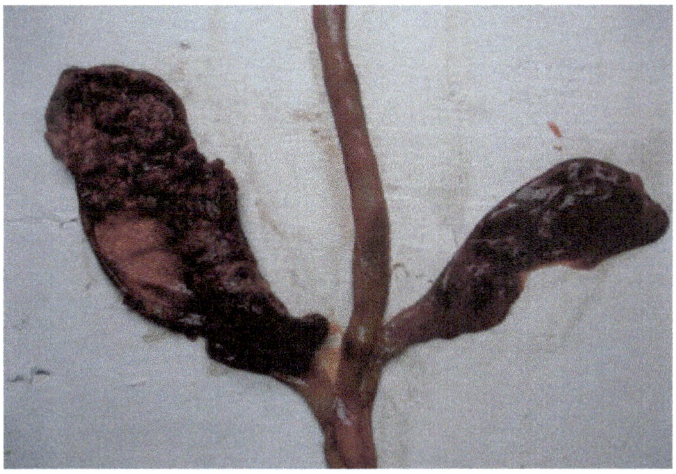

(b)

Figure 1: (a) Infected ten-week-old broiler by E. maxima (note the petechiae through the wall of the middle intestine). (b) Cecal coccidiosis in eight-week-old pullet infected by E.tenella. The ceca are distended and the wall is thickened. The erosion of the mucosa results in the accumulation of huge amount of fibrin-necrotic material noted at the opening of the cecum.

CONCLUSION

In conclusion, our findings showed that three pathogenic Eimeria species of chicken occurred in free-range poultry in Sidi Thabet, Tunisia with E. tenella and E. maxima being the most abundant. Infection occurred mainly in the wet season with high frequency in young chickens. Layer had subclinical coccidiosis. This may pose economic implication to backyard poultry farming due to poor performance of the affected birds that most often looked apparently healthy. This is the first report of coccidiosis rate in free-range poultry in Sidi Thabet, Tunisia. Coccidiosis may be an important factor in the economic losses of the free-range poultry in this region. Therefore, proper control measures must be taken in the form of strict biosecurity, disinfection, vaccination, and good use of anticoccidial drugs. In addition to this, further investigations and design appropriate control strategies in improving management of farms are necessary and strongly recommended.

ACKNOWLEDGMENTS

The authors are thankful to laboratory staff for sampling and technical help. This study has not been supported by any foundation.

REFERENCES

1. C. A. Olanrewaju and R. Y. Agbor, "Prevalence of coccidiosis among poultry birds slaughtered at gwagwalada main market, Abuja, FCT, Nigeria," The International Journal of Engineering and Science, vol. 3, no. 1, pp. 41–45, 2014.
2. M. W. Shirley, A. L. Smith, and F. M. Tomley, "The biology of avian Eimeria with an emphasis on their control by vaccination," Advances in Parasitology, vol. 60, pp. 285–330, 2005. · ·
3. S. Sharma, A. Iqbal, S. Azmi, and H. A. Shah, "Study of poultry coccidiosis in organized and backyard farms of Jammu region," Veterinary World, vol. 6, no. 8, pp. 467–469, 2013. · ·
4. J. Gharekhani, Z. Sadeghi-Dehkordi, and M. Bahrami, "Prevalence of coccidiosis in broiler chicken farms in Western Iran," Journal of Veterinary Medicine, vol. 2014, Article ID 980604, 4 pages, 2014. ·
5. L. R. McDougald and S. H. Fitz-Coy, "Coccidiosis," in Diseases of Poultry, pp. 1068–1085, Blackwell Publishing Professional, Ames, Iowa, USA, 2008.
6. M. A. Taylor, R. L. Coop, and R. Wall, Veterinary Parasitology, Blackwell, Oxford, UK, 2007.
7. D. P. Conway and M. E. McKenzie, Poultry Coccidiosis Diagnostic and Testing Procedures, Blackwell, Ames, Iowa, USA, 2007.
8. G. Gari, G. Tilahun, and P. Dorchies, "Study on poultry coccidiosis in Tiyo District, Arsi Zone, Ethiopia,"International Journal of Poultry Science, vol. 7, no. 3, pp. 251–256, 2008. · ·
9. E. J. L. Soulsby, Helminths, Arthropods, and Protozoa of Domesticated Animals, Lea & Febiger, Philadelphia, Pa, USA, 1982.
10. A. I. Lawal, I. D. Jatau, B. Musa, and U. Saleh, "Studies on the coccidian infection in local chickens (Gallus gallus domesticus) in Zaria and the implications for the commercial poultry production," Journal of Advances in Medical and Pharmaceutical Sciences, vol. 2, pp. 62–65, 2008.
11. I. D. Jatau, N. H. Sulaiman, I. W. Musa et al., "Prevalence of coccidia infection and preponderanceEimeria species in free range indigenous and intensively managed exotic chickens during hot-wet season, in Zaria, Nigeria," Asian Journal of Poultry Science, vol. 6, no. 3, pp. 79–88, 2012. · ·
12. Z. Karaer, E. Guven, A. Akcay, S. Kar, S. Nalbantoglu, and A. Cakmak, "Prevalence of subclinical coccidiosis in broiler farms in Turkey," Tropical Animal Health and Production, vol. 44, no. 3, pp. 589–594, 2012. · ·
13. D. Oljira, A. Melaku, and B. Bogale, "Prevalence and risk factors of coccidiosis in poultry farms in and around Ambo Town, Western Ethiopia," American-Eurasian

Journal of Scientific Research, vol. 7, no. 4, pp. 146–149, 2012.

14. V. S. Nikam, S. V. Kanse, N. Jadab, and E. L. Jaid, "Comparative study of seasonal incidence of chicken coccidiosis in eight districts of Marathwada region, Maharashtra state," Trends in Parasitology Research, vol. 1, no. 1, pp. 7–9, 2012.

15. A. Muazu, A. A. Masdooq, J. Ngbede et al., "Prevalence and identification of species of Eimeria causing coccidiosis in poultry within Vom, Plateau state, Nigeria," International Journal of Poultry Science, vol. 7, no. 9, pp. 917–918, 2008. · ·

16. M. Q. Khan, H. Irshad, R. Anjum, M. Jahangir, and U. Nasir, "Eimeriosis in poultry of Rawalpindi/Islamabad area," Pakistan Veterinary Journal, vol. 26, no. 2, pp. 85–87, 2006.

17. M. Q. Al-Natour, M. M. Suleiman, and M. N. Abo-Shehada, "Flock-level prevalence of Eimeria species among broiler chicks in northern Jordan," Preventive Veterinary Medicine, vol. 53, no. 4, pp. 305–310, 2002. · ·

18. L. R. McDougald, L. Fuller, and R. Mattiello, "A survey of Coccidia on 43 poultry farms in Argentina,"Avian Diseases, vol. 41, no. 4, pp. 923–929, 1997.

19. A. Györke, L. Pop, and V. Cozma, "Prevalence and distribution of Eimeria species in broiler chicken farms of different capacities," Parasite, vol. 20, article 52, 2013. · ·

20. M. M. Hadipour, A. Olyaie, M. Naderi, F. Azad, and O. Nekouie, "Prevalence of Eimeria species in scavenging native chickens of Shiraz, Iran," African Journal of Microbiology Research, vol. 5, no. 20, pp. 3296–3299, 2011. ·

21. M. Hachimi, D. Belghyti, K. E. Kharrim, and Y. E. Guamri, "Coccidioses du poulet dans la région du Gharb (maroc)," Bulletin de la Société de Pharmacie de Bordeaux, vol. 147, pp. 49–60, 2008.

22. O. M. Majaro, "Oocystes de coccidies chez les poulets de chair au Nigeria," Revue d'Elevage et de Médecine Vétérinaire des Pays Tropicaux, vol. 34, no. 1, pp. 23–25, 1981.

23. G. Reza Razmi and G. Ali Kalideri, "Prevalence of subclinical coccidiosis in broiler-chicken farms in the municipality of Mashhad, Khorasan, Iran," Preventive Veterinary Medicine, vol. 44, no. 3-4, pp. 247–253, 2000. · ·

24. M. R. Shirzad, S. Seifi, H. R. Gheisari, B. A. Hachesoo, H. Habibi, and H. Bujmehrani, "Prevalence and risk factors for subclinical coccidiosis in broiler chicken farms in Mazandaran province, Iran," Tropical Animal Health and Production, vol. 43, no. 8, pp. 1601–1604, 2011. · ·

25. P. Thebo, A. Lundén, A. Uggla, and P. Hooshmand-Rad, "Identification of seven Eimeria species in Swedish domestic fowl," Avian Pathology, vol. 27, no. 6, pp. 613–617, 1998. · ·

26. R. B. Williams, A. C. Bushell, J. M. Répérant et al., "A survey of Eimeria species in commercially-reared chickens in France during 1994," Avian Pathology, vol. 25, no. 1, pp. 113–130, 1996. · ·

27. S. Sharma, A. Iqbal, S. Azmi, I. Mushtaq, Z. A. Wani, and S. Ahmad, "Prevalence of poultry coccidiosis in Jammu region of Jammu & Kashmir State," Journal of Parasitic Diseases, vol. 39, no. 1, pp. 85–89, 2015. · ·

28. H. A. Bachaya, M. A. Raza, M. N. Khan et al., "Predominance and detection of different eimeria species causing coccidiosis in layer chickens," The Journal of Animal & Plant Sciences, vol. 22, no. 3, pp. 597–600, 2012. ·

29. A. Haug, A.-G. Gjevre, E. Skjerve, and M. Kaldhusdal, "A survey of the economic impact of subclinicalEimeria infections in broiler chickens in Norway," Avian Pathology, vol. 37, no. 3, pp. 333–341, 2008. · ·

30. M. A. A. Shah, S. Uamr, M. F. Iqbal, F. Rehman, I. Qadri, and N. He, "Recent advances in DNA vaccination against coccidiosis," World's Poultry Science Journal, vol. 70, pp. 315–328, 2014.

31. M. Raman, S. S. Banu, S. Gomathinayangam, and G. D. Raj, "Lesion scoring technique for assessing the virulence and pathogenicity of Indian field isolates of avian Eimeria species," Veterinary Archives, vol. 81, pp. 259–271, 2011.

CHAPTER 16

CRYPTOSPORIDIOSIS IN BROILER CHICKENS IN ZHEJIANG PROVINCE, CHINA: MOLECULAR CHARACTERIZATION OF OOCYSTS DETECTED IN FECAL SAMPLES

Lengmei Wang[1], Xue Xue[1], Jianqiu Li[2], Qianjin Zhou[3], Yingchao Yu[1], and Aifang Du[1]

[1]Institute of Preventive Veterinary Medicine, College of Animal Sciences, Zhejiang University, Hangzhou, Zhejiang 310058, PR China

[2] Hangzhou College of Commerce, Zhejiang Gongshang University, Hangzhou, Zhejiang 310012, PR China

[3] Faculty of Life Science and Technology, Ningbo University, Ningbo, Zhejiang 315211, PR China

ABSTRACT

Cryptosporidium is one of the most important parasites in poultry, and this pathogen can infect more than 30 avian species. The present study investigated the infection rate of Cryptosporidium among broiler chicken flocks. A total of 385 fecal samples from broiler chickens in 7 regions of Zhejiang Province collected from November 2010 to January 2012 were examined by microscopy. Thirty-eight (10%) samples were positive for Cryptosporidium infection, and 3 genotypes (Cryptosporidium baileyi, Cryptosporidium meleagridis, and avian genotype II) were identified by PCR and sequencing. A phylogenetic tree of the isolates was analyzed. These results suggest that cryptosporidiosis is widespread in poultry in Zhejiang Province, and is a potential threat to public health as well as the economy. This is the first report about the infection rate and molecular characterization of Cryptosporidium in broiler chickens in Zhejiang.

INTRODUCTION

Cryptosporidiosis is caused by *Cryptosporidium*, which has a broad range of hosts and worldwide distribution. The *Cryptosporidium* species can infect human beings as well as other animals; it is mainly located in the epithelial cells of the gastrointestinal tract, and is likely in the respiratory tract [7], particularly in the case of infection by *C. meleagridis*, a bird species. The main clinical manifestation is persistent diarrhea, and respiratory disturbances can occasionally be observed [5, 12].

Cryptosporidium is one of the most common and important parasites in poultry, and this pathogen can infect more than 30 avian species. Traditionally, three different species of *Cryptosporidium* (*C. baileyi*, *C. meleagridis*, and *C. galli*) were considered to be the major species in birds [4, 6, 17, 20, 23, 30]. Recently, more than 11 novel genotypes have been described which are genetically different from the above three species by means of molecular analysis, including avian genotypes (I–V), goose genotypes (I–IV), the Eurasian woodcock genotype and the black duck genotype [1, 9, 14–17, 20, 31]. *C. meleagridis*, *C. parvum*,*and C. hominis* carried by poultry may infect human beings through the oocysts in contaminated water or vegetables eaten uncooked [1, 13, 20, 31, 32]. Considering that the possibility of exposure to*Cryptosporidium* of human beings still exists, the prevention of Cryptosporidiosis is important for public health [10].

Up to now, there is little information regarding the distribution of *Cryptosporidium* spp. in Zhejiang Province, and also limited data about its molecular characterization in poultry, particularly in chickens. The aim of the present study was to estimate the infection rate of *Cryptosporidium* in poultry in Zhejiang Province, and to determine the genotypes in the area.

Citation: Lengmei Wang, Xue Xue, Jianqiu Li, Qianjin Zhou, Yingchao Yu, and Aifang Du, Cryptosporidiosis in broiler chickens in Zhejiang Province, China: molecular characterization of oocysts detected in fecal samples, DOI: 10.1051/parasite/2014035.

MATERIALS AND METHODS

Sample collection

Three hundred and eighty-five fecal samples were randomly collected from broiler chickens that were around 90 days old in seven regions (Hangzhou, Huzhou, Jiaxing, Jinhua, Ningbo, Quzhou, and Shaoxing) in Zhejiang Province during the period from November 2010 to January 2012. Chickens were reared in steel cages; each contained 5 ~ 7 birds whose feces were collected on the tray under the cages gathered as a mixture. Therefore, the feces in one cage were considered as one sample, collected by the use of disposable plastic gloves, marked with the region name, serial number, and collection date. The sampling process was conducted to collect the fresh droppings to the best of our ability. The weight of each sample was approximately equal to about 50 g. Samples were kept in ice boxes until they were transported to the laboratory, then stored in the refrigerator at 4 °C and processed as soon as possible.

Microscopy detection

Samples were handled by Sheather's sugar flotation method as previously described by Huber et al. [8], and*Cryptosporidium* oocysts were examined by optical microscopy observation under 400× magnification based on the shape of oocysts and the shape index measured. Subsequently, the positive samples containing oocysts were stored in 2.5% potassium dichromate and kept at 4 °C until DNA extraction.

DNA extraction

Oocysts in positive samples were purified by discontinuous sucrose density gradient centrifugation [3]. For genomic DNA extraction, 100 μL of suspension liquid containing oocysts was frozen-thawed for 5 min in liquid nitrogen and then kept in a 65 °C water bath kettle for 5 min. The process was repeated three times, then the treated samples were centrifuged at 12 000 × g for 5 min. The genomic DNA was extracted using a Genomic DNA Extraction Kit (TaKaRa Biotechnology (Dalian) Co. Ltd., Dalian, China) in accordance with the manufacturer's instructions, and kept at −20 °C until detected by the PCR method.

Nested-PCR amplification and sequencing

A nested PCR was done in order to amplify a fragment of approximately 830 bp [30]. Then, the secondary purified PCR product was sequenced (BGI sequencing) to confirm the species/genotype identification.

Cryptosporidium genotyping and phylogenetic analysis

The acquired sequences were submitted to a BLAST search (http://blast.ncbi.nlm.nih.gov/Blast.cgi) to initially define the species/genotypes and to confirm the high similarity and homology with other known sequences of *Cryptosporidium* spp. in GenBank. All sequences were multiple-aligned and analyzed by Bioedit and MEGA 4.0 software (http://www.mbio.ncsu.edu/BioEdit/bioedit.html andhttp://www.megasoftware.net/). A neighbor-joining cladogram was built using MEGA 4.0. To assess the reliability of this tree, bootstrap analysis was done with 1000 replicates using the Kimura 2-parameter logarithm.

The partial 18S rRNA nucleotide sequences obtained in this study have been deposited in the GenBank database under accession numbers JX548291–JX548300.

Statistical analysis

The infection rate of *Cryptosporidium* was analyzed using the chi-square test. Differences were considered significant when $P < 0.05$.

RESULTS

Infection rate of *Cryptosporidium* in Zhejiang Province

Of the 385 fecal samples from broiler chickens examined in this study, 38 samples were positive, and the overall infection rate of *Cryptosporidium* was 9.9%. The infection rate of *Cryptosporidium* varied among the seven regions. The highest infection rate was 16.9% in Huzhou, followed by 16.7% in Hangzhou, 12.1% in Ningbo, 7.7% in Shaoxing, 5.3% in Jiaxing, 4.0% in Quzhou, and 2.3% in Jinhua (Table 1). Significant statistical differences were not found in relation to the geographical provenance of chickens and infection rates in each region.

Table 1: Infection rate of *Cryptosporidium* in different source supplied for the native chicken

Region	No. of cages examined	No. of cages *Cryptosporidium* positive	Infection rate (%)	*Cryptosporidium* species/genotypes (No. of isolates)
Hangzhou	66	11	16.7	*C. baileyi* (10), *C. meleagridis* (1)
Huzhou	59	10	16.9	*C. baileyi* (7), *C. meleagridis* (1), Avian genotype II (2)
Shaoxing	52	4	7.70	*C. baileyi* (4)
Ningbo	58	7	12.1	*C. baileyi* (6), Avian genotype II (1)
Jiaxing	57	3	5.26	*C. baileyi* (3)
Jinhua	43	1	2.33	*C. baileyi* (1)
Quzhou	50	2	4.00	*C. baileyi* (2)
Total	385	38	9.87	*C. baileyi* (33), *C. meleagridis* (2), Avian genotype II (3)

Distribution of *Cryptosporidium* species

Two species and one genotype, including *C. baileyi*, *C. meleagridis*, and the avian genotype II, were identified through morphological observation and sequencing. *C. baileyi* was widely distributed in the seven areas. 33 of 38 positive samples were for *C. baileyi* infection (86.8%), only two samples for *C. meleagridis*infection (5.3%), and three samples for avian genotype II infection (7.9%). Moreover, the average size of oocysts for *C. baileyi* was 5.96 μm × 4.73 μm by measuring 35 oocysts, for *C. meleagridis* it was 4.96 μm × 4.15 μm, and for avian genotype II it was 6.02 μm × 5.47 μm. The neighbor-joining among these species/genotypes and other previously described species and genotypes of *Cryptosporidium* is shown in Figure 1.

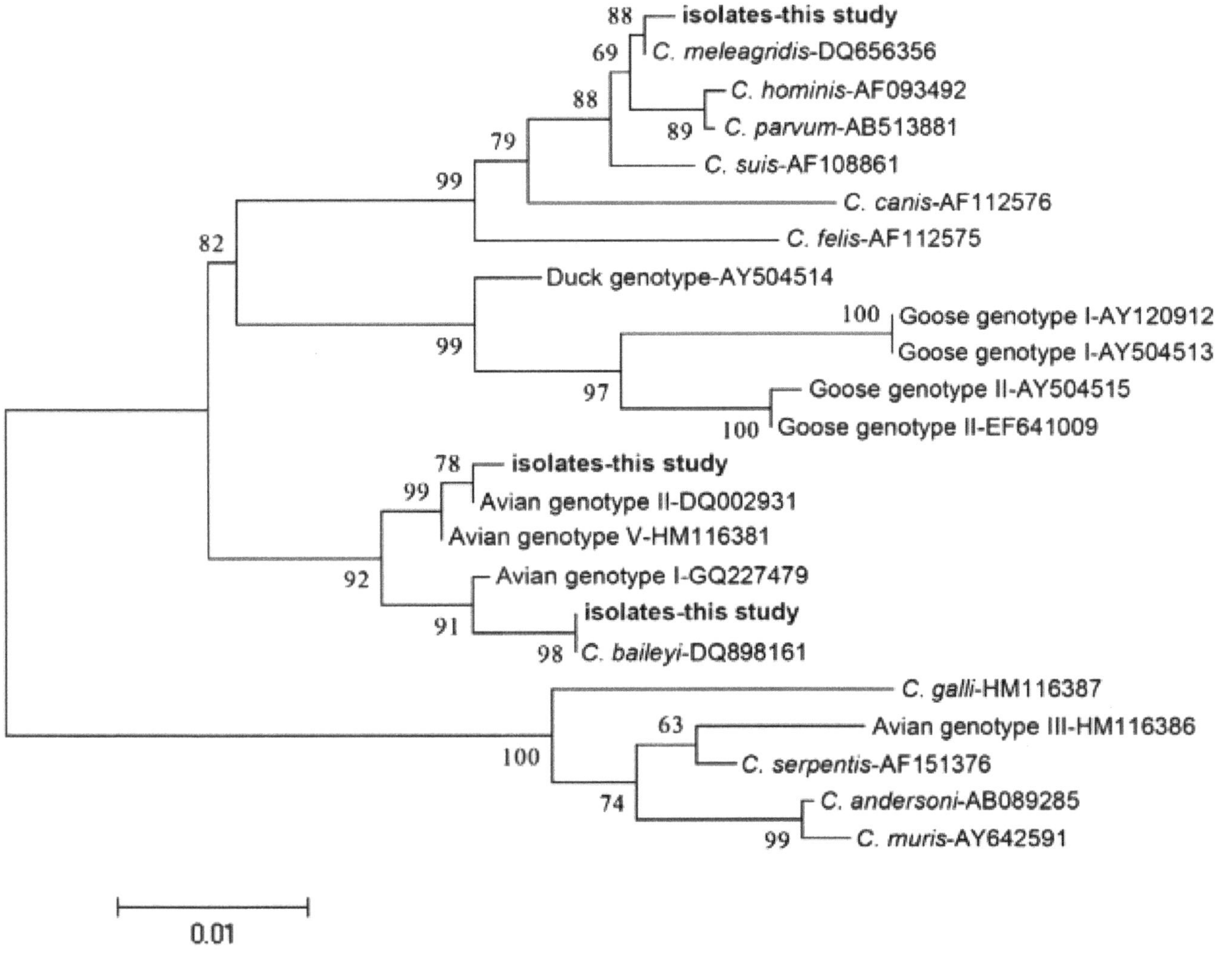

Figure 1: Phylogenetic tree of *Cryptosporidium* spp. built by the neighbor-joining method using Mega 4.0, based on 18S rRNA. To assess the reliability of this tree, bootstrap analysis was done with 1000 replicates.

Sequence and phylogenetic analysis

The 18S rRNA gene of *C. baileyi* isolates showed high sequence homology with each other by direct sequence alignment, and exhibited 99% sequence similarity with a GenBank sequence of quail origin (DQ898161). Two *C. meleagridis* isolates showed 99.5% sequence similarity with a GenBank sequence from Iran (DQ656356). Three avian genotype II isolates showed 99.2% sequence similarity with a GenBank sequence (DQ002931).

DISCUSSION

Cryptosporidium is widespread around the world except Antarctica, and is most common in developing countries and less developed countries [22]. Thus far, there are few data available about the infection rate of*Cryptosporidium* in poultry, especially in chickens in China. It was reported that the infection rate of*Cryptosporidium* was 3.4% in Henan and 23.8% in Shandong, China [26, 27]. Moreover, the rate was 3.75% in the Garmsar region, Iran, and 4.5% in Tunisia [21, 24]. It was clear that the overall rate in this study was much higher than in other countries. We speculate that this difference may be attributed to the different approaches in the sample collection. In our study, the fecal sample was collected from a pool of animals; thus, it is possible to find a higher rate of infection when compared with individual samples. Moreover, the various environmental factors and host species may also account for the difference [2]. The differences between different studies may be due to various factors such as seasonality, the age of chickens, the breeding environment, etc. Given the similar climate of the regions in Zhejiang Province, the interregional variation in infection rates observed could be due to the nutrient levels, breeding conditions and the density of animals [11–25].

In China, the infection rate of *Cryptosporidium* derived from poultry has been reported so far in almost 10 provinces. However, most researchers were focused on the prevalence in the region through traditional morphological observation, rather than identifying the species or genotypes of the *Cryptosporidium* by modern molecular biology approaches. One exception is Henan Province. In more recent studies, the prevalence of *Cryptosporidium* spp. has been reported in detail in quails, chickens, Pekin ducks, pet birds, and ostriches in Henan, and most species have been identified as *C. baileyi* and *C. meleagridis* [18, 27–29]. The epidemiological investigation of *Cryptosporidium* in poultry in Zhejiang Province was carried out in our research.

Among the three *Cryptosporidium* species/genotypes identified in this study, *C. baileyi* was the primary species of the broiler chickens, for the reason that it was not only widely distributed in the seven areas, but also had the highest percentage of positive samples (33/38). Thus, the phenomenon of *C. baileyi* infection in broiler chickens in this study confirmed the following views. *C. baileyi*, which is the most common species in poultry, has more than 20 kinds of hosts including chickens [19]. In addition, studies in China showed that most cases in chickens were diagnosed as *C. baileyi* infections, which can slow down the growth rate in broilers and decrease egg production of layer chickens. Because the poultry industry plays a critical role in the agricultural economy in China, it is essential to pay sufficient attention to this pathogen. Only two isolates were identified as *C. meleagridis* in our investigation. Meanwhile, *C. meleagridis* had extensive hosts too, and it could cause deadly diseases in immunocompromised persons [19]. People could be infected with *C. meleagridis* by potential zoonotic transmission when the chickens carry the pathogen. Therefore, it has a great influence on public health. Three isolates were identified as avian genotype II in the present study. Avian genotype II was first described in turkey and was reported in parrot in the same year [14, 16]. Afterward, avian genotype II was found in ostriches [17]. Recently, chickens have also appeared to be a new host for avian genotype II. Perhaps we could make a bold conjecture that avian genotype II also has a range of hosts like *C. baileyi* and *C. meleagridis*. In addition, according to the phylogenetic analyses of 18S rRNA, together with the analysis based on actin and HSP70 in a previous study by Abe and Makino [1], it is further assumed that avian genotype II has a close relationship with avian genotype V at a genetic level. The cladogram in the present study proved the above points, which demonstrated the reliability of the tree.

In conclusion, this is the first report about the infection rate and molecular characterization of*Cryptosporidium* in broiler chickens in Zhejiang. The results suggest that *Cryptosporidium* is widespread in poultry in Zhejiang Province, and may pose a potential threat to public health as well as the economy.

ACKNOWLEDGMENTS

This work was supported by a grant from the Science and Technology Department of Zhejiang Province (Grant number 2012C12009-2). The authors thank the team of the Parasite Laboratory, College of Animal Sciences, Zhejiang University.

REFERENCES

1. Abe N, Makino I. 2010. Multilocus genotypic analysis of *Cryptosporidium* isolates from cockatiels, Japan. Parasitology Research, 106, 1491–1497
2. Amer S, Zidan S, Adamu H, Ye J, Roellig D, Xiao L, Feng Y. 2013. Prevalence and characterization of*Cryptosporidium* spp. in dairy cattle in Nile River delta provinces, Egypt. Experimental Parasitology, 135, 518–523
3. Arrowood MJ, Donaldson K. 1996. Improved purification methods for calf-derived *Cryptosporidium parvum* oocysts using discontinuous sucrose and cesium chloride gradients. Journal of Eukaryotic Microbiology, 43, S89–S89
4. Current WL, Upton SJ, Haynes TB. 1986. The life cycle of *Cryptosporidium baileyi* n. sp. (Apicomplexa, Cryptosporidiidae) infecting chickens. Journal of Protozoology, 33, 289–296
5. Das G, Changkija B, Sarkar S, Das P. 2011. Genotyping of *Cryptosporidium parvum* isolates in bovine population in Kolkata and characterization of new bovine genotypes. Research in Veterinary Science, 91, 246–250
6. Fayer R. 2010. Taxonomy and species delimitation in *Cryptosporidium*. Experimental Parasitology, 124, 90–97
7. Gomes RS, Huber F, da Silva S, do Bomfim TC. 2012. *Cryptosporidium* spp. parasitize exotic birds that are commercialized in markets, commercial aviaries, and pet shops. Parasitology Research, 110, 1363–1370
8. Huber F, Bomfim TC, Gomes RS. 2005. Comparison between natural infection by *Cryptosporidium* sp.,*Giardia* sp. in dogs in two living situations in the West Zone of the municipality of Rio de Janeiro. Veterinary Parasitology, 130, 69–72
9. Jellison KL, Distel DL, Hemond HF, Schauer DB. 2004. Phylogenetic analysis of the hypervariable region of the 18S rRNA gene of *Cryptosporidium* oocysts in feces of Canada geese (*Branta canadensis*): evidence for five novel genotypes. Applied and Environmental Microbiology, 70, 452–458
10. Karanis P, Kourenti C, Smith H. 2007. Waterborne transmission of protozoan parasites: a worldwide review of outbreaks and lessons learnt. Journal of Water and Health, 5, 1–38
11. Lai M, Zhou RQ, Huang HC, Hu SJ. 2011. Prevalence and risk factors associated with intestinal parasites in pigs in Chongqing, China. Research in Veterinary Science, 91, e121–e124
12. Langsley G, van Noort V, Carret C, Meissner M, de Villiers EP, Bishop R, Pain A. 2008. Comparative genomics of the Rab protein family in Apicomplexan parasites. Microbes and Infection, 10, 462–470
13. Majewska AC, Graczyk TK, Slodkowicz-Kowalska A, Tamang L, Jedrzejewski S, Zduniak P, Solarczyk P, Nowosad A, Nowosad P. 2009. The role of free-ranging, captive, and domestic birds of Western Poland in environmental contamination with *Cryptosporidium parvum* oocysts and *Giardia lamblia*cysts. Parasitology Research, 104, 1093–1099
14. Meireles MV, Soares RM, dos Santos MM, Gennari SM. 2006. Biological studies and molecular characterization of a *Cryptosporidium isolate* from ostriches (*Struthio camelus*). Journal of Parasitology, 92, 623–626
15. Morgan UM, Monis PT, Xiao L, Limor J, Sulaiman I, Raidal S, O'Donoghue P, Gasser R, Murray A, Fayer R, Blagburn BL, Lal AA, Thompson RC. 2001. Molecular and phylogenetic characterisation of*Cryptosporidium* from birds. International Journal for Parasitology, 31, 289–296
16. Ng J, Pavlasek I, Ryan U. 2006. Identification of novel *Cryptosporidium* genotypes from avian hosts. Applied and Environmental Microbiology, 72, 7548–7553
17. Nguyen ST, Fukuda Y, Tada C, Huynh VV, Nguyen DT, Nakai Y. 2013. Prevalence and molecular characterization

of *Cryptosporidium* in ostriches (*Struthio camelus*) on a farm in central Vietnam.Experimental Parasitology, 133, 8–11

18. Qi M, Wang R, Ning C, Li X, Zhang L, Jian F, Sun Y, Xiao L. 2011. *Cryptosporidium* spp. in pet birds: genetic diversity and potential public health significance. Experimental Parasitology, 128, 336–340
19. Ryan U. 2010. *Cryptosporidium* in birds, fish and amphibians. Experimental Parasitology, 124, 113–120
20. Ryan UM, Xiao L, Read C, Sulaiman IM, Monis P, Lal AA, Fayer R, Pavlasek I. 2003. A redescription of *Cryptosporidium galli* Pavlasek, 1999 (Apicomplexa: Cryptosporidiidae) from birds. Journal of Parasitology, 89, 809–813
21. Shemshadi B, Rangbar Bahadori S, Mozafari A. 2010. Study on cryptosporidiosis incidence in broilers in Garmsar region, Iran. Comparative Clinical Pathology, 20, 143–149
22. Shirley D, Moonah S, Kotloff K. 2012. Burden of disease from cryptosporidiosis. Current Opinion in Infectious Diseases, 25, 555–563
23. Slavin D. 1955. *Cryptosporidium meleagridis* (sp. nov.). Journal of Comparative Pathology, 65, 262–266
24. Soltane R, Guyot K, Dei-Cas E, Ayadi A. 2007. Prevalence of *Cryptosporidium* spp. (Eucoccidiorida: Cryptosporiidae) in seven species of farm animals in Tunisia. Parasite, 14, 335–338
25. Taylor M, Webster K. 1998. Recent advances in the diagnosis in livestock of *Cryptosporidium*,*Toxoplasma*, *Giardia* and other protozoa of veterinary importance. Research in Veterinary Science, 65, 183–193
26. Ti-sen X. 2009. Epidemiological investigation of *Cryptosporidium* from poultry in Shandong province. Chinese Journal of Veterinary Medicine, 4, 3–5
27. Wang R, Jian F, Sun Y, Hu Q, Zhu J, Wang F, Ning C, Zhang L, Xiao L. 2010. Large-scale survey of*Cryptosporidium* spp. in chickens and Pekin ducks (*Anas platyrhynchos*) in Henan, China: prevalence and molecular characterization. Avian Pathology, 39, 447–451
28. Wang R, Qi M, Zhu J, Sun D, Ning C, Zhao J, Zhang L, Xiao L. 2011. Prevalence of *Cryptosporidium baileyi* in ostriches (*Struthio camelus*) in Zhengzhou, China. Veterinary Parasitology, 175, 151–154
29. Wang R, Wang F, Zhao J, Qi M, Ning C, Zhang L, Xiao L. 2012. *Cryptosporidium* spp. in quails (*Coturnix coturnix japonica*) in Henan, China: Molecular characterization and public health significance. Veterinary Parasitology, 187, 534–537
30. Xiao L, Fayer R, Ryan U, Upton SJ. 2004. *Cryptosporidium* taxonomy: recent advances and implications for public health. Clinical Microbiology Reviews, 17, 72–97
31. Zhou L, Kassa H, Tischler ML, Xiao L. 2004. Host-adapted *Cryptosporidium* spp. in Canada geese (*Branta canadensis*). Applied and Environmental Microbiology, 70, 4211–4215
32. Zhou P, Chen N, Zhang R-L, Lin R-Q, Zhu X-Q. 2008. Food-borne parasitic zoonoses in China: perspective for control. Trends in Parasitology, 24, 190–196

CHAPTER 17

HISTOMONOSIS - AN EXISTING PROBLEM IN CHICKEN FLOCKS IN POLAND

Beata Dolka[1] & Artur Żbikowski [1] & Izabella Dolka[1] & Piotr Szeleszczuk[1]

[1]Department of Pathology and Veterinary Diagnostics, Faculty of Veterinary Medicine, Warsaw University of Life Sciences-SGGW, Nowoursynowska 159c St., 02-776 Warsaw, Poland

ABSTRACT

Histomonosis (histomoniasis, blackhead), beside coccidiosis, belongs to the most important parasitic protozoan diseases in poultry. So far Histomonas meleagridis infections with varied mortality rates have been mainly diagnosed in young turkeys. Recently an increasing number of cases have been reported in chicken flocks in Europe resulting in economic losses. It is thought that this situation is predominantly caused by a complete withdrawal of the effective antihistomonals in the EU. Authors listed the selected outbreaks of histomonosis in 10 chicken flocks originated from different farms of 4 regions in Poland: 8 broiler breeder flocks (at mean age of 33 weeks) and 2 commercial layers flocks (at mean age of 38 weeks). This study reported here naturally occurring case of H.meleagridis infection in commercial broiler breeder (BB) flock line ROSS 308 at the age of 16 weeks. We showed acute form of infection with characteristic necrotic foci in the liver, and ulcerative typhilitis. Beside the liver and caeca, the multiple histomonads, lymphoid tissue depletion and heavy destruction in the bursa of Fabricius were observed. Additionally, the absence of systemic diffuse histomonads and lack of Heterakis gallinarum, caecal worm eggs in faecal samples were noted. PCR technique enabled to detect the presence of H.meleagridis genetic material in the investigated tissue samples. Authors indicate that histomonosis can be considered as re-emerging infectious diseases in chicken flocks of intensive production system.

INTRODUCTION

Histomonosis (also known as Blackhead) is one of the most important diseases in poultry caused by the flagellated protozoon *Histomonas meleagridis*. The diseases is mainly associated with the turkeys, due to their susceptibility to *H. meleagridis* and economic importance, however other bird species, such as: chickens, pheasant, peafowl, quail, partridge, guinea fowl, duck and ostrich may also be prone to infection. Although the first cases were described in 1895 in turkeys and in 1900 in chickens, the disease still poses a serious threat to the poultry industry due to the mortality (McDougald 2005; Hess and McDougald 2013). For many years chemotherapeutics have been used in histomonosis prevention and treatment, especially nitroimidazoles (metronidazole, dimetridazole, ronidazole), nitrofurans (furazolidone), arsenical derivatives (e.g., nitarsone, roxarsone, acetarsol). However, their use in poultry has been banned in countries belonging to the European Union (EU), due to the serious risk to public health (possible toxic and cancerogenic effects). The ban of these products in combination with the changes in animal husbandry were followed by an upsurge in reported cases in poultry (CEC 2003; Hess et al. 2006; Callait-Cardinal et al. 2007; EFSA 2013; Hess et al.2015). As a consequence, the problem of histomonosis has escalated in chickens. Histomonosis

Citation: Beata Dolka & Artur Żbikowski & Izabella Dolka & Piotr Szeleszczuk, Histomonosis - an existing problem in chicken flocks in Poland, DOI 10.1007/s11259-015-9637-2.

in chickens has been noted in some European countries i.a. Belgium (layers, Esquenet et al. 2003), Austria (layers, Grafl et al. 2011), in the Netherlands (layers, Van der Heijden and Landman 2011), in Denmark (layers, Stokholm et al. 2010), Germany (broilers, Popp et al. 2011; layers, Hafez et al. 2001; chickens, Hauck et al. 2010), also in the USA (leghorn pullets, Homer and Butcher 1991) and in Asia: Malaysia (broilers; Ganapathy et al.2000), India (broiler breeder flock; Banerjee et al. 2006), (broilers; Patra et al. 2013). Moreover, the serological evidences for *H.meleagridis* distribution in layer chicken flocks kept in different housing systems (Grafl et al. 2011; Van der Heijden and Landman 2011) and genotypic variations of parasite isolates have been shown (Bilic et al. 2014). It is considered that the type of poultry farming and hygienic conditions significantly influence the spread of the disease (Esquenet et al. 2003; Grafl et al. 2011). Renewed efforts in histomonosis investigations have led to new insights into the epidemiology and molecular characterization of*H. meleagridis* (Grabensteiner et al. 2006; Hess et al. 2006; Hu et al. 2006; Bilic et al. 2014; Lotfi et al. 2014; Hess et al. 2015). In order to improve control strategies, the research studies have boosted to develop of new treatment and prophylactic strategies including vaccination (Hu and McDougald 2002; Bleyen et al. 2009; Hafez et al. 2010; Van der Heijden et al. 2011; Liebhart et al. 2013; Hess et al. 2015).

The main goal of current study was to investigate the prevalence of natural infection of *Histomonas meleagridis* in commercial broiler breeder flock as well as highlight the problem of histomonosis involving chickens raised in the intensive farming systems.

MATERIALS AND METHODS

Case presentation, clinical history, treatment

Six 16-weeks-old chickens from affected broiler breeder flock line ROSS 308 which showed clinical signs before death were submitted to the Division of Avian Diseases, Faculty of Veterinary Medicine at the Warsaw University of Life Sciences. Case history revealed that the chicken farm was situated about 100 m from a road which was used to transport feed, chickens and poultry manure; 1 km from other broiler breeder farm, and about 2 km from a commercial turkey farm. In the investigated farm the parent stock was kept for the third time with the initial chickens number of 30 081. The farm was operated according to the all-in all-out system. There was 2 weeks interval between each introduction of new chickens to the production house, during which the hot cleaning and disinfection were performed with the use of Rapicid solution (Evans Vanodine International, UK), liquid ammonia, sodium hypochlorite solution, Aldekol Des® 03 (Ewabo, Germany), formaldehyde fumigation (used twice), and thermal disinfection (open flame). The flocks had no access to outdoor areas. The breeding conditions, vaccination program and feeding were conducted in accordance with the standards for this type of poultry production system. Chickens were vaccinated (at 3 days of age) against coccidiosis and they were routinely dewormed at 8 and 14 weeks of age through the administration levamisole in drinking water. At the beginning of rearing period the birds were kept in three grow-out houses (two facilities held 24 000 hens, one 6 000 roosters) and one house remained empty. In the 5th week of rearing the hens were divided into two flocks by moving 15 819 birds into the empty production house. In this house, the onset of disease was noted in 16-weeks-old chickens. Serum samples were randomly collected from 23 chickens at the age of 16 weeks and tested using ELISA (Idexx, USA) for antibodies against infectious bursal disease virus (IBDV) and infectious anemia virus (CIAV). Before the onset of disease, the flock was vaccinated against IBD according to the immunoprophylaxis program. Vaccination against CIA was planned at 19 weeks of age. Serological investigation showed 100 and 95.5 % positive samples for antibodies against IBDV (geometric mean titer 6371) and CIAV (S/N 0.081) respectively.

The owner of the investigated poultry farm was advised to treat the infected flock with herbal preparation composed of natural extracts from plants and aromatic substances (Fitotril, Chemifarma, Italy) in a dose of 200 mL/100 L of water for 7 days. Additionally, flubendazol (Solubenol, Janssen Animal Health, Belgium) was used for deworming the chickens at 19 weeks of age in a dose of 1.43 mg/kg body weight daily, administered orally in drinking water for 7 days. Moreover, the disinfectants used for foot mats in front of chicken house were replaced with the solution contained glutaraldehyde. The litter used to cover the losses was replaced with a new one free from soil and earthworms.

Necropsy and histopathological examination

During necropsy, tissue samples (liver, spleen, small intestines, caeca, kidney, bursa of Fabricius) were collected for histopathological examination. After fixation in 10 % buffered formalin, tissue specimens were processed, embedded in paraffin and finally stained with hematoxylin and eosin (H-E).

Parasitological examination

The faecal samples were collected for examination by using normal saline solution direct smear wet preparation technique. The liver and caeca samples were stained with Hemacolor® kit (Merck, Germany) and observed under microscope (Olympus, Japan). The visual inspection for intestinal parasites, including*Heterakis gallinarum* in the caeca was undertaken.

Microbiological examination

Microbiological examination were performed on samples from liver, spleen and caeca, which were cultured in standard and selective media (Columbia agar with 5 % sheep blood, MacConkey agar).

Polymerase chain reaction (PCR)

PCR technique was used to detect the presence of *Histomonas meleagridis* genetic material in the liver and intestinal samples. A 25 mg of organ material was taken for DNA extraction using Chelex 100 (Biorad, Poland) and Sherlock AX kit (A&A Biotechnology, Poland) according to manufacturers' instructions. Amplification of *H. meleagridis* DNA was done using a species specific pair of primers Hmf 5′-GAAAGCATCTATCAAGTGGAA-3′, Hmr 5′ GATCTTTTCAAATTAGCTTTAAA-3′ previously described by Grabensteiner and Hess (2006). The each reaction mixture consisted of 25 μl DreamTaq PCR Master Mix (2X), 0.5 μM of each primer, 4 μl DNA and PCR-clean water (added up to a volume of 50 µl). PCR conditions were used in accordance with Grabensteiner and Hess (2006): initial denaturation at 95 °C for 5 min, followed by 35 cycles: denaturation at 95 °C for 60 s, annealing at 50 °C for 45 s, extension at 72 °C for 120 s. Thereafter, the samples were maintained at 72 °C for 10 min for final extension step. Amplification products (10 µl) were analyzed by agarose gel (1.2 %) electrophoresis after ethidium bromide staining and visualized under UV light (UVP, USA). Fragment sizes were determined with reference to a 100 bp ladder (Thermo Fisher Scientific Inc., USA). The expected PCR product size was 574 bp.

RESULTS

Clinical signs and mortality

For the first 15 weeks of rearing period, the chickens showed no obvious clinical signs, even though mortality was recorded (1.2 %). In details, between 1 and 4 week the mortality was 1.33 % (99.8 birds/per week), then 1.05 % between 5 and 15 week (15.1 birds/per week, after moving to the new house). Beginning from 16 weeks of age, the symptoms were noticed. The chickens showed untypical behaviour, manifested by aversion to moving, sitting on hocks, depression, ruffled feathers, drooping wings. Additionally, decreased of feed and water uptake were noted. The mortality reached 5.01 % (49.6 birds/per day; 347.2 birds/per week) within approx. 2 weeks with a peak on day 114 (102 birds/per day). After the peak the fluctuations in daily losses were observed (gradual reduction to 63 birds at 116 day, then increase up to 82 birds at 118 day). In total, 6.6 % (74.1 birds/per week) of chickens have died in this house between 5 and 19 weeks of age.

In Table 1 we presented the list of 10 selected outbreaks of histomonosis in commercial chicken flocks: 8 broiler breeder (BB) and 2 commercial layers flocks (CL). All flocks originated from different farms located on 4 of 16 voivodeships in Poland. Total of 4 voivodeships were located nearby and represented areas with intensive chicken (Mazovian and Greater Poland voivodeship) and turkey production in Poland (Warmian-Masurian, Lubusz and Greater Poland voivodeship). The histomonosis was diagnosed based on clinical data, pathological lesions (including histopathological examination in cases from three flocks) and PCR (in cases from five flocks). The mean age at onset of clinical signs was 33 weeks in BB and 38 weeks in CL flocks. The age of each flock was showed in Table 1.

Table 1: The list of selected outbreaks of histomonosis in commercial chicken flocks in Poland

Case	Date of diagnosis (month, year)	Type of production	Age of birds (weeks) at which clinical signs were noticed	Farm location (voivodeship)	Clinical & postmortem diagnosis (Yes/No)	Confirmation by PCR (Yes/No)	Undertaken therapy (Yes/No)
1	11.2002	BB	40	Mazovian	Yes	No	No
2	01.2010	BB	16	Mazovian	Yes	Yes	Nd
3	01.2010	BB	16	Lubusz	Yes	Yes	Yes
4	02.2010	BB	44	Mazovian	Yes	No	Nd
5	12.2010	BB	44	Warmian-Masurian	Yes	No	Yes
6	03.2011	BB	40	Mazovian	Yes	No	Yes
7	03.2011	CL	25	Greater Poland	Yes	Yes	Nd
8	03.2011	CL	51	Mazovian	Yes	Yes	Yes
9	08.2012	BB	19	Warmian-Masurian	Yes	No	Yes
10	02.2014	BB	42	Mazovian	Yes	Yes	Nd

BB Broiler Breeders, *CL* Commercial Layers, *Nd* no data

Necropsy and histopathological examination

The external inspection of carcasses revealed severe emaciation, mat feathers and cloaca covered with faeces. During necropsy, an advanced liver damage manifested with enlargement, congestion with numerous yellow necrotic foci were noted (Fig. 1a). Additionally, we noted spleen congestion with beige rounded areas of necrosis, pulmonary congestion and obliterated structure of folds bursa of Fabricius. The kidneys were pale brown with increased urates in the ureters. We noted haemorrhagic inflammation of small intestine, thickening of the caecal wall with caseous inflammation and the ulceration of the mucosa (Fig. 1b).

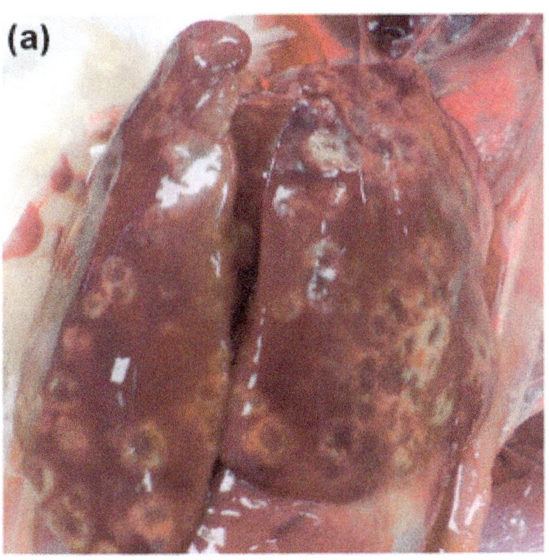

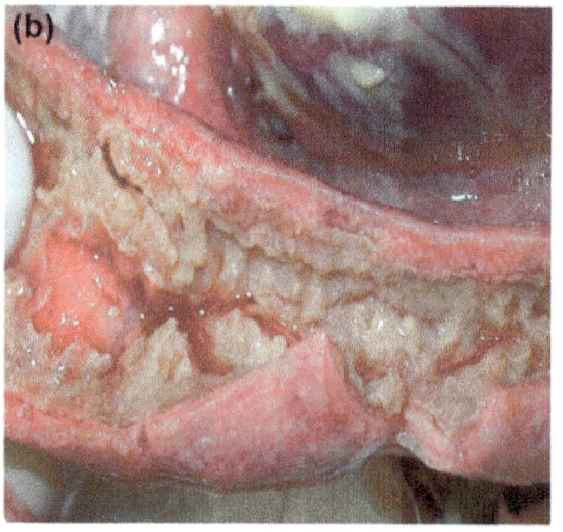

Figure 1: Macroscopic lesions in liver (**a**) and in caeca (**b**) in chickens.

Histopathological examination showed massive multifocal necrosis and haemorrhages in the liver, moderate infiltration of mononuclear cells and multiple flagellated forms of the trophozoite dispersed within the organ (Fig. 2a). Furthermore, in the caeca were found trophozoites under the layer of exudation and multiple bacteria. Haemorrhage lesions were noted in kidneys, together with parenchyma degeneration and necrosis. Bursa of Fabricius showed depletion of lymphoid tissue and focal localization of trophozoites in the cytoplasm of phagocytes (Fig. 2b).

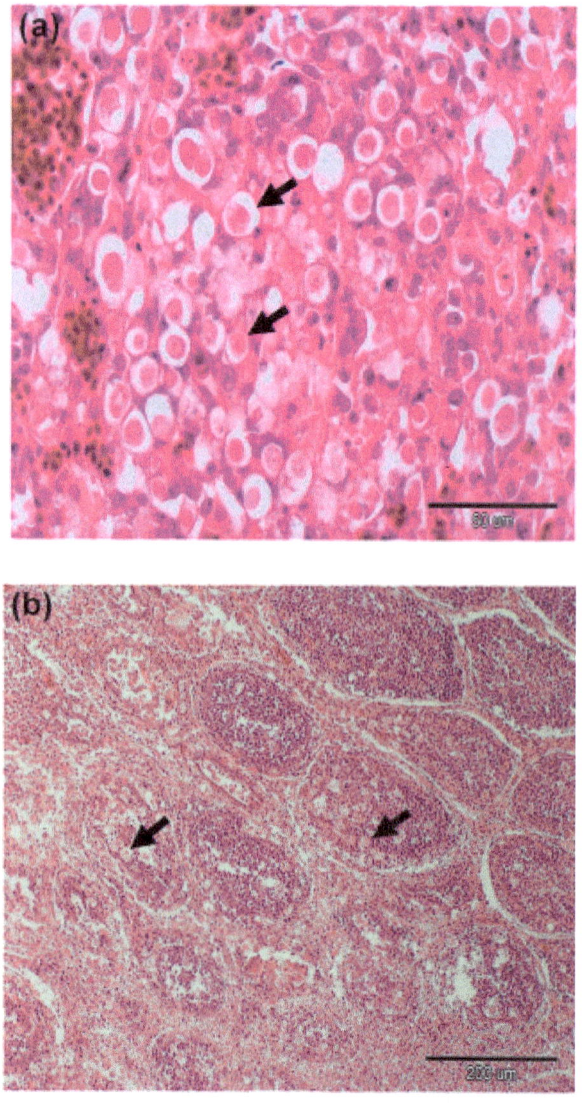

Figure 2: Histopathology of liver (**a**) and bursa of Fabricius (**b**) with multiple oval-shaped histomonads (*arrows*). Original magnifications: 400x (**a**), 100x (**b**); hematoxylin-eosin staining (H-E).

Parasitological examination

The parasitological examination showed no presence of oocysts, nematodes or their eggs in faecal samples. Direct microscopic examination of the caecal contents as well as stained preparations did not reveal the presence of protozoa.

Microbiological examination

Microbiological cultures enabled to identify numerous bacteria of *Gallibacterium* spp.

PCR

The parasite *H.meleagridis* DNA was detected in analyzed liver and caecal samples (Fig. 3).

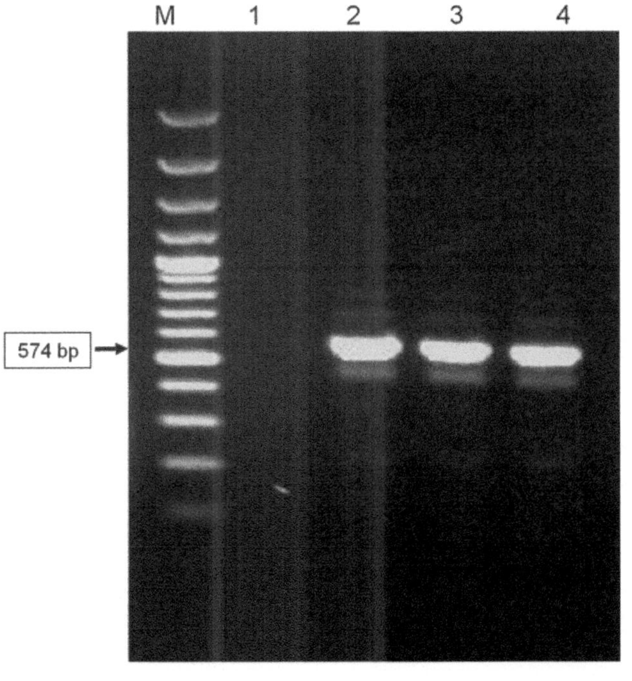

Figure 3: Agarose gel electrophoresis showing PCR amplification of fragment DNA Histomonas meleagridis. From left: M-molecular size marker (100 bp ladder); 1-negative control, 2-positive control; 3-liver sample; 4-caeca sample. The length of PCR product was 574 bp.

DISCUSSION

Although several previous studies have investigated the prevalence of *H.meleagridis* infections in chickens (Tyzzer 1934; Gerth et al. 1985; Homer and Butcher 1991; McDougald 2005), the recent reports placed these birds next to the turkeys as the main affected poultry species (Callait-Cardinal et al. 2007; EFSA 2013; Hess and McDougald 2013; Hess et al. 2015). Many outbreaks of histomonosis in chickens have been reported in free-range systems, including organic flocks (Hafez et al. 2001; Esquenet et al. 2003; Stokholm et al. 2010; Popp et al. 2011). The present study supports the findings that chicken flocks in intensive production systems may be seriously affected. In contrast to the turkeys, histomonosis in chickens is known as usually less fatal, may be unnoticed and cause decrease in the performance indicators (McDougald 2005; Hess and McDougald 2013). Other reports documented more severe clinical signs, characterized by decrease in egg production and increased mortality in chicken flocks (Ganapathy et al. 2000; Esquenet et al. 2003; Popp et al. 2011). In comparison to above reports, experimental studies indicated on the role of chickens as an asymptomatic parasite carriers (Hess et al. 2006). Clinically, in our study the affected chickens exhibited mortality with apparent clinical signs. The observed symptoms were nonspecific, generalized and similar to those described in the literature (Popp et al. 2011; Hess and McDougald 2013). However, chickens showed no cyanosis of the head opposited to other reports (Ganapathy et al. 2000; Esquenet et al. 2003) and did not suffer from foamy or yellow diarrhoea, which is more typical for infected turkeys (Ganapathy et al. 2000; Cortes et al. 2004; McDougald 2005). In our study mortality rate was lower than recorded in chickens (Ganapathy et al. 2000; McDougald 2005; Popp et al. 2011) also after experimental infection (Desowitz1951). On the other hand the noted mortality was higher than in pullets (Homer and Butcher 1991) or in commercial broilers (Cortes et al. 2004). In the examined flock, between 5 and 15 weeks, when no signs were observed the mortality was 1.05 % (0.1 % birds died/per week). After that, mortality in the flock reached 5.01 % in the period of disease spreading (2.2 % birds died/per week). Our results were similar to data obtained by Esquenet et al. (2003). However, according to the above authors, at time when no problems were observed mortality in the flock was approximately 0.20 % per week, then gradually rose to reach a peak of 1.05 %. Based on the field reports, mortality tends to be moderate (10–40 birds/week), but lingers for several weeks (McDougald 2005). Similarly to above author, chicken deaths were recorded constantly for many weeks. On the other hand, in our study, a rapid increase in mortality with the highest losses (347.2 birds/per week) was observed only during approx. 2 weeks of the disease (at 16 and 17 week).

Interestingly, we noted that older chickens were more likely to be affected by acute histomonosis than reported in previous literature (Desowitz 1951; Homer and Butcher 1991; Ganapathy et al. 2000; Popp et al.2011). Zahoor et al. (2011) showed in experimental studies, that chickens may show frequently milder course of infection without clinical signs and mortality, despite of significant lesions in caeca. It is connected with the mechanism of early immune response activated in the intestinal mucosa, especially in caecal tonsils (Powell et al. 2009; Windisch and Hess 2010). Lotfi et al. (2014) suggested that, the genetic background of the chickens influences the reaction to infection with *H. meleagridis*.

It has been shown that hot and humid weather may exacerbated the histomonosis severity in chickens (Ganapathy et al. 2000). The field outbreaks in turkeys have occurred more frequently in the hottest months (Callait-Cardinal et al. 2007). Although in the present study, the outbreak of diseases occurred in winter month, the environmental conditions including microclimatic might be involved on manifestation of the disease.

According to the previous reports, the most prominent histomonosis-associated gross lesions were localised in the liver and caeca of chickens (Stokholm et al. 2010; Patra et al. 2013). The presence of multiple diffuse necrotic foci in the whole liver indicated on advanced and massive damage process. Our results were opposed by the general opinion, that rounded necrotic liver lesions are more typical for turkeys and often absent in chickens (Homer and Butcher 1991; Esquenet et al. 2003). The post mortem lesions in caeca, spleen and kidneys were characteristic for the disease (Homer and Butcher 1991;

Ganapathy et al. 2000; Esquenet et al. 2003; Popp et al. 2011; Hess and McDougald 2013). Powell et al. (2009) found, that formation of pathological lesions in the course of histomonosis was less severe in chickens than turkeys, due to limited migration of protozoa from intestines to the liver. According to these authors, at 6–8 days post infection in chickens, regeneration of damaged caecal mucosa takes place and within a month the birds may recover, gain immunity, however they remain the transmitters of the parasite. We demonstrated multiple histomonads and destruction of the bursa of Fabricius in chickens. No histomonads were detected in spleen, kidneys, lungs. Although the spread of *H.meleagridis* to bursa was observed in chickens during a field outbreaks (Marx 1973; Cortes et al. 2004), the data obtained after experimental infections of chickens were not ambiguous (Grabensteiner et al. 2006; Zahoor et al. 2011). Many aspects of the pathogenesis of*H.meleagridis* infection have not yet been fully clarified and further studies are needed to investigate the parasite impact on the bursa of Fabricius in chickens.

Despite of histopathological lesions typical for histomonosis and detection DNA *H.meleagridis*, direct microscopic parasitological examination did not confirm the presence of protozoan parasites. Probably this could have been caused by a relatively long period that had passed after the death of birds, as identification of protozoa requires fresh material. Similarly to our results, other authors reported outbreaks of histomonosis in chickens without the presence of the gastrointestinal worms (Ganapathy et al. 2000; Cortes et al. 2004).

Histomonosis in chickens may be more severe by the co-infections which contribute significantly to the mortality (Stokholm et al. 2010; Popp et al. 2011). The degree of intestinal lesions depends on *Histomonas*virulence and factors damaging the intestinal mucosa, i.e., coccidia (*Eimeria tenella)*, nematode, bacteria (*E.coli, Clostridium perfringens*) and mycotoxicoses (Ganapathy et al. 2000; McDougald and Hu 2001; McDougald 2005). Authors suggested that *Gallibacterium* spp. might be involved in the disease picture. Previous studies showed that chickens may serve as the preferable host for those bacteria. *Gallibacterium*spp. may constitute a part of their normal flora of the respiratory and genital tracts. However, *Gallibacterium*isolates have also been recovered from various pathological lesions in chickens (Bojesen et al. 2003; Stokholm et al. 2010). Bojesen et al. (2003) reported higher prevalence of *Gallibacterium* spp. in chickens from production systems with moderate or low levels of biosecurity. Although the source of infection in the presented case was not known, the possible deterioration in hygienic conditions could not be excluded. Moreover, the introduction of CIAV to the flock, may indicated on the break in biosecurity. We suggested, that the presence of anti-CIAV antibodies may resulted from an early infection, from which chickens recovered spontaneously. This infection could weakened birds' immune system.

The fight against *H.meleagridis* infections is based mainly on prevention and non-specific prophylactic methods (e.g., quarantine, hygienic practices, disinfection of litter and soil) (McDougald 2005). Authors suggested that the introduced treatment, and improvement of sanitary conditions might have contributed to gradual limitation of losses and control of histomonosis in the examined flock. The divergences in the epidemiology of *H.meleagridis* in chickens and turkeys (Hu et al. 2006) underline the importance of*H.gallinarum* as a vector for *H.meleagridis* in chickens. Chickens can usually become infected through the ingestion of *Histomonas*-infected eggs of caecal worm *Heterakis gallinarum* (intermediate host) or the earthworm (McDougald 2005; Hu et al. 2006). In contrast to the turkeys, direct transmission (via"cloacal drinking") has not been showed (Hu et al. 2006) or it may occur to a lesser extent than observed in turkeys (Hess et al. 2006). Therefore, it is still recommended to perform deworming (especially against *Heterakis gallinarum*) and rear chickens and turkeys separately. In general, management practices were found as very important in preventing outbreaks, but not always sufficient.

CONCLUSIONS

All findings described in this case strongly support the interpretation that chickens have become important host for *Histomonas meleagridis.* Previously it was thought that chickens constitute mainly a reservoir and source of infection for other birds. The present study, together with the recognized lack of effective therapeutics available on the market, and limitations in prophylactics indicate that histomonosis is a re-emerging poultry disease which can pose serious health threat, decrease animal welfare and considerable economic losses in poultry production. The histomonosis will remain a formidable challenge in the years ahead.

ACKNOWLEDGMENTS

The authors thank Division of Bacteriology and Molecular Biology, Warsaw University of Life Sciences – SGGW for microbiological examination. Preliminary data was presented during an oral session at the Scientific Conference "Current problems in the poultry pathology with particular emphasis on parasitic diseases" in Wroclaw, Poland, 01 – 02.07.2011.

REFERENCES

1. Banerjee PS, Garg R, Singh VS, Shukla SK, Yadav CL. An outbreak of histomonosis in a broiler breeder flock in Uttaranchal. Indian J Anim Sci. 2006;76:922–924.
2. Bilic I, Jaskulska B, Souillard R, Liebhart D, Hess M. Multi-locus typing of *histomonas meleagridis*isolates demonstrates the existence of two different genotypes. PLoS ONE. 2014;9(3) doi: 10.1371/journal.pone.0092438.
3. Bleyen N, Ons E, De Gussem M, Goddeeris BM. Passive immunization against *Histomonas meleagridis* does not protect turkeys from an experimental infection. Avian Pathol. 2009;38(1):71–76. doi: 10.1080/03079450802641255.
4. Bojesen AM, Nielsen SS, Bisgaard M. Prevalence and transmission of haemolytic *Gallibacterium*species in chicken production systems with different biosecurity levels. Avian Pathol. 2003;32(5):503–510. doi: 10.1080/0307945031000154107.
5. Callait-Cardinal MP, Leroux S, Venereau E, Chauve CM, Le Pottier G, Zenner L. Incidence of histomonosis in turkeys in France since the bans of dimetridazole and

nifursol. Vet Rec.2007;161(17):581–585. doi: 10.1136/vr.161.17.581.

6. CEC Regulation (EC) No 1831/2003 of the European Parliament and of the Council of 22 September 2003 on additives for use in animal nutrition. OJ EU. 2003;L268:29–43.
7. Cortes PL, Chin RP, Bland MC, Crespo R, Shivaprasad HL. Histomoniasis in the bursa of Fabricius of chickens. Avian Dis. 2004;48:711–715. doi: 10.1637/7175-030404R.
8. Desowitz RS. Age as a factor influencing fatal infections of histomoniasis in chickens. J Comp Pathol.1951;61:231–236. doi: 10.1016/S0368-1742(51)80022-5.
9. EFSA European food safety authority event report. technical meeting on histomonosis in turkeys.EFSA Support Publ. 2013;EN-464:1–12.
10. Esquenet C, De Herdt P, De Bosschere H, Ronsmans S, Ducatelle R, Van Erum J. An outbreak of histomoniasis in free-range layer hens. Avian Pathol. 2003;32:305–308. doi: 10.1080/0307945031000097903.
11. Ganapathy K, Salamat MH, Lee CC, Johara MY. Concurrent occurrence of salmonellosis, colibaccillosis and histomoniasis in a broiler flock fed with antibiotic-free commercial feed. Avian Pathol. 2000;29:639–642. doi: 10.1080/03079450020016000.
12. Gerth C, Rudiger-Boesch B, Schmidt U, Mumme J, Friedhoff KT. Histomoniasis in pullet stock and its effect on later laying performance. Tierarztl Prax. 1985;13:519–527.
13. Grabensteiner E, Hess M. PCR for the identification and differentiation of *Histomonas meleagridis*,*Tetratrichomonas gallinarum* and *Blastocystis* spp. Vet Parasitol. 2006;142:223–230. doi: 10.1016/j.vetpar.2006.07.011.
14. Grabensteiner E, Liebhart D, Weissenböck H, Hess M. Broad dissemination of *Histomonas meleagridis* determined by the detection of nucleic acid in different organs after experimental infection of turkeys and specified pathogen-free chickens using a mono-eukaryotic culture of the parasite. Parasitol Int. 2006;55(4):317–322. doi: 10.1016/j.parint.2006.07.004.
15. Grafl B, Liebhart D, Windisch M, Ibesich C, Hess M. Seroprevalence of *Histomonas meleagridis* in pullets and laying hens determined by ELISA. Vet Rec. 2011;168:160. doi: 10.1136/vr.c6479.
16. Hafez HM, Hauck R, Gad W, De Gussem K, Lotfi A. Pilot study on the efficacy of paromomycin as a histomonostatic feed additive in turkey poults experimentally infected with *Histomonas meleagridis*.Arch Anim Nutr. 2010;64:77–84. doi: 10.1080/17450390903478851.
17. Hafez HM, Mazaheri A, Prusas C, Bohland K, Poppel M, Schulze D. Actual infectious diseases in layer flocks kept in alternative rearing systems. Tierarztl Prax. 2001;29:168–174.
18. Hauck R, Balczulat S, Hafez HM. Detection of DNA of *Histomonas meleagridis* and*Tetratrichomonas gallinarum* in German poultry flocks between 2004 and 2008. Avian Dis.2010;54:1021–1025. doi: 10.1637/9261-012910-Reg.1.
19. Hess M, Grabensteiner E, Liebhart D. Rapid transmission of the protozoan parasite *Histomonas meleagridis* in turkeys and specific pathogen free chickens following cloacal infection with a mono-eukaryotic culture. Avian Pathol. 2006;35(4):280–285. doi: 10.1080/03079450600815507.
20. Hess M, Liebhart D, Bilic I, Ganas P. *Histomonas meleagridis*-New insights into an old pathogen. Vet Parasitol. 2015;208(1-2):67–76. doi: 10.1016/j.vetpar.2014.12.018.
21. Hess M, McDougald LR. Histomoniasis (blackhead) and other protozoan diseases of the intestinal tract. In: Swayne DE, Glisson JR, McDougald LR, Nolan LK, Suarez DL, Nair V, editors. Diseases of poultry. 13. Ames: Wiley; 2013. pp. 1172–1178.
22. Homer BL, Butcher GD. Histomoniasis in leghorn pullets on a Florida farm. Avian Dis. 1991;35:621–624. doi: 10.2307/1591231.
23. Hu J, Fuller L, Armstrong PL, McDougald LR. *Histomonas meleagridis* in chickens: attempted transmission in the absence of vectors. Avian Dis. 2006;50:277–279. doi: 10.1637/7431-090605R.1.
24. Hu J, McDougald LR. Effect of anticoccidials and antibiotics on the control of blackhead disease in broiler breeder pullets. J Appl Poult Res. 2002;11:351–357. doi: 10.1093/japr/11.4.351.
25. Liebhart D, Sulejmanovic T, Grafl B, Tichy A, Hess M. Vaccination against histomonosis prevents a drop in egg production in layers following challenge. Avian Pathol. 2013;42(1):79–84. doi: 10.1080/03079457.2012.760841.
26. Lotfi A, Hauck R, Olias P, Hafez HM. Pathogenesis of histomonosis in experimentally infected specific-pathogen-free (SPF) layer-type chickens and SPF meat-type chickens. Avian Dis.2014;58:424–432. doi: 10.1637/10782-012814-Reg.1.
27. Marx DJ. A turkey bursa of Fabricius infected with *Histomonas meleagridis*. J Protozool.1973;20:519.
28. McDougald LR. Blackhead disease (histomoniasis) in poultry: a critical review. Avian Dis.2005;49:462–476. doi: 10.1637/7420-081005R.1.
29. McDougald LR, Hu J. Blackhead disease (*Histomonas meleagridis*) aggravated in broiler chickens by concurrent infection with cecal coccidiosis (*Eimeria tenella*) Avian Dis. 2001;45:307–312. doi: 10.2307/1592969.
30. Patra G, Prasad H, Lalsiamthara J, Kataria JL, Malsawmkima D, Lalrinkima H. Prevalence of*histomonas meleagridis* in broiler chicken in different parts of Mizoram. India Int J Poult Sci.2013;12(2):98–101. doi: 10.3923/ijps.2013.98.101.
31. Popp C, Hauck R, Balczulat S, Hafez HM. Recurring histomonosis on an organic farm. Avian Dis.2011;55:328–330. doi: 10.1637/9596-110810-Case.1.

32. Powell FL, Rothwell L, Clarkson MJ, Kaiser P. The turkey, compared to the chicken, fails to mount an effective early immune response to *Histomonas meleagridis* in the gut. Parasite Immunol.2009;31:312–327. doi: 10.1111/j.1365-3024.2009.01113.x.

33. Stokholm NM, Permin A, Bisgaard M, Christensen JP. Causes of mortality in commercial organic layers in Denmark. Avian Dis. 2010;54(4):1241–1250. doi: 10.1637/9375-041910-Reg.1.

34. Tyzzer EE. Studies on histomoniasis or blackhead infection in the chicken and the turkey. Proc Am Acad Arts Sci. 1934;69:189–264. doi: 10.2307/20023041.

35. Van der Heijden HM, De Gussem K, Landman WJ. Assessment of the antihistomonal effect of paromomycin and tiamulin. Tijdschr Diergeneeskd. 2011;136(6):410–416.

36. Van der Heijden HM, Landman WJ. High seroprevalence of *Histomonas meleagridis* in Dutch layer chickens. Avian Dis. 2011;55:324–327. doi: 10.1637/9609-120610-ResNote.1.

37. Windisch M, Hess M. Experimental infection of chickens with *Histomonas meleagridis* confirms the presence of antibodies in different parts of the intestine. Parasite Immunol. 2010;32:29–35. doi: 10.1111/j.1365-3024.2009.01159.x.

38. Zahoor MA, Liebhart D, Hess M. Progression of histomonosis in commercial chickens following experimental infection with an *in vitro* propagated clonal culture of *Histomonas meleagridis*. Avian Dis. 2011;55:29–34. doi: 10.1637/9508-082110-Reg.1.

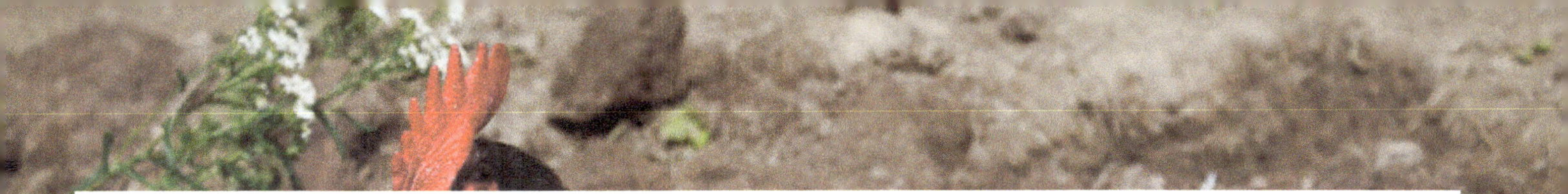

CHAPTER 18

SEROPREVALENCE OF TOXOPLASMA GONDII INFECTION IN SLAUGHTERED CHICKENS, DUCKS, AND GEESE IN SHENYANG, NORTHEASTERN CHINA

Na Yang[1], Ming-Yang Mu[1], Hong-Kui Li[2], Miao Long[1] and Jian-Bin He[1]

[1] College of Animal Science and Veterinary Medicine, Shenyang Agricultural University, Shenyang, Liaoning Province 110866, China

[2] Liaoning Center for Animal Disease Control and Prevention, Shenyang, Liaoning Province 110164, China

ABSTRACT

Background

In recent years, investigations of Toxoplasma gondii infection in poultry (chickens, ducks, and geese) have been reported worldwide, including China. However, little is known about the prevalence of T. gondii infection in poultry in northeastern China. Therefore, the present study was performed to determine the prevalence ofT. gondii infection in slaughtered chickens, ducks, and geese in Shenyang, northeastern China.

Methods

In the present study, the seroprevalence of T. gondii in 502 adult chickens, 268 adult ducks, and 128 adult geese was surveyed using the modified agglutination test (MAT).

Results

The seroprevalences of T. gondii were 5.8%, 7.8%, and 4.7% in chickens, ducks, and geese, respectively. Prevalence was higher in free-range groups (11.2%, 12.3%, and 8.9%) than caged groups (4.7%, 7.5%, and 6.0%), and there was a statistically significant difference only between free-range chickens and caged chickens, but no significant difference was found between free-range ducks, geese and caged ducks, geese.

Conclusions

The present study shows the prescence of T. gondii infection in slaughtered chickens, ducks, and geese in Shenyang, northeastern China, which suggests that consumption of poultry meat in Shenyang may pose a potential threat to human health and should be given attention.

Citation: Na Yang, Ming-Yang Mu, Hong-Kui Li, Miao Long and Jian-Bin He, Seroprevalence of Toxoplasma gondii infection in slaughtered chickens, ducks, and geese in Shenyang, northeastern China, DOI: 10.1186/1756-3305-5-237.

BACKGROUND

Toxoplasmosis is a widely prevalent zoonotic disease, caused by *Toxoplasma gondii*[1, 2, 3, 4, 5]. Domestic cats and other felids are the only definitive hosts for the parasite, and almost all warm-blooded animals and birds, including humans, are intermediate hosts. Humans can be infected by ingestion of raw, or undercooked, meat from the infected animals, and by consuming food or water contaminated with oocysts excreted by cats[1]. Meat from *T. gondii*-infected poultry (including chickens, ducks, geese, and pigeons) is consumed widely in many countries, including China, and is known to be the primary source of infection for humans[1, 6]. Moreover, the prevalence of *T. gondii* in chickens and ducks is a good indicator of soil contamination with *T. gondii* oocysts[7].

Worldwide seroprevalences of *T. gondii* in chickens, ducks, and geese are summarized by Dubey[1]. In recent years, there have several reports of *T. gondii* infection in chickens, ducks, and geese in China[8, 9, 10, 11]. However, there is no information regarding *T. gondii* infection in ducks and geese, and only limited information on seroprevalence of *T. gondii* in chickens in Liaoning, China, therefore, an investigation of the seroprevalence of *T. gondii* infections in chickens, ducks, and geese was undertaken.

METHODS

The study area

The study was conducted in Shenyang City, the capital of Liaoning Province, northeastern China. Shenyang is located in the southern part in northeastern China, covering an area of 1, 2948 km^2 and a population of approximately 8.19 million. Its geographical position is at east longitude 122°25′ - 123°48′ and at north latitude 41°11′ - 43°2′. The area has a temperate monsoon climate, with abundant sunshine, a long winter and summer, with a brief spring and autumn. The average annual temperature is 8.3°C, with a mean annual rainfall of 600–800 mm.

Three different poultry abattoirs located in Dadong, Heping, and Shenbei in Shenyang, were selected for sample collections. All of the above abattoirs are the main suppliers of poultry meat to Shenyang and the neighboring regions.

Blood samples

A total of 502 blood samples from adult chickens, 268 blood samples from adult ducks, and 128 blood samples from adult geese were collected from the above three poultry abattoirs in Shenyang between February and July 2012. Free range birds and caged birds were separated to slaughter in the same abattoirs and sold to market. The blood samples were sent to the laboratory for serological examination and centrifuged at 3,000 rpm for 10 min, and the sera were stored at −20°C until tested for antibodies to *T. gondii*.

Serological assay

Sera were tested for *T. gondii* antibodies using 2-fold serial dilutions from 1:25 to 1:3,200 with the modified agglutination test (MAT), as described previously[12]. Briefly, the harvested parasites were kept in 6% formaldehyde solution at 4°C overnight, and suspended in the alkaline buffer at 20,000 parasites/mL. Two-fold dilutions of sera were performed using the serum diluting buffer, and agglutination was performed in U-bottom 96-well microtiter plates using a mixture of 50 µL antigen and 50 µL diluted sera. The plates were incubated at 37°C overnight. The test was considered positive when a layer of agglutinated parasites was formed in wells at dilutions of 1:25 or higher; positive and negative controls were included in each test.

Statistical analysis

Statistical analysis of *T. gondii* prevalence between free-range (FR) and caged groups was performed using a Chi square test with SPSS (SPSS Inc., Chicago, Illinois). A *P*-value < 0.05 was considered statistically significant.

Ethics statement

All animals were handled in strict accordance with good animal practice according to the Animal Ethics Procedures and Guidelines of the People's Republic of China, and the study was approved by the Animal Ethics Committee of Shenyang Agricultural University (Permit No. SYXK<Liao>2011-0001).

RESULTS AND DISCUSSION

Overall, the seroprevalences of *T. gondii* were 5.8%, 7.8%, and 4.7% in chickens, ducks, and geese, respectively (Table 1).

Table 1: Seroprevalence of *Toxoplasma gondii* infection in chickens, ducks, and geese in Shenyang, northeastern China by the modified agglutination test (MAT)

Animal species		No. tested	No. with anti-*T. gondii*antibodies 1:25	1:50	1:100	1:200	1:400	Total positive	Prevalence (%)
Chicken	FR	206	16	4	0	0	3	23	11.2
	Caged	296	13	1	0	0	0	14	4.7
	Total	502	29	5	0	0	3	37	5.8
Duck	FR	122	12	1	1	1	0	15	12.3
	Caged	146	9	2	0	0	0	11	7.5
	Total	268	21	3	1	1	0	26	7.8
Goose	FR	45	2	2	0	0	0	4	8.9
	Caged	83	4	0	0	1	0	5	6.0
	Total	128	6	2	0	1	0	9	4.7

FR: Free-range.

In the present study, 37 (5.8%) of 502 chickens were seropositive to *T. gondii*, with titers of 1:25 in 29, 1:50 in 5, and 1:400 in 3 (Table 1). The seroprevalence of *T. gondii* from 3 different abattoirs ranged from 6.2% to 8.9% (Table 2). High prevalence was found in FR chickens (11.2%), compared with caged chickens (4.7%) (χ^2=7.37, P<0.01), indicating that FR chickens are more likely to be infected by *T. gondii* oocysts since they feed on the ground. The present study showed that the overall seropositivity (5.8%) for *T. gondii* infection in chickens was lower than those tested in other countries[13]. In China, it was also lower than the 25.2% prevalence reported for chickens in a study conducted in Jinzhou[11], 8.4% in Guangzhou[8], 7.4% in Zhangjiakou[9], and 7.3% in Lanzhou[14].

Table 2: Seroprevalence of *Toxoplasma gondii* infection in chickens, ducks, and geese in different poultry abattoirs in Shenyang, northeastern China by the modified agglutination test (MAT)

Animal species	Poultry abattoir	No. tested	No. positive	Prevalence (%)
Chicken	Dadong	167	11	6.6
	Heping	145	9	6.2
	Shenbei	190	17	8.9
Duck	Dadong	101	10	9.9
	Heping	79	9	11.4
	Shenbei	88	7	8.0
Goose	Dadong	45	3	6.7
	Heping	24	2	8.3
	Shenbei	59	4	6.8

Antibodies to *T. gondii* were found in 26 of 268 (7.8%) ducks with titres of 1:25 in 21, 1:50 in 3, 1:100 in 1, and 1:200 in 1 (Table 1). The seroprevalence in the present study was lower than those reported in other countries[1], and also lower than 16.0% in Guangzhou[8], 11.4% in Lanzhou[14] in China. The seroprevalence (12.3%) in FR ducks was higher than 7.5% in caged ducks, but no significant difference was found between FR ducks and caged ducks. Seroprevalence of *T. gondii* infection from 3 poultry abattoirs ranged from 8.0% to 11.4% (Table 2).

T. gondii antibodies were detected in 9 (4.7%) of 128 tested geese with titers of 1:25 in 6, 1:50 in 2, and 1:200 in 1 (Table 1), and the seroprevalences in FR and caged geese were 8.9% and 6.0%, respectively, but the difference was not statistically significant (P>0.05). To our knowledge, there was only one report regarding *T. gondii* infection in geese in Guangdong, China[10], and the seroprevalence (4.7%) in Shenyang in this study was lower than 15.0% in Gungdong. Seroprevalence of *T. gondii* infection from 3 poultry abattoirs ranged from 6.7% to 8.3% (Table 2).

The seroprevalences in chickens, ducks, and geese, were lower than those in other regions in China, which may be affected by ecological and geographical factors, as well as feeding conditions. The average annual temperature in Shenyang is 8.3°C, a rather cold climate, with typically dry conditions, which may be unfavorable for the survival of *T. gondii* oocysts.

The modified agglutination test (MAT) has been evaluated extensively in experimentally and naturally infected birds, and is sensitive and specific for assay of *T. gondii* antibodies[1, 10, 13, 14], compared to other serologic methods. However, the test needs to be validated by bioassays of viable *T. gondii* from meat consumed by humans in China.

CONCLUSIONS

The present study shows the *T. gondii* infection in slaughtered chickens, ducks, and geese in Shenyang, northeastern China, which suggests that consumption of poultry meat in Shenyang may pose a potential threat to human health and should be given attention.

DECLARATIONS

Acknowledgements

This study was supported by National Natural Science Foundation of China (NSFC, Grant No. 31201894).

Authors' contributions

JBH and NY conceived and designed the study, and critically revised the manuscript. NY, MYM, HKL and ML performed the experiments, analysed the data and drafted the manuscript. All authors read and approved the final manuscript.

REFERENCES

1. Dubey JP: Toxoplasmosis of animals and humans. 2010, CRC Press Inc, Boca Raton, Florida, New York, 1-313. 2
2. Yang N, Li HK, He JB, Mu MY, Yang SH: Seroprevalence of Toxoplasma gondii infection in domestic sheep in Liaoning province, northeastern china. J Parasitol. 2012, -http://dx.doi.org/10.1645/GE-3201.1.
3. Zhou P, Chen ZG, Li HL, Zheng HH, He SY, Lin RQ, Zhu XQ: Toxoplasma gondii infection in humans in China. Parasit Vectors. 2011, 4: 165-10.1186/1756-3305-4-165.
4. Wu SM, Huang SY, Fu BQ, Liu GY, Chen JX, Chen MX, Yuan ZG, Zhou DH, Weng YB, Zhu XQ, Ye DH: Seroprevalence of Toxoplasma gondii infection in pet dogs in Lanzhou, Northwest China. Parasit Vectors. 2011, 4: 64-10.1186/1756-3305-4-64.
5. Zhao GH, Zhang MT, Lei LH, Shang CC, Cao DY, Tian TT, Li J, Xu JY, Yao YL, Chen DK, Zhu XQ: Seroprevalence of Toxoplasma gondii infection in dairy

goats in Shaanxi Province, Northwestern China. Parasit Vectors. 2011, 4: 47-10.1186/1756-3305-4-47.

6. Dubey JP, Webb DM, Sundar N, Velmurugan GV, Bandini LA, Kwork OC, Su C: Endemic avian toxoplasmosis on a farm in Illinois: Clinical disease, diagnosis, biologic and genetic characteristics of Toxoplasma gondii isolates from chickens (Gallus domesticus), and a goose (Anser anser). Vet Parasitol. 2007, 148: 207-212. 10.1016/j.vetpar.2007.06.033.

7. El-Massry A, Mahdy OA, El-Ghaysh A, Dubey JP: Prevalence of Toxoplasma gondii antibodies in sera of turkeys, chickens, and ducks from Egypt. J Parasitol. 2000, 86: 627-628.

8. Yan C, Yue CL, Yuan ZG, He Y, Yin CC, Lin RQ, Dubey JP, Zhu XQ: Toxoplasma gondii infection in domestic ducks, free-range and caged chickens in southern China. Vet Parasitol. 2009, 65: 337-340.

9. Tian PR, Cui P: Investigation on Toxoplasma gondii infection in chickens in Zhangjiakou city. Ani Husbandry Feed Sci. 2010, 31: 172-173. in Chinese

10. Yan C, Yue CL, Zhang H, Yin CC, He Y, Yuan ZG, Lin RQ, Song HQ, Zhang KX, Zhu XQ: Serological Survey of Toxoplasma gondii infection in the Domeastic Goose (Anser domestica) in Southern China. Zoonoses public Health. 2011, 58: 299-302. 10.1111/j.1863-2378.2010.01349.x.

11. Xu P, Song XS, Wang W, Wang FY, Cao LL, Liu Q: Seroprevalence of Toxoplasma gondii Infection in Chickens in Jinzhou, Northeastern China. J Parasitol. 2012,-http://dx.doi.org/10.1645/GE-3164.1.

12. Dubey JP, Desmonts G: Serological responses of equids fed Toxoplasma gondii oocysts. Equine Vet J. 1987, 19: 337-339. 10.1111/j.2042-3306.1987.tb01426.x.

13. Dubey JP: Toxoplasma gondii infections in chickens (Gallus domesticus): prevalence, clinical disease, diagnosis and public health significance. Zoonoses public Health. 2010, 57: 60-73.

14. Cong W, Huang SY, Zhou DH, Xu MJ, Wu SM, Yan C, Zhao Q, Song HQ, Zhu XQ: First report of Toxoplasma gondii infection in market-sold adult chickens, ducks and pigeons in northwest China. Parasit Vectors. 2012, 5: 110-10.1186/1756-3305-5-110.

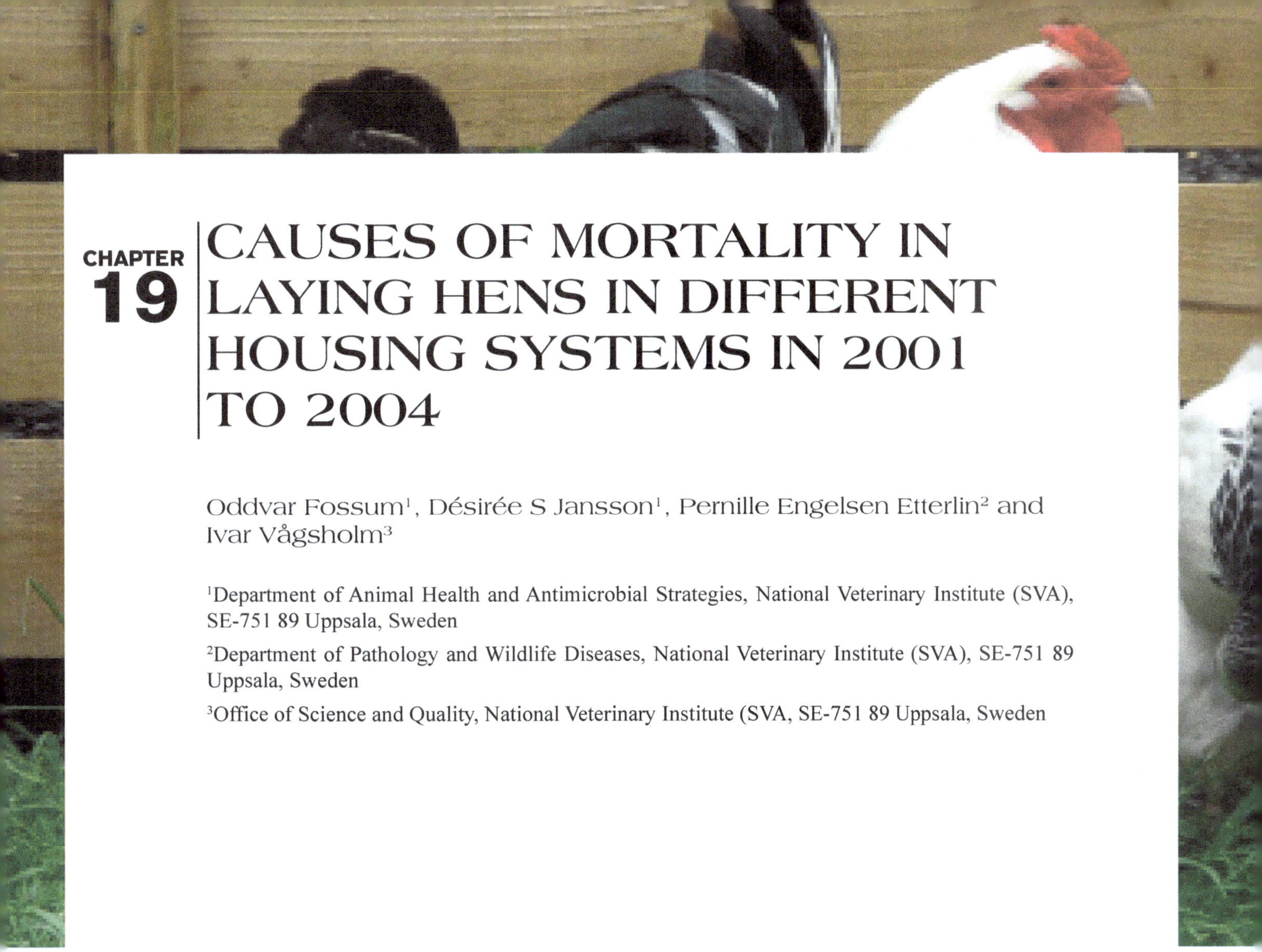

CHAPTER 19 CAUSES OF MORTALITY IN LAYING HENS IN DIFFERENT HOUSING SYSTEMS IN 2001 TO 2004

Oddvar Fossum[1], Désirée S Jansson[1], Pernille Engelsen Etterlin[2] and Ivar Vågsholm[3]

[1]Department of Animal Health and Antimicrobial Strategies, National Veterinary Institute (SVA), SE-751 89 Uppsala, Sweden

[2]Department of Pathology and Wildlife Diseases, National Veterinary Institute (SVA), SE-751 89 Uppsala, Sweden

[3]Office of Science and Quality, National Veterinary Institute (SVA, SE-751 89 Uppsala, Sweden

ABSTRACT

Background

The husbandry systems for laying hens were changed in Sweden during the years 2001 – 2004, and an increase in the number of submissions for necropsy from laying hen farms was noted. Hence, this study was initiated to compare causes of mortality in different housing systems for commercial laying hens during this change.

Methods

Based on results from routine necropsies of 914 laying hens performed at the National Veterinary Institute (SVA) in Uppsala, Sweden between 2001 and 2004, a retrospective study on the occurrence of diseases and cannibalism, i.e., pecking leading to mortality, in different housing systems was carried out. Using the number of disease outbreaks in caged flocks as the baseline, the expected number of flocks with a certain category of disease in the other housing systems was estimated having regard to the total number of birds in the population. Whether the actual number of flocks significantly exceeded the expected number was determined using a Poisson distribution for the variance of the baseline number, a continuity correction and the exact value for the Poisson distribution function in Excel 2000.

Results

Common causes of mortality in necropsied laying hens included colibacillosis, erysipelas, coccidiosis, red mite infestation, lymphoid leukosis and cannibalism. Less common diagnoses were Newcastle Disease, pasteurellosis and botulism. Considering the size of the populations in the different housing systems, a larger proportion of laying hens than expected was submitted for necropsy from litter-based systems and free range production compared to hens in cages ($P < 0.001$). The study showed a significantly higher occurrence of bacterial and parasitic diseases and cannibalism in laying hens

Citation: Oddvar Fossum, Désirée S Jansson, Pernille Engelsen Etterlin and Ivar Vågsholm, Causes of mortality in laying hens in different housing systems in 2001 to 2004, DOI: 10.1186/1751-0147-51-3.

kept in litter-based housing systems and free-range systems than in hens kept in cages ($P < 0.001$). The occurrence of viral diseases was significantly higher in indoor litter-based housing systems than in cages ($P < 0.001$).

Conclusion

The results of the present study indicated that during 2001–2004 laying hens housed in litter-based housing systems, with or without access to outdoor areas, were at higher risk of infectious diseases and cannibalistic behaviour compared to laying hens in cages. Future research should focus on finding suitable prophylactic measures, including efficient biosecurity routines, to reduce the risk of infectious diseases and cannibalism in litter-based housing systems for laying hens.

BACKGROUND

The Swedish Animal Welfare Act from 1988 mandated a switch from conventional battery cages for laying hens to alternative housing systems i.e. litter-based housing systems, including free range, and enriched cages. A fundamental requirement according to the new Swedish legislation was that laying hens should be able to behave naturally, e.g. have access to nests, perches and dust baths.

The change of housing systems started slowly, but during the years 2001–2004 practically all the remaining conventional battery cages, equivalent to about 80 % of the population of layers in 2001, were exchanged for alternative housing systems. During the same period, the number of routine necropsies of laying hens submitted to The National Veterinary Institute (SVA) in Uppsala, Sweden increased noticeably compared to the years before. Results from necropsies from this period have for that reason been compiled in an effort to analyse the effects of the change in housing systems on bird health. The results will probably have relevance outside Sweden, as a decision has been taken in the European Union to ban conventional battery cages by 2012 [1].

METHODS

The study was based on results from necropsies of commercial laying hens submitted to SVA for routine examinations from all parts of Sweden in connection with disease associated with increased mortality in the flocks. Other diseases, parasite infections or lesions not leading to a manifest increase of mortality are not included in this study. During the study period (January 1, 2001 to December 31, 2004) four different hybrids were used; Lohmann Selected Leghorn, Lohmann Brown, Hy-Line White and Hy-Line Brown. At the time of the study, laying hens in Sweden were vaccinated against Marek's disease, avian encephalomyelitis and infectious bronchitis during the rearing period and against infectious bronchitis regularly during the laying period. Most laying hens intended for litter-based housing systems were also immunised against coccidiosis early during the rearing period.

In Sweden, there were three veterinary diagnostic laboratories, including SVA, which performed necropsies on farm animals during the study period. Numbers of poultry necropsies performed by the other laboratories (Kallay TB and Linder A, AnalyCen Nordic AB, personal communication) were compared to those of SVA. The share of SVA was 78% of all chicken necropsies during the period 2001 to 2004. During the study period, SVA's share of laying hen necropsies remained stable.

The criteria for inclusion in this study were the following: 1) The laying hens must come from a flock with increased mortality. 2) The number of submitted hens should be three or more. 3) There should be information about the housing system, age of the birds, flock size, and disease history in the flock. All birds were necropsied according to a routine protocol of SVA. Histological, bacteriological, virological, parasitological and chemical examinations were performed having regard to disease history and gross pathological findings. These examinations were performed according to routine methods used at SVA. In some cases additional diagnostic tests were required such as PCR and virus isolation for Newcastle Disease virus, and serology to detect antibodies against avian leukosis virus. The protocols for necropsy, microbiological and chemical examinations (in Swedish) are available from the corresponding author upon request.

The housing systems used in Sweden during the study period were: 1) single-tiered floor systems with manure bins, with or without regular removal of manure, 2) multi-tiered floor systems (aviaries) with litter belts for regular removal of manure, 3) conventional battery cages, and 4) furnished cages (cages with perches, nests and dust bathing areas). A review of housing systems in use is given by R. Tauson [2]

In the single-tiered floor systems the maximum bird density allowed was 7.5 or 9 birds per m^2 available area (depending on the body weight) while the maximum density in aviaries was 7 birds per m^2 available area or 20 birds per m^2 floor area. The required area in single nests was 0.0125 m^2 per bird and in colony nests 0.010 m^2per bird. For all housing systems at least 15 cm perch per hen was required. The conventional cages should according to the regulations in force during the time of the study offer an available area of at least 600 cm^2per bird while furnished cages in addition should have a nest and a dust bathing area of 200 cm^2each [3]. Ten birds per cage was the largest group size in furnished cages at the time of the study. Hens in free-range systems, including organic laying hens, were housed in either single-tiered floor systems or multi-tiered aviary systems, and the birds had access to outside pens and/or pasture. In organic production the maximal number of hens allowed during the study period was 7 per m^2 available floor area [4].

Submitted birds were divided into three categories: 1) birds housed in conventional and furnished cages 2) birds housed indoors in litter-based housing systems (single-tiered floor systems and multi-tiered aviary systems), and 3) birds in free range systems with access to outdoor pens and/or pasture, including organic laying hens. Since the numbers of submissions from conventional cages and furnished cages were small we considered birds from these two systems as one category. Birds from indoor single-tiered floor systems and multi-tiered aviary systems were also regarded as one category since the available annual reports showing the hen populations in Sweden made no distinction between these systems. These two systems are henceforward called litter-based systems. The sizes of flocks included in the study varied from 400 birds to 37,000 birds, and the age of the laying hens ranged from 18 to 78 weeks.

During the study period there was a change in housing systems for Swedish laying hens with a decrease of hens in conventional cage systems and an increase of hens in enriched cages and in litter-based housing systems including organic production. The total number of laying hens per year and the proportions of hens in different housing systems [5] are presented in Table 1.

Table 1: Percentage of commercial laying hens in different housing systems in Sweden in 2001–2004[1]. The total number of hens varied between 5,042 to 5,904 million birds per year

Year/Housing system	2001	2002	2003	2004	2001–2004
Conventional battery cages	66.5	52.3	26.0	13.5	38.6
Furnished cages	7.5	12.6	24.2	24.8	17.6
Litter-based systems [2]	22.6	31.2	43.8	55.0	38.7
Free range [3]	3.4	3.9	6.0	6.7	5.1
Total	100	100	100	100	100

[1]The table is based on data collected in May to August each year [5].

[2]Includes single-tiered floor systems and multi-tiered aviary systems.

[3]Flocks housed in litter-based systems indoors, with access to outdoor pens and pasture, including organic flocks.

The length of the egg production period for laying hens in Sweden during the study period was approximately 12 months. For the analysis, we therefore assumed that approximately four production periods were completed for each category during the four-year period. The categories of populations that we compared were the total number of birds in each of the main housing systems (cages, litter based systems and free range) during the four-year period.

Statistical analysis

In this study, the epidemiological units of interest were the flocks from which birds were submitted for necropsy. Thus, the effects of variable numbers of birds in some of the submissions and of repeated submissions from some flocks were reduced. The results of necropsies were divided into major diagnostic categories i.e. bacterial, viral, parasitic diseases, and cannibalism. As more than one diagnosis was observed in some of the flocks, these flocks were represented in two or more diagnostic categories. On the other hand, several submissions from one single flock showing the same disease were considered as a single "outbreak". Using flocks of laying hens kept in cages from which birds were submitted for necropsy as the baseline, the expected number of flocks with submissions with each of the major diagnoses was estimated for indoor litter based systems and for free-range systems. We assumed that the number of flocks would be proportionate to the total number of birds in the different systems during the four year period. Since the submission of laying hens for necropsy was a rare occasion given the total number of birds, we chose to compare the number of flocks from indoor litter based systems with cage systems, and free-range systems with cage systems. Whether these numbers significantly exceeded the expected numbers was determined looking at the upper 95% confidence level for the expected number assuming a Poisson distribution for the variance of the expected baseline number, a continuity correction, and the exact value for the Poisson distribution function in Excel 2000 [6].

RESULTS

Causes of mortality

Altogether 914 laying hens from 172 flocks were included in the study (Table 2). In most submissions one specific disease was predominant i.e. was observed in more than 50% of the submitted laying hens. Less common were cases in which two (or more) diseases contributed substantially to the mortality in a flock (observed in 12% of the flocks) which was usually noticed when birds were submitted from the same flock several times with long intervals. The main disease categories of the included flocks are given in Table 3. Diseases or problems of other aetiologies than mentioned in the table were infrequent, and were usually not the main cause of increased mortality on flock level at the time of investigation. A summary of these findings is presented in Table 4.

Table 2: Numbers and percentage of commercial laying hen flocks submitted for necropsy to SVA and included in the study

	2001		2002		2003		2004	
Housing systems	*N*	%	*N*	%	*N*	%	*N*	%
Cages [1]	5	41.7	6	9.1	4	9.5	5	9.6
Litter-based systems [2]	5	41.7	54	81.8	32	76.2	38	73.1
Free range [3]	2	16.6	6	9.1	6	14.3	9	17.3
Total	12	100	66	100	42	100	52	100

[1]Includes conventional battery cages and enriched cages.

[2]Includes single-tiered floor systems and multi-tiered aviary systems.

[3]Flocks housed in litter-based systems indoors, with access to outdoor pens and pasture, including organic flocks.

Table 3: Occurrence of diseases (divided into main categories) in laying hen flocks submitted to SVA in 2001–2004

		Bacterial diseases		Viral	diseases	Parasitic diseases		Cannibalism	
Housing system	**Total no. of flocks** [1]	*N*	%	*N*	%	*N*	%	*N*	%
Cages [2]	20	13	65.0	6	30.0	2	10.0	1	5.0
Litter-based systems [3]	129	94	72.9	15	11.6	23	17.8	24	18.6
Free range [4]	23	17	73.9	1	4.4	5	21.7	6	26.1

[1]No. of examined flocks. Note that each flock may have several diagnoses.

[2]Includes conventional battery cages and enriched cages.

[3]Includes single-tiered floor systems and multi-tiered aviary systems.

[4]Flocks housed in litter-based systems indoors, with access to outdoor pens and pasture, including organic flocks.

Table 4: List of miscellaneous diagnoses in 173 necropsied laying hens, not included in main diagnostic categories and the statistical analysis

		Housing of the birds (no. of flocks)		
Diagnosis	**No. of hens**	**Cages** [1]	**Litter-based systems** [2]	**Free range** [3]
Visceral gout	29	1	10	1
Unknown cause of death	23	6	17	0
Dehydration and cachexia	17	0	6	0
Trauma	16	2	12	2
Hepatic lipidosis and liver rupture	11	3	2	0
Circulatory disturbances[4]	16	0	3	0
Anaemia and haemorrhages, suspected intoxication	11	0	0	1
Osteoporosis	10	4	0	0
Egg bound	7	3	4	0
Hepatitis	5	0	4	1
Obstipation (straw)	5	0	1	2
Miscellaneous neoplasms[5]	4	1	3	0
Other causes of death[6]	19	2	17	0

[1]Includes conventional battery cages and enriched cages.

[2]Includes single-tiered floor systems and multi-tiered aviary systems.

[3]Flocks housed in litter-based systems indoors, with access to outdoor pens and pasture, including organic flocks.

[4]Botulism was later diagnosed from hens in the same flocks.

[5]Neoplasms other than lymphoid leukosis.

[6]Including egg yolk peritonitis (n = 4), gastritis (n = 2), ovarian cyst (n = 2), air sacculitis (n = 2), enteritis (n = 2), chronic salpingitis (n = 1), endocarditis (n = 1), intestinal volvulus (n = 1), myositis (n = 1) ruptured ovary and abdominal hemorrhage (n= 2). hepatitis (n = 1).

Bacterial diseases

Bacterial diseases appeared to be the most common causes of mortality during the study period (Table 3). The predominating disease in all housing systems was infections caused by *Escherichia* (*E.*) *coli*, i.e. colibacillosis, which was found in 85 flocks. The pathological findings were usually acute or subacute fibrinous salpingitis, oophoritis and peritonitis, or more infrequently pericarditis, perihepatitis, pneumonia and air sacculitis. A relatively high proportion (52%) of the cases of colibacillosis occurred between start of lay and 30 weeks of age. In 50% of the infected flocks cloacal cannibalism or vent pecking was observed in one or more birds submitted for necropsy. Severe cloacal injuries were observed in 19% (out of 312) of the layers with colibacillosis.

Outbreaks of erysipelas, caused by *Erysipelothrix* (*E.*) *rhusiopathiae*, were observed in ten of 129 flocks from indoor litter-based housing systems and in six of 23 flocks from free-range systems but not in any caged flock. The post mortem examinations showed birds with acute, septicaemic disease with splenomegaly and hepatomegaly as the most prominent lesions. Valvular endocarditis, necrotic hepatitis, and necrotic splenitis were observed sporadically.

In four flocks kept in litter-based systems indoors, infections with *Pasteurella multocida* were diagnosed. No cases of pasteurellosis were observed in caged birds or free-range birds.

Botulism type C/D was diagnosed on one farm with laying hens kept in aviaries. The birds had shown signs of paralysis and high mortality. Birds from two houses on the farm were submitted for necropsy. Signs of circulatory disturbances/ failure such as pale musculature and congested abdominal organs were observed in most of the laying hens and no other gross or microscopic lesions were noted.

Parasitic diseases

Coccidiosis was observed in 18 of 129 flocks housed in litter-based systems indoors, in five of 23 free-range flocks and in two of 20 flocks from cage systems. Most of the outbreaks (76%) occurred in birds younger than 24 weeks.

In five of 129 flocks kept in indoor litter-based housing systems, increased mortality caused by infestation with the poultry red mite (*Dermanyssus* (*D.*) *gallinae*) was demonstrated. In addition, *D. gallinae* were found in the plumage of birds from another seven flocks from litter-based housing systems including free range. Mites were not detected in birds submitted from cages.

Viral diseases

In total, 22 outbreaks of viral diseases were diagnosed within the frame of the study. Lymphoid leukosis was diagnosed in ten of 129 flocks housed in litter based housing systems, and in six of 20 flocks housed in cages. These outbreaks were observed in birds in the age interval 20–39 weeks during 2001 and 2002. No case of lymphoid leukosis was observed in free-range birds. Marek' s disease was diagnosed in two of 129 flocks in litter-based housing systems and in one of 23 free-range flocks during 2001–2002. Newcastle Disease was diagnosed 2004 in three flocks housed in litter-based housing systems indoors from two closely situated, but separate farms.

Cannibalism

The most common traumatic injuries in the necropsied birds leading to increased mortality were wounds in the cloacal region indicative of vent pecking (cannibalism). Cannibalism was observed in all housing systems and was the main cause of mortality in five of 129 flocks housed in litter based systems indoors and in four of 23 free range flocks. Cannibalism was not observed as the main cause of death in any of the flocks housed in cages.

Differences in occurrence of diseases between housing systems

The results from the statistical analyses are shown in tables 5 and 6.

Table 5: Risk analysis regarding main disease categories between laying hen flocks in cages[1] and litter-based systems[2]

Disease category	Observed no. of flocks from litter-based systems	Expected no. of flocks if same risk as in cages	Excess no. of flocks in litter-based systems compared to cages
Bacterial diseases	94	9	85***
Viral diseases	15	4	11***
Parasitic diseases	23	1	22***
Cannibalism	24	1	23***
Total	129	14	115***

[1]Includes conventional battery cages and enriched cages.

[2]Includes single-tiered floor systems and multi-tiered aviary systems.

Level of significance is denoted by *** $P < 0.001$.

Table 6: Risk analysis regarding main disease categories between laying hen flocks in cages[1] and free range housing[2]

Disease category	Observed no. of flocks from free range housing	Expected no. of flocks if same risk as in cages	Excess no. of flocks in free range housing compared to cages
Bacterial diseases	17	1	16***
Viral diseases	1	1	0
Parasitic diseases	5	0	5***
Cannibalism	6	0	6***
Total	23	2	21***

[1]Includes conventional battery cages and enriched cages.

[2]Flocks housed in litter-based systems indoors, with access to outdoor pens and pasture, including organic flocks.

Levels of significance are denoted by *** $P < 0.001$

DISCUSSION

The results of the present study showed that there was a significant difference between housing systems concerning the diagnostic categories and number of flocks from which laying hens were submitted for necropsy to SVA during 2001–2004. Compared to caged flocks, more submissions than expected arrived for necropsy from indoor litter-based housing systems and from farms with hens in free-range systems. Supporting evidence for assuming that the presented results reflected the true health situation of Swedish laying hens during the time of study would be: 1) That the readiness of the poultry farmers to submit laying hens for necropsy was independent of their choice of housing system, and 2) That the farms with different housing systems were evenly distributed in the country. Based on our long experience from routine diagnostics, we cannot exclude that there may be differences in the owners′ willingness to submit birds for necropsy from different housing systems. Available information indicates, however, that the primary cause of the increase of submissions to SVA during the study period were health problems connected to the change in housing systems as there were no other known major changes in the egg production industry during that time. Furthermore, the cost of necropsies remained stable and the market share of SVA did not change substantially. In the second case, regional differences were known to exist, i.e. in some areas of the country litter-based housing systems were more common than in other regions. However, SVA received laying hens for necropsy from all regions of the country, which to some extent reduced the risk for biases due to regional differences.

Bacterial diseases were the most common causes of mortality in laying hens submitted to SVA for necropsy. Similar results have been reported from surveys on health of commercial layers in other countries [7, 8, 9]. Bacterial infections seem to be more common in laying hens in litter-based housing systems including free-range birds, than in caged birds [8, 10]. Furthermore, *Kreienbrock et al.* (2003) found that antibiotics were more commonly used in German laying hens kept in litter-based housing systems than in caged birds [10].

The most common bacterial infection diagnosed in this study was colibacillosis, which has been reported from many countries as a frequent cause of disease in commercial laying hens, as well as in hens in experimental trials [7, 9, 11, 12, 13, 14]. The dominating lesions observed in our cases were in agreement with reports from other countries [12, 13, 14, 15]. An interesting finding in this study was that a high proportion of the birds infected with *E. coli* showed wounds or purulent inflammation in the cloacal region, which indicates that vent pecking was an important predisposing factor. Mortality caused by cannibalism was also common in these flocks. Similar observations have been reported from commercial flocks, as well as from experimental trials [9,16, 17, 18].

Infections with *E. rhusiopathiae* and *P. multocida* were observed in hens in litter-based systems, with or without free-range, but not from hens in cages. Erysipelas has previously been reported sporadically in laying hens in different housing systems from several countries [8, 19, 20, 21, 22]. Our finding concur with reports from Germany indicating that there is a higher risk of erysipelas in laying hens housed in litter-based housing systems (including free-range) than in caged birds [10, 19].

The first case of botulism in laying hens in Sweden was diagnosed in hens housed in an aviary system in 2003. Worldwide, reports of botulism in laying hens are very rare with only a few outbreaks reported in the literature [23, 24], whereas the disease has more often been observed in broilers [25]. *Huin and Sakaguchi*showed that keeping broilers on litter increased the risk of botulism compared to housing in cages [26], and this may explain the difference between laying hens and broilers concerning the number of reports in recent years. The Swedish outbreak of botulism may indicate an increased risk associated with litter-based housing systems for laying hens.

This study showed an apparent difference between litter-based housing systems and cages concerning submissions due to coccidiosis. During the study period many commercial pullets were reared in cages because of a shortage of litter-based rearing systems. The fact that these cage-reared birds usually were not vaccinated against coccidiosis may explain many of the outbreaks during the study period. However, it cannot be excluded that suboptimal administration of the vaccine may explain some of the cases. Probably, the risk of coccidiosis can be further reduced by adjusting the way pullets are reared to the conditions they meet in the production units. It is also very important to ensure that the vaccination of pullets intended to produce in litter based systems offers sufficient immunity.

The poultry red mite, *D. gallinae*, caused increased mortality in several flocks in the litter-based systems. This parasite is widespread on poultry farms in Europe [27, 28, 29, 30, 31, 32], and mortality as a consequence of mite infestation occurs sporadically [27, 28, 30, 31]. However, the most common effects of mite infestation are the reduced welfare of the birds and the economic loss due to reduced egg production [29, 31]. Free range systems have been reported to be more commonly affected by mites than other housing systems [30, 32]. Kreienbrock et al. 2003, observed a more frequent use of acaricides in German laying hen farms with litter-based systems than in farms with cages [10] which concur with our results.

With the exception of lymphoid leukosis, the occurrence of viral diseases leading to mortality was low in the Swedish population of commercial laying hens during the study period. Probably, this was a consequence of vaccination and other prophylactic measures, including screening and eradication of viruses from the breeder population. The differences in occurrence of viral diseases between cage and litter-based housing systems were not as obvious as for parasitic and bacterial diseases. Concerning lymphoid leukosis, the occurrence in the adult laying hens was probably not influenced by the housing system, considering the importance of vertical transmission of the virus, and the development of age resistance [33]. The number of flocks affected by lymphoid leukosis during the study period was unusually high for Sweden, since this disease is not normally present in the Swedish commercial breeding population and commercial laying hens. The outbreaks reported in this study reflect an accidental infection of parents flock of one laying hen hybrid prior to the start of the study.

Cannibalism was one of the main causes of death in laying hens housed in indoor litter-based systems and in free range systems in this study, but it appeared to be a minor problem in caged laying hens. Data from both experimental and commercial flocks from several countries have shown that cannibalism is one of the most severe threats to egg production in both litter-based housing systems and in cages [8, 9, 10, 16, 17, 18, 27, 34,35]. Several workers have shown that there is a greater risk for a cannibalistic behaviour to occur in larger groups [16, 18, 36, 37, 38]. On Swedish laying hen farms with aviary housing systems, flock sizes between 20,000 and 35,000 birds are not uncommon. Beak trimming, which is a common prophylactic measure against cannibalism in many countries, is not allowed in Sweden according to the Swedish Animal Welfare Act. Consequently, cloacal pecking and cannibalism must be considered to be important health risks in large flocks. The low occurrence of cannibalism in the Swedish cage systems may, at least partly, be explained by the small average group size at the time of study.

Overall, laying hens from flocks housed in litter-based systems and free-range systems were comparatively more frequently submitted for necropsy to SVA during the years 2001–2004, indicating a higher risk for increased mortality in these systems than in cages. Comparisons of mortality, health and performance of laying hens housed in cages and litter-based systems have been performed on an experimental basis (small scale experiments and experimental farms with up to 10 000 birds) by several workers [16, 34, 39, 40, 41, 42] in different countries and results from large-scale investigations comprising commercial laying hens in different housing systems have been reported from Germany [8, 10], Switzerland [35, 43], Denmark [44] and The Netherlands [45]. The results from the experimental trials show great variations, but the field surveys generally point to increased risk of disease and mortality in litter-based and free-range systems compared to cages agreeing with the findings in this study.

In this study, we have identified several disease problems being associated with the different housing systems. It is, however, important to emphasize that the results reflect the unique situation in Sweden during the years 2001–2004, when the change of housing systems from conventional battery cages was at its peak. Several new types of aviary systems were introduced, and the knowledge and experience of keeping large flocks of laying hens in aviaries was limited. Additionally, during the study period many new egg laying farms were established by people with no or little prior experience of keeping commercial laying hens, and these producers often chose the new aviary systems. Hence, the health status of birds in free range and litter based systems should improve as more experience and knowledge are gained. Preliminary results of necropsies of laying hens after 2004 (not included in this study) indicate that the health situation in the laying hen population has markedly improved [46].

CONCLUSION

Data from the present study suggested that during the change in housing systems for laying hens in Sweden in 2001–2004, there were significant differences in bird health between housing systems, with birds in litter-based housing systems and free-range systems showing more health problems than caged laying hens. To increase the safety of the egg production in litter-based housing systems and free-range systems it is necessary to pay much attention to management and preventive measures, such as biosecurity and vaccinations. Adequate education of personnel responsible for running the operations is crucial.

DECLARATIONS

Authors' contributions

PEE participated in necropsy work. IV participated in the design of the study and performed the statistical analyses. DSJ and OF participated in designing the study, performed necropsies and drafted the manuscript. All authors read, edited and approved the final manuscript.

REFERENCES

1. Communities Council of Europe. Council Directive 1999/74/EC. Official Journal of the European Communities L 203/53. 1999, [http://eur-lex.europa.eu/en/index.htm]
2. Tauson R: Management and housing systems for layers – effects on welfare and production. Worlds Poult Sci J. 2005, 61: 477-487. 10.1079/WPS200569.
3. Jordbruksverkets författningssamling. SJVFS. 2003, 6: L100-
4. Krav. [http://krav.se/regler]
5. EuroEgg and Business AB. [http://eurobusiness.se/egg/prodhonsdia-egg.htm]
6. Armitage P, Berry G: Statistical methods in medical research. 1987, Blackwell Scientific Publications, London, UK, 559-2
7. Van Emous RA, Fiks-Van Niekerk Th GCM: Inventory on commercial layer farms with aviaries and free range. Animal Research – Animal Sciences Group-Wageningen UR. Practical Scientific Report 7. 2003
8. Petermann S: Legehennen in alternativen Haltungssystemen- Prachtische Erfahrungen. Dtsch Tierärztl Wschr. 2003, 110: 220-224.
9. Hegelund L, Hermansen JE, Sörensen JT, Horsted T: Ökologisk aegproduktion: Produktion, sundhed, velfaerd og naeringsstofhusholdning. DJF rapport Husdyrbrug nr.71. 2006
10. Kreienbrock L, Schneider B, Schäl J, Glaser S: EpiLeg – Orientierende epidemiologische Untersuchung zum Leistungsniveau und Gesundheitsstatus in Legehennenhaltungen verschiedener Haltungssysteme. Zwischenbericht: Deskriptive Auswertung. Institut fur Biometrie, Epidemiologie und Informationsverarbeitung (IBEI), Hannover, (Stand: 1. September 2003)
11. Dhillon AS, Jack OK: Two outbreaks of colibacillosis in commercial caged layers. Avian Dis. 1996, 40: 742-746. 10.2307/1592290.
12. Jordan FT, Williams NJ, Wattret A, Jones T: Observations on salpingitis, peritonitis and salpingoperitonitis in a layer breeder flock. Vet Rec. 2005, 5: 573-77.
13. Vandekerchove D, De Herdt P, Laevens H, Pasmans F: Colibacillosis in caged layer hens: characteristics of the disease and the etiological agent. Avian Pathol. 2004, 33: 117-127. 10.1080/0307945031000l642149.
14. Bisgaard M, Dam A: Salpingitis in poultry. II Prevalence, bacteriology, and possible pathogenesis in egg-laying chickens. Nord Vet Med. 1981, 33: 81-89.
15. Landman WJ, Cornelissen RA: *Escherichia coli* salpingitis and peritonitis in layer chickens: an overview. Tijdschr Diergeneeskd. 2006, 15: 814-822.
16. Abrahamsson P, Tauson R: Aviary Systems and conventional cages for laying hens. Acta Agric Scand. 1995, 45: 191-203.
17. Abrahamsson P, Fossum O, Tauson R: Health of laying hens in an aviary system over five batches of birds. Acta Vet Scand. 1998, 39: 367-379.
18. Weitzenburger D, Vitz A, Hamann H, Distl O: Effect of furnished small group housing systems and furnished cages on mortality and causes of death in two layer strains. Br Poult Sci. 2005, 46: 553-559. 10.1080/00071660500303206.
19. Mazaheri A, Lierz M, Hafez HM: Investigation on the pathogenicity of *Erysipelothrix rhusiopathiae* in laying hens. Avian Dis. 2005, 49: 574-576. 10.1637/7362-040805R.1.
20. Mutalib AA, King JM, McDonough PL: Erysipelas in caged laying chickens and suspected erysipeloid in animal caretakers. J vet Diagn Invest. 1993, 5: 198-201.
21. Bisgaard M, Norrung V, Tornoe N: Erysipelas in poultry. Prevalence of serotypes and epidemiological investigations. Avian Pathol. 1980, 9: 355-362. 10.1080/03079458008418419.
22. Eriksson H, Jansson D, Fossum O, Chirico J, Gunnarsson A: Erysipelas in layers – a growing problem in aviary and organic housing systems. Proceedings of the XIII Congress of the World Veterinary Poultry Association: 19–23. 2003, 130-July , Denver
23. Cygan Z, Barcz I, Sikorski T: Enzootia botulizmu w stadzie kur – niosek. Med Wet. 1981, 37: 583-586.
24. Gama NMSQ, Nagamatsu M, Baldassi L, Gama JRQ: Botulismo em aves de postura na regiâo noroeste do estado Sâo Paulo. Ars vet. 1992, 8: 58-63.
25. Dohms JE: Botulism. Diseases of Poultry. Edited by: Saif YM, Barnes HJ, Glisson JR, Fadly AM, McDougald

LR, Swayne DE. 2003, Iowa State Press, Ch. 23: 785-791. 11

26. Hyun SH, Sakaguchi G: Implication of coprophagy in pathogenesis of chicken botulism. Nippon Juigaku Zasshi. 1989, 51: 582-586.
27. Swarbrick O: Clinical problems in "free range layers". Vet in Rec. 1986, 118: 363-
28. Guy JH, Khajavi M, Hlalel MM, Sparagano O: Red mite (*Dermanyssus gallinae*) prevalence in laying units in Northern England. Br Poult Sci. 2004, 45 (Suppl 1): 15-16. 10.1080/00071660410001698001.
29. Kilpinen O, Roepstorff A, Permin A, Norgaard-Nielsen G, Lawson LG, Simonsen HB: Influence of *Dermanyssus gallinae*and *Ascaridia galli* infections on behaviour and health of laying hens (*Gallus gallus* domesticus). Br Poult Sci. 2005, 46: 26-34. 10.1080/00071660400023839.
30. Fiddes MD, Le Gresly S, Parsons DG, Epe C, Coles GC, Stafford KA: Prevalence of the poultry red mite (*Dermanyssus gallinae*) in England. Vet Rec. 2005, 157: 233-235.
31. Wojcik AR, Grygon-Frankiewicz B, Zbikowska E, Wasielewski L: Invasion of *Dermanyssus gallinae* (De Geer, 1778) in poultry farms in the Torun region. Wiad Parazytol. 2000, 46: 511-515.
32. Höglund J, Nordenfors H, Uggla A: Prevalence of the red poultry mite, *Dermanyssys gallinae*, in different types of production systems for egg layers in Sweden. Poult Sci. 1995, 74: 1793-1798.
33. Fadly AM, Payne LN: Leukosis/sarcoma group. Diseases of Poultry. Edited by: Saif YM, Barnes HJ, Glisson JR, Fadly AM, McDougald LR, Swayne DE. 2003, Iowa State Press, 465-516. 11, Ch.15
34. Hansen I: Ethological studies of laying hens in aviaries and cages. PhD thesis. 1993, Dept. Animal Sci. Agricultural University of Norway
35. Morgenstern R, Lobsieger CH: Health of laying hens in alternative systems in practice. Proceedings of the 4th Europeen Symposium on Poultry Welfare. Edinburgh. 1993, 81-86.
36. Nicol CJ, Gregory NG, Knowles TG, Parkman ID, Wilkens LJ: Differential effects of increased stocking density, mediated by increased flock size, on feather pecking and aggression in laying hens. Appl Anim Behav Sci. 1999, 65: 137-152. 10.1016/S0168-1591(99)00057-X.
37. Keeling LJ: Feather pecking and Cannibalism in layers. Poult Int. 1995, 34: 46-50.
38. Allen J, Perry GC: Feather pecking and cannibalism in a caged layer flock. Br Poult Sci. 1975, 16: 441-51. 10.1080/00071667508416212.
39. Amgarten M: Swiss layers perform well in alternative housing. Poultry Misset. 1989, April/May: 8-9.
40. Tanaka T, Hurnik JF: Comparison of behaviour and performance of laying hens housed in battery cages and an aviary. Poult Sci. 1992, 71: 235-243.
41. Taylor AA, Hurnik JF: The long-term productivity of hens in battery cages and an aviary. Poult Sci. 1996, 75: 47-51.
42. Michel V, Huonnic D: A comparison of welfare, health and production performance of laying hens in cages and aviaries. Br Poult Sci. 2003, 44: 775-776. 10.1080/00071660410001666691.
43. Meierhans D, Amgarten M, Guler HP, Strasser M: The economical consequences of the introduction of alternative housing systems for laying hens in Switzerland. Proceedings XIX WPSA Poultry Congress, Amsterdam, The Netherlands. 1992, 190-
44. Bang Jensen H: Effektivitetskontrollen. Det Danske Fjerkraeråd- beretning. 2006
45. Van Horne PLM: Production and economic results of commercial flocks with white layers in aviary systems and battery cages. Br Poult Sci. 1996, 37: 255-261. 10.1080/00071669608417857.
46. Engström B: Health situation in poultry in the Nordic Countries 2007. Nordic Poultry Conference 2007 Nov. 21–23 Uppsala, Sweden (Report). 2007, Nov. 21–23 Uppsala, Sweden (Report)

INDEX

P

R

S

T

U

V